# Progress in Inflammation Research

## Series Editor

Prof. Dr. Michael J. Parnham
PLIVA
Research Institute
Prilaz baruna Filipovica 25
10000 Zagreb
Croatia

**Forthcoming titles:**
*Nitric Oxide and Inflammation*, D. Salvemini, T.R. Billiar, Y. Vodovotz (Editors), 2001
*Migraine: A Neuroinflammatory Disease?* E.L.H. Spierings, M. Sanchez del Rio (Editors), 2001
*NMDA Antagonists as Potential Analgesic Drugs*, R.G. Hill, D.J.S. Sirinathsinghji (Editors), 2001
*Disease-modifying Therapy in Vasculitides*, C.G.M. Kallenberg, J.W. Cohen Tervaert (Editors), 2001
*Neuroinflammatory Mechanisms in Alzheimer's Disease*, J. Rogers (Editor), 2001
*Mechanisms and mediators of neuropathic pain*, A.B. Malmberg, S.R. Chaplan (Editors), 2001

(Already published titles see last page.)

# TGF-β and Related Cytokines in Inflammation

Samuel N. Breit
Sharon M. Wahl

Editors

Springer Basel AG

Editors

Samuel N. Breit
Centre for Immunology
St. Vincent's Hospital & University of NSW
Victoria St.
Sydney, NSW 2010
Australia

Sharon M. Wahl
Oral Infection and Immunity Branch
National Institute of Dental and Craniofacial Research
National Institutes of Health
30 Convent Drive
Bethesda, MD 20878-4352
USA

A CIP catalogue record for this book is available from the Library of Congress, Washington D.C., USA

Deutsche Bibliothek Cataloging-in-Publication Data
TGF-β and related cytokines in inflammation / Samuel N. Breit ; Sharon M. Wahl, ed..
- Basel ; Boston ; Berlin : Birkhäuser, 2001
    (Progress in inflammation research)
    ISBN 978-3-0348-9531-6      ISBN 978-3-0348-8354-2 (eBook)
    DOI 10.1007/978-3-0348-8354-2

ISBN 978-3-0348-9531-6

Printed on acid-free paper produced from chlorine-free pulp. TCF ∞
Cover design: Markus Etterich, Basel
Cover illustration: Crystal structure of TGF-$\beta_2$, with friendly permission of Samuel N. Breit

ISBN 978-3-0348-9531-6

9 8 7 6 5 4 3 2 1

# Contents

# List of contributors

Asne R. Bauskin, Centre for Immunology, St. Vincent's Hospital and University of New South Wales, Victoria St., Sydney NSW, 2010, Australia

Samuel N. Breit, Centre for Immunology, St. Vincent's Hospital and University of New South Wales, Victoria St., Sydney NSW, 2010, Australia; e-mail: s.breit@cfi.unsw.edu.au

Peter K. Brown, Centre for Immunology, St. Vincent's Hospital and University of New South Wales, Victoria St., Sydney NSW, 2010, Australia

W. Douglas Fairlie, Centre for Immunology, St. Vincent's Hospital and University of New South Wales, Victoria St., Sydney NSW, 2010, Australia

Mark W.J. Ferguson, Division of Cells Immunology and Development, School of Biological Sciences, University of Manchester, 3.239 Stopford Building, Oxford Road, Manchester M13 9PT, UK; e-mail: Mark.Ferguson@man.ac.uk

Jennifer R. Gamble, Division of Immunology, Hanson Centre for Cancer Research, Institute of Medical & Veterinary Science and The University of Adelaide, Frome Road, Adelaide 5000, South Australia; e-mail: Jennifer.Gamble@imvs.sa.gov.au

Don M. Gash, Department of Anatomy and Neurobiology, University of Kentucky Medical Center, 800 Rose Street, MN 224, Lexington, KY 40536-0298, USA; e-mail: dongash@pop.uky.edu

David J. Grainger, Dept of Medicine, Box 157, Addenbrooke's Hospital, Hills Road, Cambridge CB2 2QQ, UK; e-mail: djg15@mde.bio.cam.ac.uk

Carl-Henrik Heldin, Ludwig Institute for Cancer Research, Box 595, Biomedical Center, 751 24 Uppsala, Sweden; e-mail: C-H.Heldin@LICR.uu.se

Susumu Itoh, The Netherlands Cancer Institute, Antoni van Leeuwenhoek Hospital, Division of Cellular Biochemistry, H3, Plesmanlaan 121, 1066 CX Amsterdam, The Netherlands; e-mail: sitoh@nki.nl

Nancy L. McCartney-Francis, Oral Infection and Immunity Branch, National Institute of Dental and Craniofacial Research, National Institutes of Health, 30 Convent Drive, Building 30, Room 326, Bethesda, MD 20892-4352, USA; e-mail: nfrancis@dir.nidcr.nih.gov

Navin Maswood, Department of Anatomy and Neurobiology, University of Kentucky Medical Center, 800 Rose Street, MN 224, Lexington, KY 40536-0298, USA; e-mail: nmasw1@pop.uky.edu

Anthony G. Moore, Centre for Immunology, St. Vincent's Hospital and University of New South Wales, Victoria St., Sydney NSW, 2010, Australia

David E. Mosedale, Dept of Medicine, Box 157, Addenbrookes Hospital, Hills Road, Cambridge CB2 2QQ, UK; e-mail: dem@mole.bio.cam.ac.uk

Aristidis Moustakas, Ludwig Institute for Cancer Research, Box 595, Biomedical Center, 751 24 Uppsala, Sweden; e-mail: Aris.Moustakas@LICR.uu.se

Carola U. Niesler, Division of Cells Immunology and Development, School of Biological Sciences, University of Manchester, 3.239 Stopford Building, Oxford Road, Manchester M13 9PT, UK; e-mail: carola.niesler@man.ac.uk

A. Hari Reddi, Center for Tissue Regeneration and Repair and Department of Orthopaedic Surgery, University of California, Research Building I, Room 2000, 4635 Second Avenue, Sacramento, CA 95817, USA; e-mail: ahreddi@ucdavis.edu

Patricia K. Russell, Centre for Immunology, St. Vincent's Hospital and University of New South Wales, Victoria St., Sydney NSW, 2010, Australia

Serhiy Souchelnytskyi, Ludwig Institute for Cancer Research, Box 595, Biomedical Center, 751 24 Uppsala, Sweden; e-mail: Serhiy.Souchelnytskyi@LICR.uu.se

Peter ten Dijke, The Netherlands Cancer Institute, Antoni van Leeuwenhoek Hospital, Division of Cellular Biochemistry, H3, Plesmanlaan 121, 1066 CX Amsterdam, The Netherlands; e-mail: ptdijke@nki.nl

Mathew A. Vadas, Division of Immunology, Hanson Centre for Cancer Research, Institute of Medical & Veterinary Science and The University of Adelaide, Frome Road, Adelaide 5000, South Australia

Sharon M. Wahl, Oral Infection and Immunity Branch, National Institute of Dental and Craniofacial Research, National Institutes of Health, 30 Convent Drive, Bethesda, MD 20878-4352, USA; e-mail: smwahl@dir.nidcr.nih.gov

Pu Xia, Division of Immunology, Hanson Centre for Cancer Research, Institute of Medical & Veterinary Science and The University of Adelaide, Frome Road, Adelaide 5000, South Australia

Hong-Ping Zhang, Centre for Immunology, St. Vincent's Hospital and University of New South Wales, Victoria St., Sydney NSW, 2010, Australia

# Introduction

The TGF-β superfamily is a large and expanding multigene family which in vertebrates includes the TGF-β proteins themselves, the bone morphogenetic proteins (BMPs), the growth and differentiation factors (GDF), the activins/inhibins (INH), Mullerian inhibitory substance (MIS), glial derived neurotropic factor (GDNF) and more recently macrophage inhibitory cytokine 1 (MIC-1). They are characterised by conserved structural elements and a broad commonality of function.

## Major structural elements

All members of the TGF-β superfamily contain as their major structural hallmark a conserved spacing and distribution of seven cysteine residues. This structure is known as the cysteine knot and tethers together regions of the peptide as well as binding the two chains of the dimer to each other. High resolution structures are now available on proteins from three families within this group including glial derived neurotropic factor (GDNF), BMP-7 and several of the TGF-βs. Despite low similarity between some of these proteins (eg, TGF-βs and GDNF are only 13% identical) they share a strikingly similar three dimensional conformation (Fig. 1). These structural elements imbue the protein with some of its familial characteristics. These include its physico-chemical stability due to tight tethering of portions of the peptide chain via criss-crossing disulphide bonds. Much of its surfaces are coated with hydrophobic patches leading to a propensity to bind non-specifically to other proteins as well as to its self. This also causes a marked propensity for aggregation when the recombinant protein is present at high concentration.

TGF-β superfamily proteins are characterised by the presence of a long pro-peptide and a mature bioactive protein that is dimeric (110 and 120 amino acids in length). It is non-glycosylated and separated from the longer pro-peptide by a conserved dibasic RXXR motif that is the substrate for furin-like proteases. Most of the mature protein is bounded by the seven cysteine domain which is the major structurally homologous element of proteins within this family. It has similarities and dif-

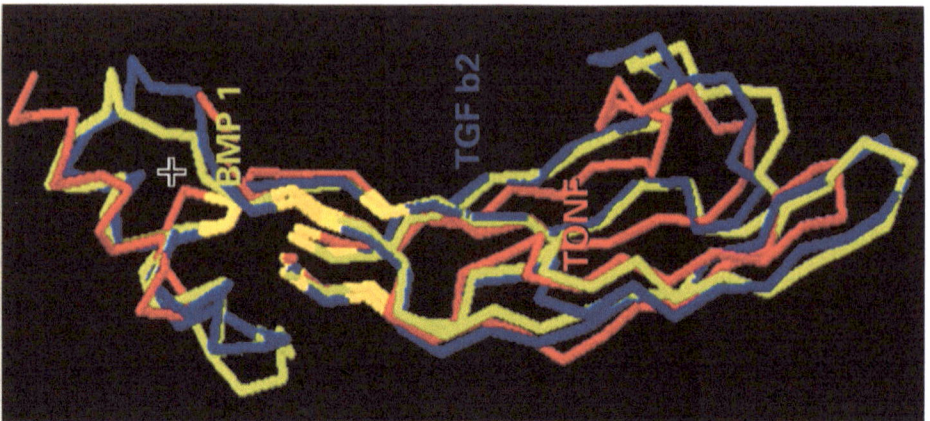

*Figure 1*

ferences within this region that are used to categorise TGF-β superfamily proteins into family groups (Fig. 2). In general, identity between different members of the one family vary between 40% and 90%. Identity between protein members of different families is lower and is usually between 13% and 30%. The level of identity in the seven cysteine domain is not shared throughout most of the rest of the protein. Whilst there is some similarity in the pro-peptide region between different members of a individual family, there is almost no similarity in this region across families.

## Functional properties of TGF-β superfamily members

Over the last decade large numbers of proteins belonging to this superfamily have been identified and a wide variety of different functions have been ascribed. However, many unique properties of the superfamily members have been revealed in the recent development of gain-of-function and loss-of-function transgenic mouse models. Despite this variety there appeared to be certain common themes which constrain the broad functional properties of these molecules. These can be broadly classified under three general headings: wound healing and repair; regulation of inflammation and immunity; cell growth and differentiation. Many, if not all, proteins within the superfamily have major elements that can be ascribed in varying proportions to the three categories. Ongoing dissection of the intracellular signal transduction pathways engaged by these ligands provides new insight into the shared and unique functional consequences of the receptor engagement by superfamily members

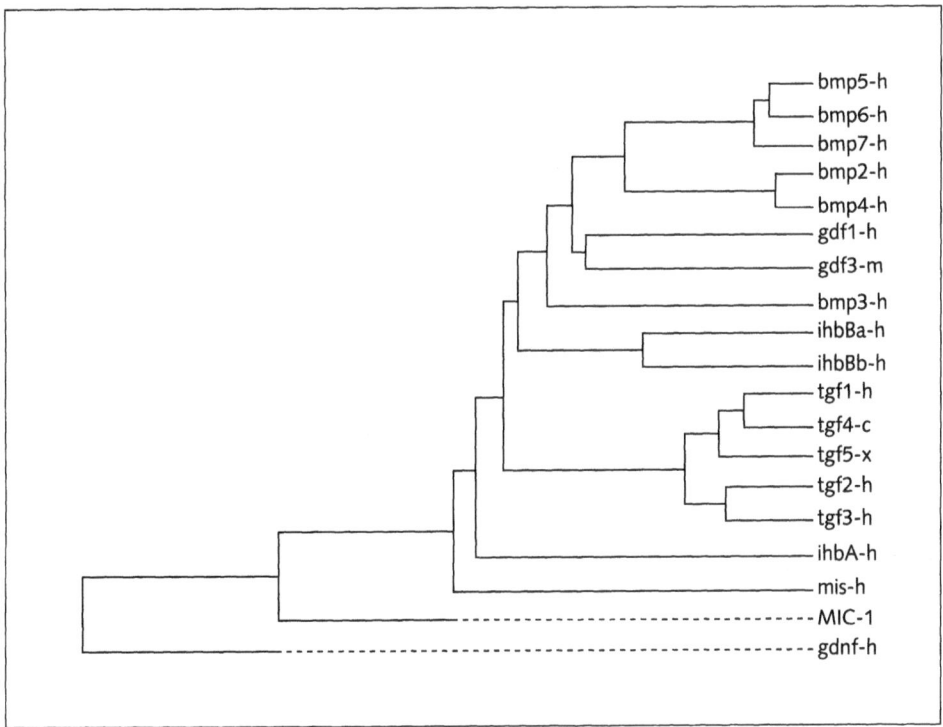

*Figure 2*

*Relationships within the TGF-β superfamily.*

## Conclusion

In this publication we have sought to provide an overall assessment of the TGF-β superfamily focusing more heavily on proteins that have a role in inflammation, wound healing and repair. TGF-β was the first identified protein in this superfamily and is by far the best analysed and studied within this group. Because of this, the largest proportion of papers relate to this protein. We trust that the large amount of information all relating to this group of proteins, collected within this one book, will be a ready source of information for the scientific community.

Samuel N. Breit
Sharon M. Wahl

# MIC-1 and other TGF-β superfamily members in inflammation

*Anthony G. Moore, W. Douglas Fairlie, Asne R. Bauskin, Peter K. Brown,*
*Patricia K. Russell, Hong-Ping Zhang and Samuel N. Breit*

Centre for Immunology, St. Vincent's Hospital and University of NSW, Victoria St., Sydney
NSW 2010, Australia

## Introduction

The TGF-β superfamily consists of an expanding number of structurally similar proteins which have been implicated in the regulation of a variety of cellular processes such as growth, motility, and differentiation. Members of the TGF-β superfamily have been classified into major family groupings on the basis of homologies within a seven cysteine domain which encompasses most of the mature protein [1–4]. These include TGF-β, bone morphogenetic protein (BMP), growth and differentiation factor (GDF), inhibin-b/activin (inhB), inhibin-α (inhA), mullerian inhibitory substance (MIS), and glial derived neurotrophic factor (GDNF). The highly characteristic secondary and tertiary structure of TGF-β superfamily proteins occurs within the seven cysteine domain [1–4], even though the level of sequence homology between disparate family members can be low [5]. The knotted structure generated by the highly conserved pattern and spacing of cysteine residues leads to dimeric proteins of remarkable stability. This highly conserved structure also makes it relatively simple to identify new members of this superfamily.

## Structure of the MIC-1 gene and protein

In 1997 a cDNA was cloned from a subtraction library enriched for transcripts associated with macrophage activation. We have named this gene macrophage inhibitory cytokine 1 (MIC-1) [5]. MIC-1 expression, however, is not restricted to macrophages and is expressed particularly strongly within placenta and weakly in prostate, kidney, pancreas and colon [6, 7] Multiple sequence alignments indicate that all cysteine residues which characterise the TGF-β superfamily are present in MIC-1 (Fig. 1). This and other structural features argue strongly that MIC-1 is a new member of the TGF-β superfamily [5]. Two additional cysteine residues located close to the amino terminus of the mature protein are present in MIC-1. These additional cysteines are also found in TGF-$\beta_{1-3}$ and inhibin $\beta_a$ and $\beta_b$ [5]. As is the

TGF-β and Related Cytokines in Inflammation, edited by Samuel N. Breit and Sharon M. Wahl
© 2001 Birkhäuser Verlag Basel/Switzerland

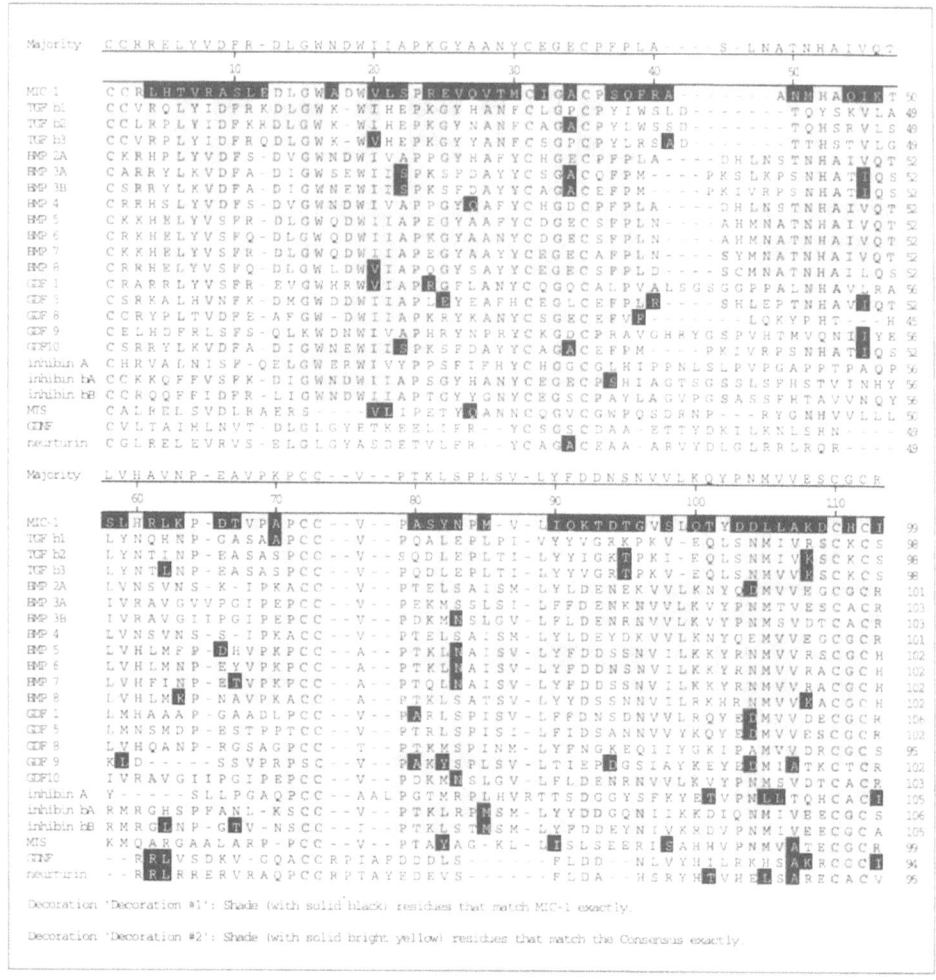

*Figure 1*

*Multiple sequence alignment of the seven cysteine domain of a representative group of human TGF-β superfamily proteins. Residues identical to the consensus are shaded in gray. Residues identical to MIC-1 (other than those identical to the consensus) are shaded in black.*

case with TGF-β₂, the additional cysteines may confer extra stability to the molecule [8]. Members of the TGF-β superfamily are in general considered to form part of the same family if they are 40% to 90% identical over the seven cysteine domain [1, 2, 5]. Sequence analysis indicates that MIC-1 is the second most divergent protein within this superfamily behind GDNF. The highest degree of homology of MIC-1 with other superfamily members is with BMP-5 and -6 (29%). Sequence homolo-

2

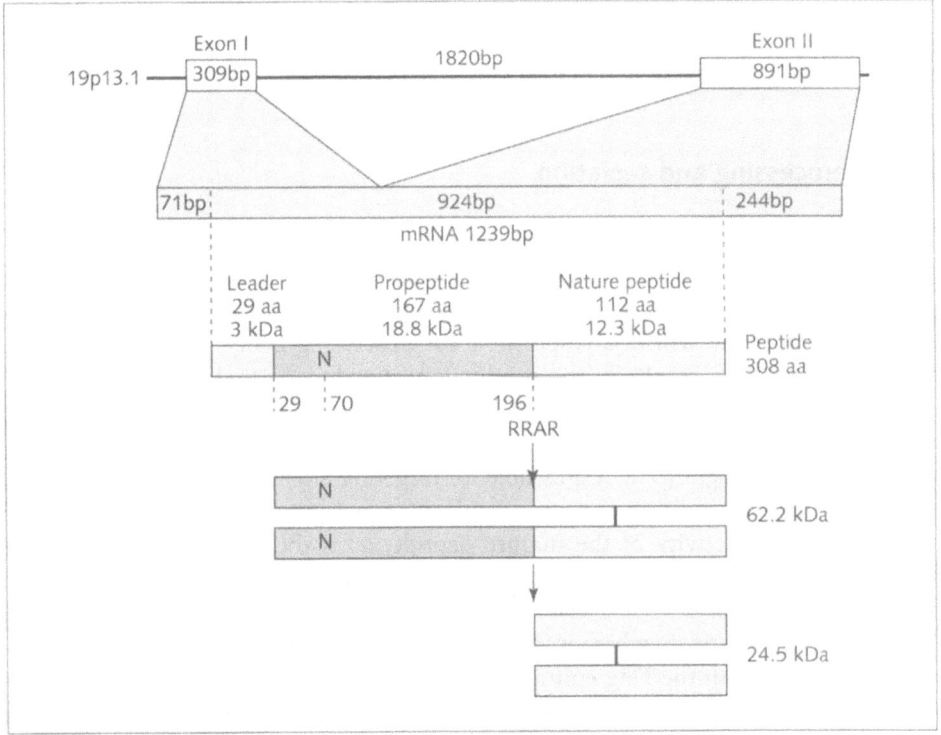

*Figure 2*
*Genomic organisation, mRNA and protein synthesis and post translational processing of MIC-1. Reproduced from [6] with permission.*

gy to other TGF-β superfamily members outside the seven cysteine domain and in the propeptide is extremely low [1, 2, 5].Therefore, MIC-1 represents a divergent member of the TGF-β superfamily and may represent the first member of a new family within this grouping.

The MIC-1 gene localises to human chromosome 19, band p12–13.1 [6, 9] and contains two coding exons. Exon I is 309 base pairs and exon II 647 base pairs in length. 71 base pairs of untranslated sequence are present at the 5' end of exon I and 244 base pairs at the 3' end of exon II. The exons are separated by one intron of approximately 1800 base pairs (Fig. 2). The 5' flanking region of the MIC-1 gene contains potential binding sites for several transcription factors, including AP-1, AP-4, TBP, SP1, Pit-1a, CAC-binding protein, and several GR elements [9]. The structure of the MIC-1 gene is similar to that of GDF-9, BMP-2 and BMP-4, all of which contain two coding exons. The GDF-9 gene contains a larger intron than the MIC-1 gene, while the BMP-2 and 4 genes contain one and three extra 5' non-coding exons respectively. The remaining members of this superfamily are less similar in gene structure to MIC-1. For example, the BMP-3 gene has three coding exons while TGF-$\beta_{1-3}$ and BMP-6–8a consist of seven coding exons.

## MIC-1 processing and secretion

The MIC-1 protein like most members of this superfamily, contains a long propeptide separated from the mature protein by a conserved di-arginine motif, RXXR, at position 193–196 [3, 6–8] (Fig. 2). This sequence is thought to be the substrate for a furin-like protease which is responsible for processing many precursor proteins. Cleavage at this site results in the production of a dimeric mature peptide of 224 amino acids [1–3, 5]. The MIC-1 propeptide contains an N-linked glycosylation consensus sequence at amino acid 70. In the case of TGF-$\beta_{1-3}$, sequences within the propeptide are thought to be responsible for targeting molecules to specific secretary compartments. In addition the propeptide may possess other functions such as inhibiting the bioactivity of the mature peptide, as is the case with TGF-$\beta_1$. The function of the MIC-1 propeptide is currently the subject of intensive investigation within our laboratory.

In order to investigate whether the MIC-1 gene encodes a secreted protein, MIC-1 cDNA tagged with the Flag epitope was cloned into a eukaryotic expression vector and transfected into CHO cells. Using immunoblot analysis it was determined that MIC-1 was secreted as a 30 kDa disulphide-linked dimer that was generated from a 62 kDa dimeric precursor. Under reducing conditions a secreted 12 kDa band was observed which correlates to the size of the mature monomer as predicted from the putative cleavage site between the propeptide and the mature peptide at position 196 [10]. This was confirmed by N-terminal sequencing of purified mature MIC-1. Interestingly, MIC-1 cDNA devoid of the sequence encoding the propeptide also resulted in the secretion of the mature 30 kDa dimer when transfected into CHO cells [10]. This characteristic makes MIC-1 unique amongst TGF-$\beta$ superfamily members which require the propeptide for secretion.

## MIC-1 and other members of the TGF-$\beta$ superfamily in inflammation

That macrophages are key cells in normal inflammatory responses is largely undisputed. Macrophages are also important mediators in orchestrating chronic inflammatory and fibrotic disorders, such as atherosclerosis and rheumatoid arthritis. When activated, macrophages are known to secrete a wide variety of bioactive molecules. Some are highly toxic to foreign organisms while others, such as cytokines, are known to modulate inflammatory processes. Many macrophage-derived immunomodulatory cytokines have been identified and cloned. Tumor necrosis factor-α (TNF-α) and interleukin-1β (IL-1β) are considered proinflammatory cytokines and form part of the chronic inflammatory response while others such as interleukin-10 (IL-10) are known for their ability to suppress the immune system.

Whilst a substantial amount is known about TGF-β isoforms in macrophage biology and inflammation (see other chapters), a lot less is known about other members of this superfamily that may well also have a role in this process. One such candidate cytokine is MIC-1. As is to be expected from a cDNA isolated from a library enriched for molecules produced by activated macrophages, its expression in resting culture-derived macrophages is minimal. A marked increase in MIC-1 expression was induced by PMA (phorbol ester) and a number of mediators associated with macrophage activation, including TNF-α, IL-1β, and macrophage-colony stimulating factor (M-CSF) [5]. Interestingly, expression was not induced by lipopolysaccharide (LPS), a potent macrophage activator. These findings indicate that MIC-1 expression is activation related in macrophages. The ability of PMA and proinflammatory cytokines but not LPS to induce the MIC-1 transcript may be due to the presence and arrangement of defined transcription factor binding sites in the 5' untranslated region of the MIC-1 gene. The MIC-1 promoter contains an AP-1 binding site but not sites for STAT and NF-κB.

Like MIC-1, TGF-$\beta_1$ and activin-A are also produced by macrophages. TGF-$\beta_1$ is secreted constitutively by circulating monocytes and tissue macrophages and can be upregulated by activating agents such as LPS and concanavalin A (CON A) [11, 12]. Activin-A is produced by macrophages predominantly after stimulation with PMA [13] and granulocyte-macrophage colony stimulating factor (GM-CSF) [14], and to a lesser extent by LPS and IFN-γ [15]. Interestingly, GM-CSF induction of activin-A is inhibited by hydrocortisone, dexamethasone, and retinoic acid [14].

TGF-$\beta_1$ is a well recognised pleotropic immunoregulator, known to be instrumental in both the initiation and regulation of inflammatory and immune events. Experimentation using culture-derived macrophages suggests that MIC-1 also possesses immunomodulatory activity. MIC-1 has been shown to inhibit the release of pro-inflammatory cytokines from LPS-activated macrophages [5]. Similar to MIC-1, TGF-$\beta_1$ has been demonstrated to suppresses macrophage activation in culture [16, 17] as well as in experimental animals [18]. At this stage MIC-1 appears to be less consistent than TGF-$\beta_1$ at inhibiting macrophage activation. The reasons for this at present are unclear. These results suggest that similar to TGF-β and IL-10, MIC-1 may act as an autocrine inhibitor of macrophage activation [5], possibly acting to limit/terminate the late phase of activation (Fig. 3). An intriguing possibility is that MIC-1, TGF-$\beta_1$, and IL-10 may act cooperatively in this manner, with differing combinations leading to variations in how long and with what potency macrophages are activated.

Other members of the TGF-β superfamily have been demonstrated to regulate macrophage function. For example, TGF-$\beta_2$ upregulates C3 gene expression in the U937 human monocyte cell line [19]. Experimental evidence suggests that activin-A

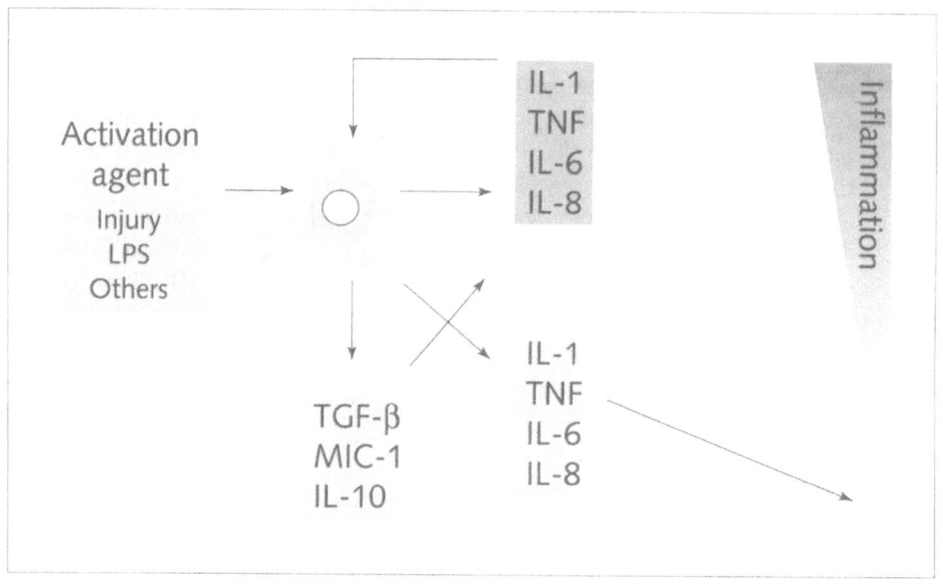

*Figure 3*
*Proposed model for the regulation of macrophage activation by inhibitory cytokines such as MIC-1, TGF-β and IL-10.*

induces the expression of the pro-inflammatory cytokines TNF-α, IL-1β, and IL-6 by purified monocytes [20], suggesting it may promote macrophage activation. In addition, activin-A has been found to reduce foam cell formation and cholesterol ester accumulation [21] while enhancing prostaglandin production by cultured macrophages [22]. It is not surprising that members of the TGF-β and activin families influence the behavior of monocyte/macrophage cell lineages, since receptors for both families are constitutively expressed by these cells [23, 24]. Interestingly, a component of the GDNF receptor (Ret) is present on the THP-1 macrophage cell line [25], suggesting that members of the GDNF family may also regulate macrophage function.

Chemotaxis is regarded as a highly specialised behavior that constitutes a fundamental precursor to several inflammatory disorders. Experimental evidence indicates that TGF-$\beta_{1-3}$ and activin are strongly chemotactic for monocytes/macrophages [26, 27], suggesting they promote the recruitment of leukocytes into sites of inflammation. This is clearly demonstrated in animals that overexpress TGF-$\beta_1$ or that have received exogenous TGF-$\beta_1$ or TGF-$\beta_2$, where several organs and tissues undergo marked leukocyte infiltration [28]. BMP-3 (also known as osteogenin), BMP-4, and BMP-7 (also known as OP-1) are also chemotactic for monocytes *in vitro*, although their effects may be due to their ability to stimulate the expression of TGF-β$_1$ [27, 29]. Further studies are necessary to determine if MIC-1 is chemotactic for cells of the monocyte/macrophage lineage.

The TGF-β superfamily historically has been centrally implicated in the regulation of cell differentiation during development. Studies employing hematopoietic progenitors have provided preliminary evidence suggesting that MIC-1 may also play some role in development. Hromas et al. [30] showed that MIC-1 suppressed the formation of erythrocyte and granulocyte/macrophage cell lineages from normal human non-adherent T-cell-depleted marrow cells. This finding suggests that MIC-1 may be a broad inhibitor of inflammation, acting to suppress the development of macrophages as well as their activation potential. MIC-1 is not exclusive in its ability to regulate hematopoiesis. TGF-β$_1$ has previously been shown to suppress the proliferation of marrow progenitors [31] while BMP-4 can induce the production of hematopoietic precursors from primitive mesoderm [32]. In addition, activin-A and TGF-β$_2$ promote the differentiation of the human promyelocytic cell line HL-60 into cells of the monocyte/macrophage lineage [33, 34]. These findings highlight the pleotropic roles of TGF-β superfamily members during development.

## Acknowledgments

This work has been funded in part by grants from St. Vincent's Hospital and by Meriton Apartments Pty Ltd through an R&D syndicate arranged by Macquarie Bank Limited. In addition, this project was partially funded by a New South Wales Health Research and Development infrastructure grant.

## References

1    Ozkaynak E, Schnegelsberg P, Jin D, Clifford G, Warren F, Drier E, Opperman H (1992) Osteogenic protein-2 A new member of the transforming growth factor-β superfamily expressed early in embryogenesis. *J Biol Chem* 267: 25220–25227

2    Burt DW, Law AS (1994) Evolution of the transforming growth factor-β superfamily. *Progr Growth Factor Res* 5: 99–118

3    Kingsley DM (1994) The TGF-β superfamily: new members, new receptors and new genetic tests of function in different organisms. *Genes Develop* 8: 133–146

4    McPherron A, Lee S (1993) GDF-3 and GDF-9: Two new members of the transforming growth factor-β superfamily containing a novel pattern of cysteines. *J Biol Chem* 268: 3444–3449

5    Bootcov MR, Bauskin A, Valenzuela SM, Moore AG, Bansal M, He C, Zhang HP, Donnellan M, Mahler S, Pryor K et al (1997) MIC-1, a novel macrophage inhibitory cytokine, is a divergent member of the TGF-β superfamily cluster. *Proc Natl Acad Sci USA* 94: 11514–11519

6   Fairlie WD, Moore AG, Bauskin AR, Russell PK, Zhang H-P, Breit SN (1999) MIC-1 is a novel TGF-β superfamily cytokine associated with macrophage activation. *J Leukocyte Biol* 65: 2–5

7   Yokoyama-Koyabashi M, Saeki M, Sekine S, Kato S (1997) Human cDNA encoding a novel TGF-β superfamily protein highly expressed in placenta. *J Biochem* 122: 622–626

8   Roberts AB, Sporn MB (1993) Physiological actions and clinical applications of transforming growth factor-β (TGF-β). *Growth Factors* 8: 1–9

9   Lawton LN, de Fatima Bonaldo M, Jelenc PC, Qiu L, Baumes SA, Marcelino RA, De Jesus GM, Wellington S, Knowles JA, Warburton D et al (1997) Identification of a novel member of the TGF-β superfamily highly expressed in human placenta. *Gene* 203: 17–26

10  Bauskin AR, Zhang H-P, Fairlie WD, He XY, Russell P, Moore AG, Brown D, Stanley KK, Breit SN (2000) The propeptide of macrophage inhibitory cytokine (MIC-1), a TGF-β superfamily member acts as a quality control determinant for correctly folded MIC-1. *EMBO J* 19: 2212–2220

11  Assoian RK, Fleurdelys BE, Stevenson HC, Miller PJ, Madtes DK, Raines EW, Ross R, Sporn MB (1987) Expression and secretion of type beta transforming growth factor by activated human macrophages. *Proc Natl Acad Sci USA* 84: 6020–6024

12  Grotendorst GR, Smale G, Pencev D (1989) Production of transforming growth factor-b by human peripheral blood monocytes and neutrophils. *J Cell Physiol* 140: 396–402

13  Nishihara T, Ohsaki Y, Ueda N, Koseki T, Eto Y (1995) Induction of apoptosis in B lineages by activin-A derivered from macrophages. *J Interferon Cytokine Res* 15: 509–516

14  Yu J, Shao YJ, Frigon NL, Logren J Schwall R (1996) Induced expression of the new cytokine, activin A, in human monocytes: inhibition by glucocorticoids and retinoic acid. *Immunol* 88: 368–374

15  Shao L, Frigon NL, Sehy DW, Yu AL, Lofgren J, Schwall R, Yu J (1992) Regulation of production of activin-A in human marrow stromal cells and monocytes. *Exp Hematol* 20: 1235–1242

16  Tsunawaki S Sporn M Ding A Nathan C (1988) Deactivation of macrophages by transforming growth factor-beta. *Nature* 334: 260–262

17  Bogdan C, Nathan C (1993) Modulation of macrophage function by transforming growth factor beta, IL-4 and IL-10. *Annal NY Acad Sci* 685: 713–739

18  Shull MM, Ormsby I, Kier AB, Pawlowski S, Diebold RJ, Yin M, Allen R, Sidman C, Proetzel G, Calvin D et al (1992) Targeted disruption of the mouse transforming growth factor-beta 1 gene results in multifocal inflammatory disease. *Nature* 359: 693–699

19  Drouin SM, Kiley SC, Carlino JA, Barnum SR (1998) Transforming growth factor-β2 regulates C3 secretion in monocytes through a protein kinase C-dependant pathway. *Molec Immunol* 35: 1–11

20  Yamashita N, Nakajima N, Takahashi H, Kaneoka H, Mizushima Y, Sakane T (1993) Effects of activin-A on IgE synthesis and cytokine production by human peripheral mononuclear cells. *Clin Exp Immunol* 94: 214–219

21  Kozaki K, Akishita M, Eto M, Yoshizumi M, Toba K, Inoue S, Ishikawa M, Hashimo-

to T, Yamada N, Orimo H et al (1997) Role of activin-A and follistatin in foam cell formation of THP-1 macrophages. *Arterioscler Thromb Vasc Biol* 17: 2389–2394

22 Nusing RM, Mohr S, Ullrich V (1995) Activin-A and retinoic acid synergise in cyclooxygenase-1 and thromboxane synthase induction during differentation of J7741 macrophages. *Eur J Biochem* 222: 130–136

23 Hilden K, Tuuri T, Eramaa M, Ritvos O (1994) Expression of type II activin receptor genes during differentiation of human K562 cells and cDNA cloning of the human type IIB activn receptor. *Blood* 83: 2163–2170

24 Brandes ME, Wakefield LM, Wahl SM (1991) Modulation of monocyte type 1 transforming growth factor beta receptors by inflammatory stimuli. *J Biol Chem* 266: 19697–19703

25 Walker DG, Beach TG, Xu R, Lile J, Beck KD, McGeer EG, McGeer PL (1998) Expression of the proto-oncogene Ret, a component of the GDNF receptor complex, persists in human substantia nigra neurons in Parkinson's disease. *Brain Res* 792: 207–217

26 Petraglia F, Sacerdote P, Cossarizza A, Angioni S, Genazzani AD, Franceschi C, Muscettola M, Grasso G (1991) Inhibin and activin modulate human monocyte chemotaxis and human lymphocyte interferon-gamma production. *J Clin Endocrinol Metab* 72: 496–502

27 Postlethwaite AE, Raghow R, Stricklin G, Ballou L, Sampath TK (1994) Osteogenic protein-1, a bone morphogenic protein member of the TGF-β superfamily, shares chemotactic but not fibrogenic properties with TGF-β. *J Cell Physiol* 161: 562–570

28 Wahl SM (1994) Transforming growth factor-β: The good, the bad and the ugly. *J Exp Med* 180: 1587–1590

29 Cunningham NS, Paralkar V, Reddi AH (1992) Osteogenin and recombinant BMP-2B are chemotatic for human monocytes and stimulate TGF-β1 expression. *Proc Natl Acad Sci USA* 89: 11740–11744

30 Hromas R, Hufford M, Sutton J, Xu D, Li Y, Lu L (1997) PLAB, a novel placental bone morphogenetic protein. *Biochim Biophys Acta* 1354: 40–44

31 Jacobsen FW, Stokke T, Jacobsen SEW (1995) Transforming growth factor-β potently inhibits the viability-promoting activity of stem cell factor and other cytokines and induces apoptosis of primitive murine hematopoietic progenitor cells. *Blood* 86: 2957–2966

32 Johansson BM, Wiles MV (1995) Evidence for involvement of activin A and bone morphogenetic protein-4 in mammalian mesoderm and hematopoietic development. *Mol Cellular Biol* 15: 141–151

33 Yamada R, Suzuki T, Hashimoto M, Eto Y, Shiokawa K, Muramatsu M (1992) Induction of differentiation of the human promyelocytic cell line HL-60 by activin/EDF. *Biochem Biophys Res Comm* 187: 79–85

34 Okabe-Kado J, Honma Y, Hayashi M, Hozumi M (1991) Effects of transforming growth factor-b and activin-A on vitamin D3-induced monocytic differentiation of myeloid leukemia cells. *Anticancer Res* 11: 181–186

# Signal transduction mechanisms for members of the TGF-β family

*Carl-Henrik Heldin[1], Aristidis Moustakas[1], Serhiy Souchelnytskyi[1], Susumu Itoh[2] and Peter ten Dijke[2]*

[1]Ludwig Institute for Cancer Research, Box 595, Biomedical Center, S-751 24 Uppsala, Sweden; [2]The Netherlands Cancer Institute, Antoni van Leeuwenhoek Hospital, Division of Cellular Biochemistry, H3, Plesmanlaan 121, 1066 CX Amsterdam, The Netherlands

## Introduction

The transforming growth factor-β (TGF-β) superfamily consists of about 30 mammalian members, including TGF-β isoforms, activins, bone morphogenetic proteins (BMPs), Müllerian inhibiting substance (MIS) and others (reviewed by [1]). These factors regulate cell growth, differentiation and apoptosis of various cell types, and have important functions during the embryonal development. TGF-β isoforms inhibit the growth of most cell types, including epithelial cells, endothelial cells and lymphocytes; however, the growth of certain connective tissue cells is stimulated. TGF-β also causes an accumulation of extracellular matrix molecules, *via* stimulation of synthesis as well as inhibition of degradation, and triggers the IgA class switch of B lymphocytes. Activins stimulate the secretion of follicle stimulating hormone secretion from pituitary cells, promote differentiation of erythropoietic cells and survival of neuronal tissue, and induce dorsal mesoderm in *Xenopus* embryos. BMPs induce bone and cartilage *in vivo*, affect the differentiation of hematopoietic stem cells and neural cells, and induce ventral mesoderm in *Xenopus*. Overactivity or loss of activity of members of the TGF-β family has been implicated in certain disorders, including fibrotic conditions, rheumatoid arthritis and cancer.

The aim of this review is to discuss the mechanisms whereby TGF-β family members exert their effects on target cells.

## Receptors for TGF-β family members

Members of the TGF-β family bind to two different types of serine/threonine kinase receptors, denoted type I and type II receptors (reviewed in [2, 3]). In addition, several cell surface binding proteins for TGF-β exist with a more indirect role in signaling, e.g. the proteoglycan TGF-β type III receptor [4] and endoglin [5]; the TGF-β type III receptor plays a role in the presentation of ligand for the signaling

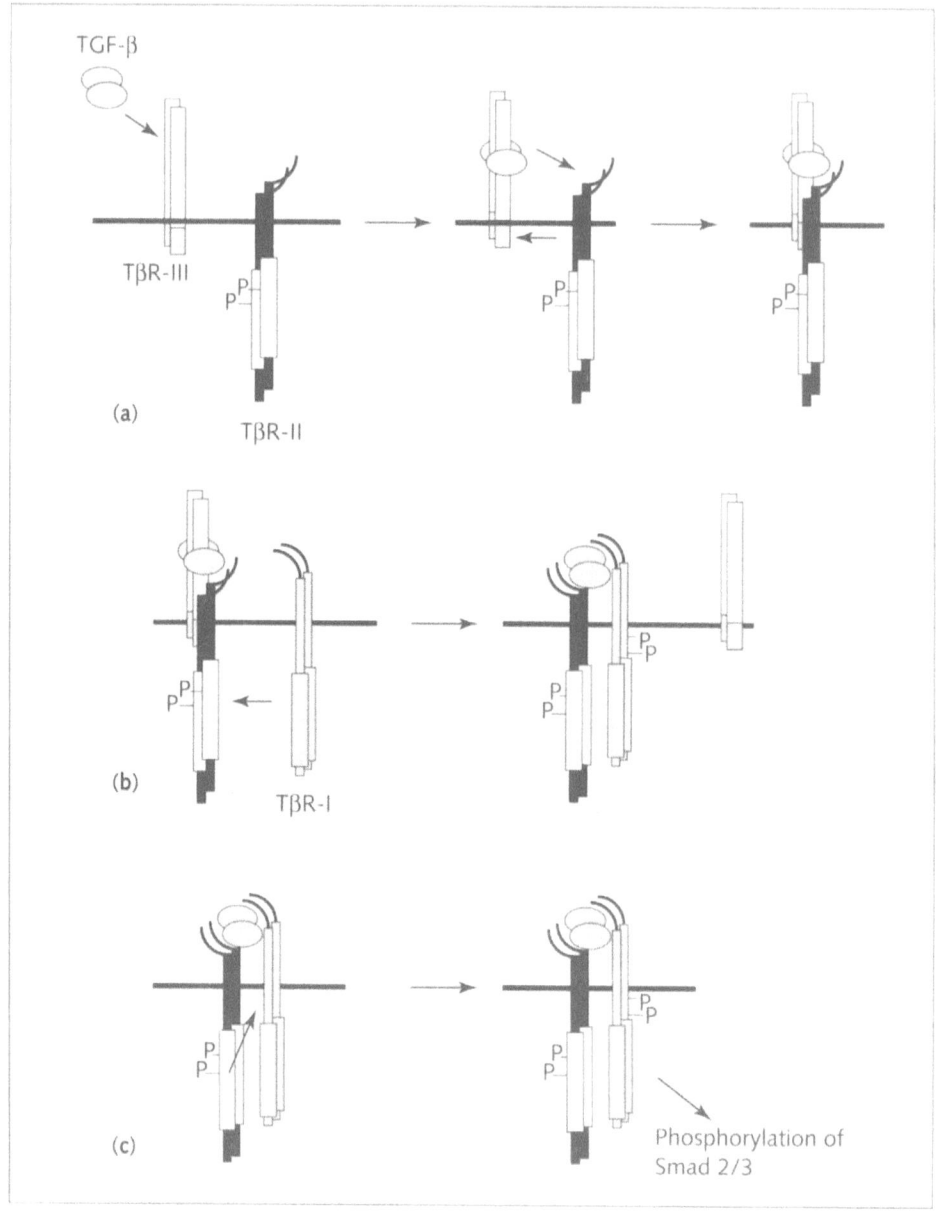

*Figure 1*

Activation of TGF-β receptors. TGF-β binds to TGF-β type III receptors (TβR-III) or, in endothelial cells, to endoglin, whereby a complex with TGF-β type II receptors (TβR-II) is formed (a).
TβR-III then "delivers" the ligand-TβR-II complex to TβR-I (b), whereafter TβR-II phosphorylates TβR-I in the GS-domain which allows phosphorylation of downstream substrates (c).

serine/threonine receptors (Fig. 1a). The TGF-β family members are dimeric molecules which induce the assembly of a signaling complex consisting of two type I and two type II receptor molecules (Fig. 1b). In the complex, the constitutively active type II receptor kinase phosphorylates the type I receptor in a region just N-terminal of the kinase domain which is referred to as the GS domain since it is rich in glycine and serine residues (Fig. 1c) [6]. This phosphorylation activates the type I receptor kinase which initiates downstream signaling. That the type I receptor is downstream of the type II receptor and determines signaling specificity has been shown using constitutively active mutants of type I receptors, e.g. the Thr204Asp mutant of the TGF-β type I receptor; such constitutively active type I receptor mutants signal in the absence of TGF-β and type II receptors [7].

Thus, the available information supports the notion that members of the TGF-β family exert their cellular effects by assembly of tetrameric complexes of characteristic combinations of type I and type II receptors. We currently know of seven type I receptors and five type II receptors in mammalian cells [2, 3]. TGF-β family members often bind to more than one member of the type I receptor family and to more than one member of the type II receptor family, and a given receptor often binds more than one ligand. Thus, TGF-β binds to TβR-II and TβR-I (ALK-5) [8, 9]. However, in endothelial cells TGF-β also binds to another type I receptor, ALK-1 (Oh et al., unpublished observations). Activin binds to two type II receptors, ActR-II and ActR-IIB, and mainly one type I receptor, ActR-1B (ALK-4) [10–12]. BMPs can use the same type II receptors as activin, i.e. ActR-II and ActR-IIB, and in addition BMPR-II; there are three type I receptors for BMPs, ActR-1 (ALK-2), BMPR-IA (ALK-3) and BMPR-1B (ALK-6) [12–15]. The individual receptor binding preferences of different members of the BMP subfamily remains to be elucidated.

The type I serine/threonine kinase receptors interact with FKBP12, an FK506 binding immunophilin, via a Leu-Pro sequence in the GS domain [16, 17]. This interaction suppresses activation of the receptor kinase and appears to protect against spontaneous ligand-independent activation. The kinase domain of TβR-I was recently crystallized in complex with FKBP12 [18]. The structure of the kinase is similar to those of other kinases with known structures, but the mechanism for regulation of the kinase activity differs. The kinase is kept inactive by interactions between the N-terminal lobe of the kinase, the activation loop and the GS domain. TβR-II phosphorylation of TβR-I in the GS domain activates the TβR-I kinase presumably by perturbing these interactions. FKBP12 stabilizes the inactive conformation by capping the phosphorylation sites in the GS domain.

There are also other phosphorylation events in the receptor complex. TβR-II autophosphorylates on certain serine residues which modulates the kinase activity positively or negatively [19], and on tyrosine residues [20], of which the significance remains to be determined. In addition to the phosphorylation in the GS domain, TβR-II also phosphorylates TβR-I at Ser165 in the juxtamembrane region which may modulate signaling since mutation of this residue leads to an enhanced TGF-β-induced growth inhibition and matrix accumulation, but to a decreased apoptosis [21].

## Smad molecules are signal transducers downstream of serine/threonine kinase receptors

The first real insight into the signaling mechanism downstream of serine/threonine receptors came through studies in *Drosophila* [22, 23] and *C. elegans* [24]. They gave genetic evidence for the involvement of *Drosophila Mad* and *C. elegans Sma* genes downstream of TGF-β and serine/threonine receptor counterparts, respectively, in these organisms. Vertebrate counterparts of *Sma* and *Mad* genes were soon found and are collectively referred to as *Smad* genes.

Smad molecules are 42 to 65 kDa transcription factors with two conserved domains, an N-terminal Mad homology (MH)1 domain and a C-terminal MH2 domain (reviewed in [2, 3]). There are three subfamilies of Smad proteins, receptor-activated Smads (R-Smads; Smad 1, 2, 3, 5 and 8), common-partner Smads (Co-Smads; Smad 4a and b) and the more distantly related inhibitory Smads (I-Smads; Smad 6 and 7).

The R-Smads have characteristic C-terminal motifs, -Ser-Ser-Xaa-Ser; the two latter serine residues are phosphorylated by activated type I receptors [25–27]. Smad 2 and 3 are substrates for TGF-β and activin receptors, whereas Smad 1, 5 and 8 are substrates for BMP receptors (reviewed in [1]). It should be noted, however, that TGF-β may also activate Smad 1 and 5 in endothelial cells through the ALK-1 receptor (Oh et al., unpublished observations; [28]). Upon activation, R-Smads form complexes with Co-Smads. In mammalian cells only one Co-Smad has been identified, Smad 4; in *Xenopus*, however, two Co-Smads have been found, Smad 4a and 4b ([29]; Howell et al., unpublished observations), also referred to as Smad 4 and Smad 10 [30]. The Smad complexes are then translocated to the nucleus where they regulate specific genes. Inhibitory Smads compete with R-Smads for receptor interaction and thereby negatively modulate Smad signaling.

The MH2 domain is well conserved in all Smads and is important for interaction with receptors, with other transcription factors and for oligomer formation (reviewed in [1]). It also contains a transcriptional transactivation activity, as was initially unravelled by the demonstration that fusion of the MH2 domain of Smads to the Gal4 DNA binding domain could activate gene expression from a Gal4-dependent reporter construct [31]. In the resting state the transactivational activity is repressed by interaction with the MH1 domain; this interaction in the R-Smads is likely to be derepressed following phosphorylation of the C-terminal serine motif [32]. Upon crystallization of the MH2 domain of Smad 4, a trimeric structure was unravelled [33]. There are observations supporting the notion that

Smad molecules can adopt oligomeric, possibly trimeric, conformations also in solution [33, 34].

The MH1 domain and the linker region are responsible for direct DNA binding [35–37] and also interact with several other nuclear proteins, including c-Jun, ATF-2 and the vitamin D receptor (see further below).

The MH1 and MH2 domains are connected with a proline-rich linker region, which in R-Smads contains consensus phosphorylation sites for MAP kinase and thus is of importance for cross-talk between the two signaling pathways (see below). The C-terminal part of the linker region of Smad 4 contains a domain, referred to as the Smad activation domain (SAD), which is necessary for signal transduction, presumably because it mediates binding of other proteins with transcriptional activity such as MSG1 [38, 39].

Regarding the mechanism whereby Smads are recognized by type I receptors, there is no evidence that R-Smads dock to phosphorylated regions of activated serine/threonine receptors. Thus, the mechanism whereby specificity in signaling is generated differs from that used by tyrosine kinase receptors. Instead, specific "presenting molecules" have been proposed to help in the recognition of specific R-Smads by receptors. One such molecule is the Smad anchor for activation (SARA), a protein anchored in the membrane *via* a FYVE domain which recognizes the membrane phospholipid phosphatidylinositol 3'-phosphate; SARA binds Smad 2 and 3 as well as the TGF-β receptor complex and thus stabilizes the interaction complex between Smad and TGF-β receptors [40] (Fig. 2a). In addition, specificity is dependent on a match between the L45 region in the kinase domain of type I receptors [41–44] and the L3 loop in the MH2 domains of R-Smads [42]. For the interaction between Smad 1/5 and ALK-1 or ALK-2, the α-helix H1 in the MH2 domain is, in addition to the L3 loop, an important determinant [45].

Upon receptor phosphorylation of R-Smads, heterooligomeric complexes with Smad 4 are formed. Smad 4 is essential for many, but not all [46], effects of TGF-β on cells. The stoichiometry of activated Smad complexes has not been firmly established. Given that Smad 4 MH2 occurs as a trimer it is, however, possible that activated Smad complexes are heteromeric complexes of different combinations of Smad 2, 3 and 4 [34] (Fig. 2b). Since the combination of Smad 2, Smad 3 and Smad 4 gives the most potent transcriptional activation [47], it is possible that all three Smads may participate in a common trimeric complex.

R-Smad phosphorylation triggers the formation of the oligomeric complex and subsequent nuclear translocation of Smads. Ligand-induced translocation of R-Smads occurs in the absence of Smad 4 [48], however, Co-Smads require R-Smads for nuclear translocation [27, 48]. Interestingly, the C-termini of R-Smads, containing the Ser-Ser-Xaa-Ser motif important for activation, are not necessary for nuclear translocation [49]. The precise mechanism for the nuclear translocation of Smads, however, remains to be elucidated. It is possible that ligand-induced heterooligomerization causes a conformational change in the Smad

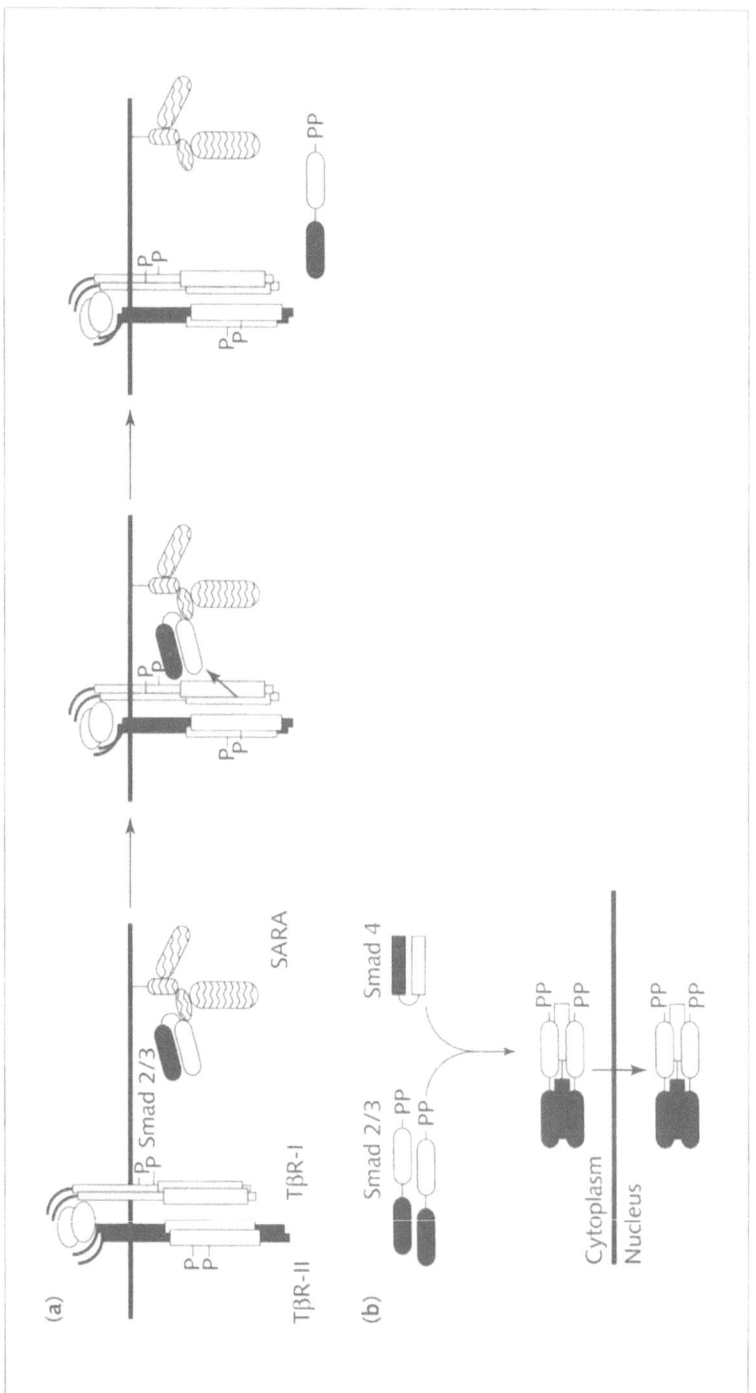

Figure 2

Activation of Smad complexes. Smad2 or 3 bound to the membrane-associated SARA molecule is presented to the activated TGF-β receptor complex, and becomes phosphorylated by TβR-I in the C-terminal Ser-Ser-Xaa-Ser motif (a). Phosphorylated and activated Smad2 or 3 molecules then forms a complex with Smad4 (b). The stoichiometry of Smad complexes has not been determined, but it is likely that they consist of trimers of different combinations of Smad2, 3 and 4.

molecules which exposes a nuclear localization signal. Alternatively, interaction with cytoplasmic anchoring proteins or transporter proteins could be involved.

## Smads interact with DNA directly

*Drosophila* Mad gave the first evidence for a Smad directly associating with DNA [36]. The Mad MH1-linker subdomain exhibits *in vitro* DNA-binding activity towards a GC-rich sequence derived from three Decapentaplegic (Dpp) target gene promoters, those of the *vestigial* (*vg*), *labial* (*lab*) and *ultrabithorax* (*ubx*) genes. Full length Mad did not associate with the DNA sequences tested and the consensus motif recognized by Mad was defined as GCCGnCGG (where n is any nucleotide). Other GC-rich sequences recognized by *Drosophila* Mad and Medea have been described in the transcription factor *tinman* and *mef2* gene promoters [50, 51]. In mammalian genes, only two GC-rich motifs have been reported to be recognized by the MH1-linker subdomains of Smad 3 and Smad 4. One belongs to the homeobox *goosecoid* (*gsc*) gene promoter and the other to the collagen VII, COL7A1 promoter [52, 53].

Subsequently, full length human Smad 4 was identified to directly associate with a chimeric sequence from a synthetic TGF-β-responsive promoter called 3TP [54]. This sequence included an activating protein-1 (AP-1) site partially overlapping the CAGACA sequence derived from the plasminogen activator inhibitor 1 (PAI-1) promoter. Thus, direct DNA-binding of Smad 4 in complex with Smad 3 and potentiation of AP-1 binding activity was proposed to explain 3TP promoter upregulation by TGF-β. Indeed, full length Smad 3 and its MH1-linker subdomain can directly bind to one half of a consensus AP-1 site and to its adjacent GC-rich sequences [55]. These DNA sequences consist of classic 12-O-tetradecanoylphorbol 13-acetate (TPA)-responsive elements and were derived from the collagenase I promoter. The PAI-1 gene is a primary target in TGF-β-mediated gene regulation. Analysis of PAI-1 promoter sequences led to the discovery of the CAGA box [56]. This is a DNA motif found in multiple interspersed copies in the PAI-1 promoter and was shown to be recognized specifically by a nuclear Smad 3/4 complex and by purified MH1-linker subdomains of Smad 3 or Smad 4, but not of Smad 1 or Smad 2. Additional Smad 3 and Smad 4-binding DNA sequences have been identified in the PAI-1 promoter, some of which consist of permutated CAGA boxes and some of non-consensus AP-1 sites [57, 58]. Mutational analyses revealed that all of the identified Smad-binding elements of the PAI-1 promoter are of importance for TGF-β-induced expression of this promoter.

An *in vitro* screen of random DNA oligonucleotides that specifically bound to MH1-linker subdomains of Smad 3 and Smad 4 resulted in the identification of an optimal, palindromic sequence motif, GTCTAGAC, which when multimerized conferred TGF-β-induced promoter activation [35]. Interestingly, this motif, which has been named Smad Binding Element (SBE), contains an inverted repeat of CAGA-like boxes. The combined analyses of the SBE and the CAGA boxes of the PAI-1 promoter led to the notion that the SBE represents the canonical mammalian DNA sequence recognized by Smad 3 and Smad 4. SBE's have also been identified in the promoter/enhancer regions of *junB*, *c-jun* and IgA genes and have been demonstrated to be responsible for TGF-β-dependent regulation of the corresponding genes ([59, 60]; Pardali et al., unpublished observations). Non-canonical SBE's have been identified in the COL7A1 promoter, the promoters of the cell cycle inhibitors p15 and p21 and in the *C. elegans myo2* gene enhancer; although these elements can associate with Smads, their exact physiological role has not yet been clarified [35, 53, 61–63].

The molecular features of Smad-DNA interactions have been analyzed in great detail by crystallization of the Smad 3 MH1 domain bound to a DNA oligonucleotide consisting of a perfect inverted repeat of the 5'GTCT3' sequence [37]. The X-ray analysis revealed that a highly conserved eleven-amino acid, β-hairpin in the center of the MH1 domain, is important for direct contact with the CAGA sequence. Interestingly, Smad 2 has two unique amino acid sequence segments on one side of the β-hairpin which are completely missing from Smad 3 and prevent binding to the SBE [35, 37, 56]. Precise deletion of the inserts from the Smad 2 sequence results in a mutant Smad 2 that has indistinguishable DNA-binding features compared to Smad 3 [64]. In addition, an alternatively spliced form of human Smad 2, which lacks exon 3 and exhibits fully competent SBE-binding properties has been isolated from various cell types [65]. Whether Smad 2 can directly associate with other, non-SBE, sequences or whether the association of Smad 2 with Smad 4 or possibly with Smad 3 or with other transcription factors such as forkhead activin signal transducer 1 (FAST-1), might alter its conformation and reveal DNA-binding activity, remain untested hypotheses.

An important issue refers to the Smad stoichiometry in the DNA-bound protein complexes. This is relevant since Smads homo- and hetero-oligomerize with each other and with other transcription factors. In one study, no cooperativity between the Smad 3 MH1 domains was identified in binding reactions with the SBE sequences [37]. In studies using full length Smad or MH1-linker subdomain, homodimeric association of Smad 3 to PAI-1 or COL7A1 sequences was identified [58, 61] and, importantly, cooperative binding of Smad 3 and Smad 4 to adjacent DNA sites was demonstrated [58]. However, the exact stoichiometry of such heteromeric Smad complexes has not been clarified.

## Smads co-operate with a large variety of transcription factors

As described above, direct DNA binding of Smads is of low affinity and can be experimentally enhanced by concatamerization of the SBE. Although promoters often contain multiple copies of SBE for most, if not all, genes, Smads mediate transcriptional responses not only through DNA interaction but also through binding and functional cooperation with other transcription factors [66].

This paradigm was initiated by studies of the promoter of the *Xenopus* homeobox gene *mix.2* which is an immediate-early response gene to activin/Vg-1 ligands [67, 68]. Activin induces the *mix.2* promoter *via* a nucleoprotein complex containing a winged helix transcription factor of the forkhead family, FAST-1, which directly binds to *mix.2* DNA sequences [67]. The complex also contains Smad 4 and Smad 2, of which the latter physically interacts with FAST-1 [68]. Interestingly, the complex of FAST-1 and Smads has been reconstituted in mammalian cells in which the *Xenopus* FAST-1 was ectopically expressed [48]. In this heterologous system it was discovered that on the one hand the Smad 4 MH1 domain promotes DNA binding of the complex *via* FAST-1 and on the other hand the Smad 4 MH2 domain serves as the transactivation domain, which presumably co-operates with components of the basal transcription machinery. Thus, Smad 2 plays the role of a protein bridge mediating FAST-1–Smad 4 communication.

More recently, two mammalian FAST-like proteins have been cloned, human FAST-1 and mouse FAST-2 [52, 69, 70]. In mammalian nuclear complexes of FASTs and Smads, DNA binding is mediated both *via* their FAST subunit and *via* their Smad 3 or Smad 4 subunits. The DNA targets tested were derived either from an artificial promoter containing a *Xenopus* FAST-binding element fused to a SBE [69], or from a small segment of the *gsc* promoter, which naturally contains Smad 3/4-binding GC-rich motifs (see above) in close proximity to FAST-2-binding DNA motifs [52]. Interestingly, whereas the FAST-2-Smad 2-Smad 4-*gsc* DNA complex activates promoter transcription, the FAST-2-Smad 3-Smad 4-*gsc* DNA complex represses transcription from the same promoter [52]. In this model system, the binding of Smad 3 or Smad 4 to the GC-rich sequences is mutually exclusive and thus represents an example of antagonistic function of the two related R-Smads, Smad 2 and 3. In addition to *Mix.2*, the *Xenopus XFKH-1* and *XFD-1* genes, also being members of the forkhead transcription factor gene family, as well as *gsc*, are also directly regulated by activin/Vg-1-like signals *via* FAST-1-containing nucleoprotein complexes [71–73].

In addition to forkhead family transcription factors, c-Jun and c-Fos physically interact with Smad 3, although the Smad 3-c-Fos association is not induced by TGF-β [55, 74]. The Smad 3 MH1-linker subdomains bind to the bZip domain of c-Jun, whereas the MH2 domain of Smad 3 interacts with c-Fos. Smad 4 does not interact directly with c-Jun or c-Fos although it participates in AP-1–Smad nucleoprotein complexes [55]. The co-operation of Smads with other cell-type-specific transcription factors provides an explanation for regulation of many TGF-β target genes in different cell types [2, 3]. One such target gene is *c-jun* itself, whose upregulation by TGF-β is mediated by the AP-1 complex associating to the corresponding DNA site in the proximal promoter and by the Smad 3/4 complex which binds to a triple CAGA motif in the first intron of the gene [60]. Thus, co-operation between Smads bound to DNA and the AP-1 complex bound to its cognate site results in a synergistic transactivation of the *c-jun* promoter.

The complex PAI-1 promoter, apart from containing SBE's and other Smad binding sequences (see above), is regulated by TGF-β *via* the action of an E-box-binding transcription factor, transcription factor E3 (TFE3), which is activated by TGF-β and synergizes with Smad 3 [75]. However, its physical interaction with Smad proteins has not yet been demonstrated.

The Smad 3 MH1 domain and in particular its N-terminal one third has been shown to physically interact with the vitamin D3 receptor (VDR) in a ligand-dependent manner which is also enhanced or stabilized by the steroid receptor co-activator (SRC1) [76]. Although this discovery has profound implications for the extensive co-operation between TGF-β's and steroids [77], no direct evidence for the convergent regulation of a common target gene by VDR and Smads has yet been provided.

Sp1 is another ubiquitous transcription factor whose binding motif, the GC-box, has been implicated in the regulation of several target genes of TGF-β, including the cell cycle inhibitors p15 and p21, TGF-$\beta_1$, TGF-β type I and II receptors, α2(I) collagen and others [78–83]. Concatamerized consensus Sp1 GC-boxes respond very potently to stimulation by TGF-β [84]. These effects can be explained by the Smad-mediated co-operation with Sp1 at least in the case of the cell cycle inhibitor p21 [85]. This promoter appears to be upregulated by Smad proteins without any requirement for Smad binding to DNA, and physical interactions between Smad 3 and Sp1 result in increased DNA binding activity of Sp1 (A. Moustakas, unpublished observations). Smad 4 also participates in nucleoprotein complexes with Smad 3 and Sp1 and potentiates or stabilizes the enhanced Sp1-DNA binding activity, but it does not interact with Sp1 directly.

Smads were also shown to functionally co-operate with NFκB in the regulation of the COL7A1 promoter [86]. Thus, one can expect that additional transcription factors will be identified to interact and synergize with Smads, especially those already implicated in the regulation of TGF-β superfamily target genes, such as CCAAT box-binding transcription factor/nuclear factor 1 (CTF/NF1) and activating transcription factor-2 (ATF2) or cAMP response element binding protein (CREB) [87, 88]. Most transcription factors that co-operate with Smads have been found to be involved in mammalian TGF-β, *Drosophila* Dpp or *C. elegans* Daf signaling pathways. Several mammalian BMP target genes have recently been identified, including the homeobox genes *gsc*, *tlx-2*, *Msx*-1 and -2, as well as members of the *Id* family [71, 89, 90]. However, a comprehensive analysis of the involvement of Smads in their regulation is still lacking.

The transcription factor Evi-1 has been shown to specifically bind to activated Smad 3, thereby preventing it from binding to DNA. This results in blocking of TGF-β-induced growth arrest and may contribute to the oncogenic properties of Evi-1 [91].

Recently, two examples of repressor proteins have been described which, upon interaction with Smads, dissociate from their promoters. The two-handed zinc-finger homeodomain protein, Smad interacting protein-1 (SIP-1), was identified as a protein which interacts with the MH2 domains of activated R-Smads [92]. Overexpression of SIP-1 prevents expression of the activin-regulated gene *Xbra*; activin-induced Smad binding to SIP-1 appears to be involved in the de-repression of the *Xbra* gene. In addition, the repression of the osteopontin gene by the homeodomain protein Hoxc-8 is relieved by BMP-induced interaction between Smad 1 and Hoxc-8 [93].

## Smads interact with co-activators, co-repressors and chromatin-modelling factors

An additional complexity has been added to the model of Smad-mediated transcriptional regulation by the discovery that the co-activators CREB-binding protein (CBP) and p300 can directly interact with phosphorylated Smad 1, 2, and 3 in a ligand-dependent manner [94-99]. The interaction is mediated by the C-terminal fifth of the Smad MH2 domain and a small subdomain of CBP/p300 around amino acid residue number 1900. Since these co-activators are known to interact and integrate transcriptional activation by a multitude of transcription factors such as c-Jun, CREB, c-Fos, p53, nuclear receptors and others [100], the interaction of Smads with CBP/p300 may explain many of the co-operative mechanisms described above [66]. Moreover, the interference of the adenoviral oncoprotein E1A with TGF-β-mediated signaling can be explained by competition with Smads for binding to p300 [94–99]. Interestingly, E1A and Smads bind to adjacent amino acid segments of p300. The CBP/p300 co-integrators could possibly mediate the bridging between the Smad MH2 transactivating domain and the basal transcriptional machinery. Alternatively, the co-integrators could mediate Smad-dependent alterations of chromatin compaction *via* their intrinsic histone acetyl transferase activity.

A different type of co-activator, MSG1, which specifically interacts with Smad 4, has been identified [38]. MSG1 potentiates the transcriptional activity of Smad 2/3-Smad 4 complexes in a TGF-β-dependent manner. However, the physiological importance of such a co-activator in TGF-β-superfamily target gene regulation remains to be elucidated.

A co-repressor, the homeobox protein TGT interacting factor (TGIF), was also recently found to directly interact with Smad 2 [101]. Recruitment of TGIF by the activated Smad 2-Smad 4 complex results in transcriptional repression of target genes such as PAI-1 or the activin response element from the *Xenopus mix.2* promoter. Repression depends on the presence of the histone deacetylase (HDAC) which interacts with TGIF and thus is also brought to the ligand-activated nuclear complex. Interestingly, p300/CBP can antagonize the interaction between TGIF and

Smad 2 when both co-regulators are provided at sufficient levels in the same nuclear environment. Another recently described repressor is the *Drosophila* protein Brinker [102–104], which appears to repress gene targets of Dpp. Signaling by Dpp-induced Mad-Medea nuclear complexes on the one hand represses *brinker* gene expression and on the other hand relieves the Brinker-dependent repression and stimulates transcription from the previously silent gene promoter.

In conclusion, Smad 2 and 3 regulate transcription by directly associating with DNA sequences, albeit with low affinity and not absolute sequence specificity. Smad proteins simultaneously interact and functionally cooperate with other transcription factors. In addition, recruitment of co-activators or co-repressors integrates the transcriptional activity of Smads and other transcription factors possibly by providing direct access to the RNA polymerase II holoenzyme or by modulating chromatin condensation and transcription factor accessibility (Fig. 3).

## Inhibitory Smads

Inhibitory Smads have been identified in mammals [47, 105–107], *Xenopus* [108] and *Drosophila* [109]. Mammalian Smad 6 and Smad 7, and *Xenopus* Smad 7 (previously termed XSmad 8; [108]), have all been shown to form stable associations with specific type I receptors, thereby preventing R-Smads from binding to, and being phosphorylated by, these receptors [47, 106, 107, 110–112]. Smad 6 has also been found to bind Smad 1, thereby preventing the formation of active Smad 4-Smad 1 signaling complexes [32].

Smad 6 and Smad 7 inhibit TGF-β-, activin- and BMP-induced responses with different potency in *Xenopus* and mammalian cells. Smad 6 can complex with many, but not all, TGF-β superfamily type I receptors, and can block phosphorylation of some, but not all, R-Smads. Smad 7 binds to all mammalian type I receptors and interferes with type I receptor-mediated R-Smad phosphorylation. Smad 7, but not Smad 6, was found to interfere with TGF-β-mediated growth arrest in mink lung epithelial cells [113], and activin-induced growth inhibition and apoptosis in B-cells [114]. Both Smad 6 and Smad 7 were found to inhibit BMP-induced growth inhibition and apoptosis in B-cells [115]. In *Xenopus*, Smad 7, and less efficiently Smad 6, inhibits TGF-β/activin-like induced responses in mesoderm induction assays. Both I-Smads inhibit BMP signaling in *Xenopus* embryos, e.g. dorsalize the ventral mesoderm and induce a (partial) secondary axis and induce the formation of neural tissue, with Smad 6 being more potent than Smad 7 [32, 47, 108, 116, 117]. Thus, Smad 7 appears to be a general inhibitor of TGF-β superfamily signaling, whereas Smad 6 preferentially inhibits BMP signaling responses (Fig. 4).

The isolated C-terminal domains of Smad 7 and Smad 6 are sufficient for association with activated type I receptor or with Smad 1, respectively [32, 110]. *Xenopus* and mouse Smad 7 are highly related in their C-terminal regions but have diver-

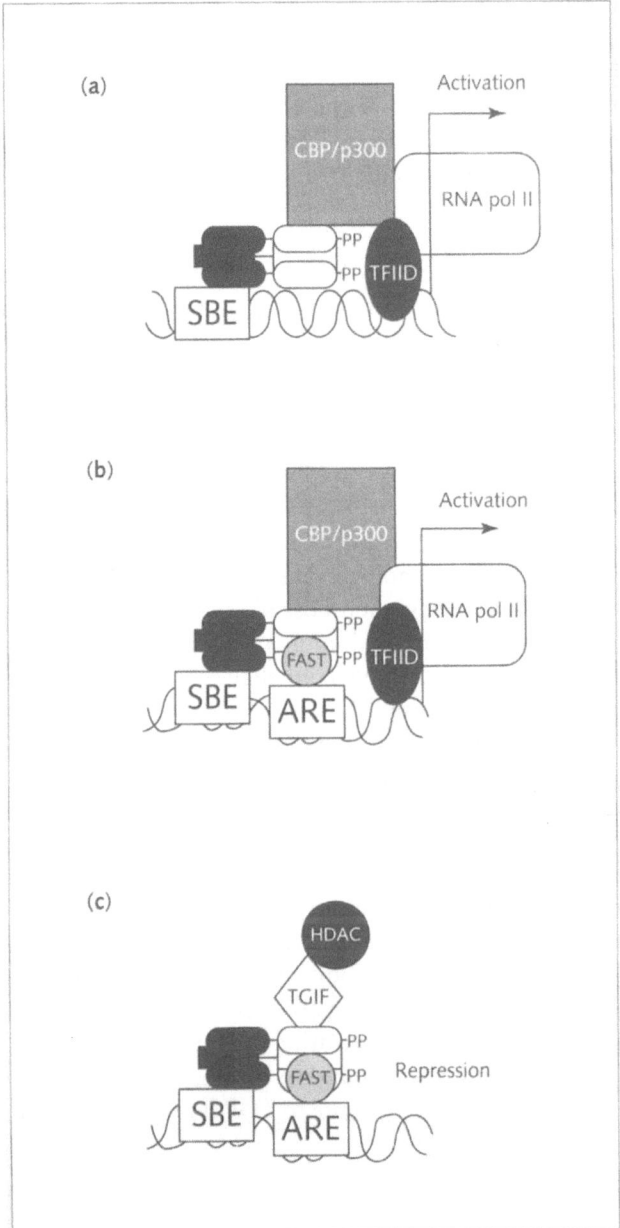

*Figure 3*
*Nuclear function of Smads. Smad complexes bind to promoter regions of specific genes*
*directly (a) or together with other transcription factors (b). The complexes also interact with*
*co-activators (a, b) or co-repressors (c), to regulate the expression of the genes.*

gent N-terminal domains. XSmad 7 was found to be a less efficient inhibitor of TβR-I-mediated responses in mammalian cells than mouse Smad 7. Furthermore, ectopic expression of XSmad 7 and mouse Smad 7 in *Xenopus* produce overlapping but different patterning defects. This suggests that these two Smad 7s may target common but also distinct signaling pathways [110]. Thus, the N-terminal region of I-Smads may play a role in determining the specificity and potency of the inhibitory actions.

XSmad 6 accumulates at the plasma membrane of many cells, but is more abundant, or restricted to, the nuclei of certain cells in *Xenopus* [108]. In mammalian cells, ectopically expressed Smad 7 was predominantly located in the nucleus and was found to redistribute to the cytoplasm upon TGF-β stimulation [113]. For TGF-β-induced nuclear export of Smad 7, an intact C-terminal domain is required [113]. The mechanism by which changes in subcellular distribution occur and whether I-Smads also have nuclear functions remain to be determined.

In mammalian cells, Smad 6 and Smad 7 are rapidly and directly induced by TGF-β, activin and BMPs [47, 114, 115, 118, 119]. In addition, *Drosophila Dad* was identified as a Dpp-inducible gene [109], and XSmad 7 was found to be inducible by BMP-4 in *Xenopus* [108]. These findings, taken together with the function of I-Smads as intracellular antagonists, suggest a possible role in negative feedback regulation. Consistent with this notion, inhibition of endogenous Smad 7 expression by anti-sense nucleotides in mink lung epithelial cells was found to potentiate the TGF-β-induced signaling response [118].

With the I-Smad expression level being a determinant for TGF-β superfamily responsiveness, stimuli that regulate their expression may provide a means for cross-talk of other signaling pathways with the TGF-β/Smad signaling pathway. In this respect it is interesting to note that epidermal growth factor (EGF) was found to induce the expression of I-Smads, and that the phorbol ester PMA potentiated the TGF-β-induced expression of Smad 7 [118]. Furthermore, Smad 6 and Smad 7 are highly expressed in vascular endothelial cells and were found to be induced by laminar shear stress [105]. The implications of this upregulated expression in endothelial cell function remain to be determined. Interferon-γ (IFN-γ) was found to upregulate Smad 7 expression, through Jak1-mediated activation of Stat1, and thereby to inhibit TGF-β/Smad signaling [120]. Smad 6 was found to be overexpressed in certain human pancreatic cells and may possibly contribute to TGF-β resistance in pancreatic cancer [121].

## Cross-talk between Smad-dependent signalling and other pathways

Several examples of cross-talk between different signaling pathways have recently been demonstrated. It is likely that such cross-talk is important to assure an appropriate response of a cell to the multitude of external signals it receives. Given the

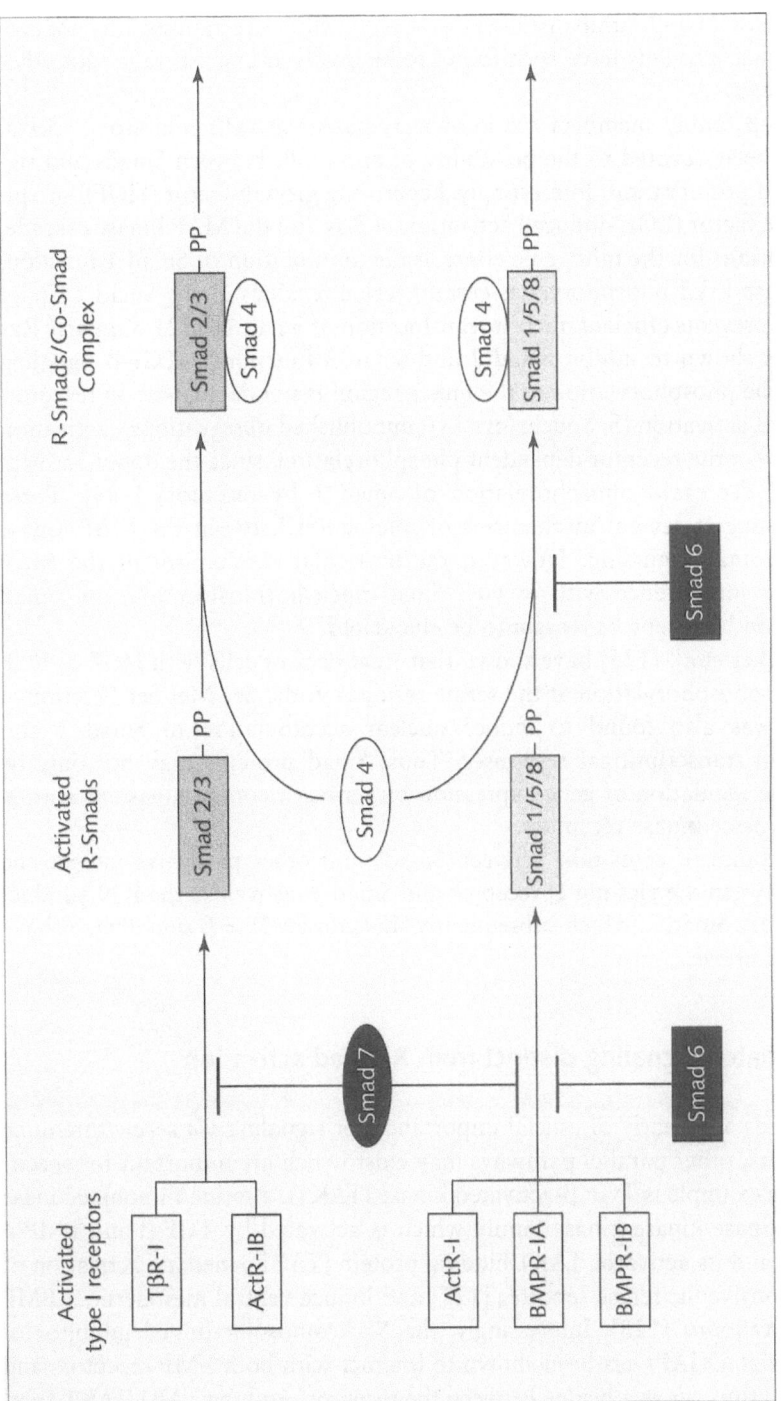

*Figure 4*
*Inhibitory effects of Smad6 and Smad7. Smad7 inhibit phosphorylation and activation of R-Smads by competition for interaction with TGF-β, activin and BMP receptors. Smad6 preferentially inhibits BMP-activated Smads by competition for interaction with receptors and with Smad4.*

important role of TGF-β family members in several cellular responses, it is not surprising that Smad proteins have been found to be involved in cross-talk with other signaling pathways.

Since TGF-β family members are known as potent growth inhibitors, special attention has been devoted to the possibility of cross-talk between Smads and signals promoting proliferation. Interestingly, hepatocyte growth factor (HGF)- or epidermal growth factor (EGF)-induced activation of Ras and the MAP kinase cascade, which is important for the mitogenic effect, leads to inhibition of Smad 1 function; the MAP kinase Erk2 phosphorylates certain serine residues in the Smad 1 linker region, which prevents efficient nuclear translocation of Smad 1 [122]. Similarly Ras activation was shown to inhibit Smad 2 and Smad 3 function in TGF-β signaling [123]. While the phosphorylation in the linker region is not dependent on receptor-mediated Smad activation (S. Souchelnytskyi, unpublished observations), activation of Ras may affect the receptor-dependent phosphorylation, since the dominant negative RasN17 decreased phosphorylation of Smad 1 by receptors [124]. These observations suggest several mechanisms of interaction between the MAP kinase pathway and Smad signaling. However, the molecular mechanism of the MAP kinase-induced interference with *in vivo* Smad nuclear translocation and Smad phosphorylation by receptors remain to be elucidated.

De Caestecker et al. [125] have shown that treatment of cells with HGF or EGF led to Smad 2 phosphorylation at the serine residues in the Ser-Met-Ser C-terminal motif. HGF was also found to induce nuclear accumulation of Smad 2 and Smad-mediated transcriptional responses. Thus, Smad proteins may not only be involved in the regulation of gene expression by serine/threonine kinase receptors, but also of tyrosine kinase receptors.

Other examples of cross-talk between Smads and other pathways include the interaction between the vitamin D receptor and Smad 3, as well as the IFN-γ-induction of inhibitory Smad 7, which subsequently shuts down TGF-β signaling, as have been discussed above.

## Receptor-initiated signaling distinct from R-Smad activation

Although Smads are clearly of crucial importance for signaling *via* serine/threonine kinase receptors, other parallel pathways may exist which are important for specific signals. One example is TGF-β-activated kinase (TAK1), a serine/threonine kinase of the MAP kinase kinase kinase family which is activated by TGF-β and BMP-4 [126]. TAK1, and its activator TAK1 binding protein (TAB1), mediate activation of a TGF-β responsive luciferase reporter [127] and induce ventral mesoderm, a BMP response, in *Xenopus* [128]. Interestingly, the X-chromosome-linked inhibitor of apoptosis protein (XIAP) has been shown to interact with both BMP receptors and TAB1, and can thus act as a bridge between the receptors and the TAB1/TAK1 complex [129]. A similar role can be played by BMP receptor associated molecule-1 (BRAM-1), which also interacts both with BMP receptors and TAB1 [130].

A downstream effector of TAK1 is MAP kinase kinase 4/stress activated protein kinase/extracellular signal regulated kinase SEK1 [131], which in turn activates the stress-activated protein kinase (SAPK)/c-Jun N-terminal kinase (JNK) which has been shown to be activated by TGF-β [132, 133]. A role for the JNK/SAPK pathway in TGF-β signaling was supported by the finding that a dominant negative JNK/SAPK molecule inhibited TGF-β-induced transcription [134]. Interestingly, the transcription factor ATF-2 which binds to the cAMP responsive element is phosphorylated and activated by JNK/SAPK and p38 kinases after TGF-β stimulation activation of TAK-1 [135]. ATF-2 interacts with the MH1 domains of Smad 3 and 4, the nuclear target of the Smad and TAK-1 pathways, and may be an example of the synergistic action of these pathways.

Signalling of TGF-β through JNK/SAPK is Smad 4-independent, at least in the case of regulation of fibronectin expression [46]. The activation of JNK by TNF-α does not interfere with Smad nuclear translocation, suggesting that this kinase does not mimic the effect of the Erk-MAP kinase. However, an upstream activator of JNK/SAPK, MEKK-1, induced Smad 2-dependent transcription by phosphorylation of Smad 2 at sites other than the C-terminal serines phosphorylated by TGF-β receptors [136]. In the same model MEK-1 and TAK1 did not activate Smad 2 transcriptional responses, illustrating the specificity of MEKK-1 action.

Certain MAP kinases, e.g. Erk1 and Erk2, have been shown to be activated by TGF-β in certain cell types [133]. Members of the Ras [137] and Rac [138] families have also been implicated in TGF-β signaling. In intestinal epithelial cells, TGF-β rapidly induces Ras activation and activation of the MAP kinase pathway [139], in contrast to the case for Ras-transformed mammary epithelial cells in which activation of the MAP kinase pathway inhibits TGF-β signaling [123]. It is thus possible that the functional consequences of interactions between the Ras/MAP kinase and Smad pathways differ between different cell types.

## Subversion of TGF-β signaling in cancer

Members of the TGF-β family have multifunctional roles in tumorigenesis. At early stages of tumor progression they may act as tumor suppressors, whereas at later stages they may promote tumor growth through effects on non-malignant cells in the tumor, causing immunosuppression and stimulation of stroma formation and angiogenesis. A biphasic role for TGF-β in tumorigenesis was demonstrated using a transgenic mouse model for skin carcinogenesis in which TGF-β expression was directed to keratinocytes [140].

A tumor suppressor role for members of the TGF-β family is supported by the finding that mice in which the gene for α-inhibin had been inactivated showed an increased frequency of gonadal tumors [141]. Moreover, during tumor progression tumor cells often escape the antimitogenic effect of TGF-β through mutation in genes for different components along the signaling pathway. Thus, the type II receptor gene is frequently mutated in an inherited form of colon cancer with a microsatellite instability phenotype [142]. In addition, mutations in the type I receptor gene has been found in prostate cancer cells [143], chronic lymphocytic leukemia [144], pancreatic and biliary carcinomas [145], and metastatic breast cancer [146]. Mutation of the Smad 4 gene occurs at high frequency in pancreatic cancers; in fact, Smad 4 was initially discovered as the DPC4 tumor suppressor gene [147]. Mutation of the Smad 4 gene has also been noticed in other tumor types, but with lower frequency [148, 149]. Genes for other Smads are not frequent targets for mutation [150], but the Smad 2 gene has been found to be mutated in colorectal and lung carcinomas [151, 152]. It is not known why the Smad 4 gene is more frequently mutated than genes for other Smads; it may reflect a more non-redundant role for the common-partner Smad 4 in TGF-β family signaling.

Whereas mice with targeted disruption of the genes for Smad 4 [153, 154] or Smad 2 [155] die during early embryonal development, Smad 3 knock-out mice are born alive [156–158]. Using the knock-out mice, Smad 3 was shown to be required for TGF-β-induced growth inhibition of primary splenocytes and embryo fibroblasts [156], as well as for T cell activation and mucosal immunity [158]. One study also reported an increased prevalence of colorectal cancer [157]; this was not found in other studies [156, 158] and may thus represent a difference between mouse strains.

## Future perspectives

During the recent few years a mechanism for signaling by members of the TGF-β family of factors has been unravelled. The ligands bind to characteristic complexes of type I and type II serine/threonine kinase receptors, whereafter the type I receptor is phosphorylated and activated by the type II receptor, leading to phosphorylation of downstream substrates including R-Smads. R-Smads then form complexes with Co-Smads, which are translocated to the nucleus where they bind, directly or indirectly, to promoter regions of specific genes. The activity of Smad pathways is controlled by a feed back mechanism involving inhibitory Smads and by cross-talk with other signaling pathways. In addition, there are indications that Smad-independent signaling pathways are also initiated downstream of serine/threonine receptors; the mechanism of activation and functional roles of these pathways deserves further attention.

Several genes that are induced by different members of the TGF-β family have been identified. An important future task will be to determine the full spectrum of genes induced or repressed by individual members of the family. The now available systematic approaches to monitor protein expression by two-dimensional gel techniques and mRNA levels by gene array techniques, will be very useful in achieving this goal.

The genes for several ligands, receptors and Smad molecules have already been targeted in mice, which has yielded important insight into the function of these components. Many of these knock-outs give embryonal lethal phenotypes, illustrating the important roles of TGF-β family members during development. In order to elucidate the functional roles of these components in the late phases of embryonal development and in the adult, it will be important to construct and study conditional knock-outs in which the respective genes are inactivated in a temporally or spatially restricted manner.

Overactivity of TGF-β has been associated with certain disorders, in particular the late phases of tumorigenesis and fibrotic conditions in the lung, kidney and liver. It is therefore possible that TGF-β antagonists will be clinically useful. The recent success in elucidating the intracellular signaling mechanism has provided numerous targets for drug discovery. However, given that TGF-β has such a multitude of effects on most cell types, severe side-effects are anticipated from total systemic blockage of TGF-β signaling. Therefore it may be necessary to develop inhibitors that specifically inhibit only certain effects of TGF-β, or to administer antagonists locally in the affected tissue.

## Acknowledgements

We thank Ingegärd Schiller for valuable help in the preparation of this manuscript.

## References

1    Piek E, Heldin C-H, ten Dijke P (1999) Specificity, diversity and regulation in TGF-β superfamily signaling. *FASEB J* 13: 2105–2124
2    Heldin C-H, Miyazono K, ten Dijke P (1997) TGF-β signalling from cell membrane to nucleus through SMAD proteins. *Nature* 390: 465–471
3    Massagué J (1998) TGF-β signal transduction. *Annu Rev Biochem* 67: 753–791
4    López-Casillas F, Wrana JL, Massagué J (1993) Betaglycan presents ligand to the TGF-β signaling receptor. *Cell* 73: 1435–1444
5    Gougos A, Letarte M (1990) Primary structure of endoglin, an RGD-containing glycoprotein of human endothelial cells. *J Biol Chem* 265: 8361–8364
6    Wrana JL, Attisano L, Wieser R, Ventura F, Massagué J (1994) Mechanism of activation of the TGF-β receptor. *Nature* 370: 341–347
7    Wieser R, Wrana JL, Massagué J (1995) GS domain mutations that constitutively acti-

vate TβR-I, the downstream signaling component in the TGF-β receptor complex. *EMBO J* 14: 2199–2208

8   Franzén P, ten Dijke P, Ichijo H, Yamashita H, Schulz P, Heldin C-H, Miyazono K (1993) Cloning of a TGFβ type I receptor that forms a heteromeric complex with the TGFβ type II receptor. *Cell* 75: 681–692

9   Lin HY, Wang X-F, Ng-Eaton E, Weinberg RA, Lodish HF (1992) Expression cloning of the TGF-β type II receptor, a functional transmembrane serine/threonine kinase. *Cell* 68: 775–785

10  Mathews LS, Vale WW (1991) Expression cloning of an activin receptor, a predicted transmembrane serine kinase. *Cell* 65: 973–982

11  Attisano L, Wrana JL, Cheifetz S, Massagué J (1992) Novel activin receptors: Distinct genes and alternative mRNA splicing generate a repertoire of serine/threonine kinase receptors. *Cell* 68: 97–108

12  ten Dijke P, Yamashita H, Ichijo H, Franzén P, Laiho M, Miyazono K, Heldin C-H (1994) Characterization of type I receptors for transforming growth factor-β and activin. *Science* 264: 101–104

13  Liu F, Ventura F, Doody J, Massagué J (1995) Human type II receptor for bone morphogenic proteins (BMPs): Extension of the two-kinase receptor model to the BMPs. *Mol Cell Biol* 15: 3479–3486

14  Nohno T, Ishikawa T, Saito T, Hosokawa K, Noji S, Wolsing DH, Rosenbaum JS (1995) Identification of a human type II receptor for bone morphogenetic protein-4 that forms differential heteromeric complexes with bone morphogenetic protein type I receptors. *J Biol Chem* 270: 22522–22526

15  Rosenzweig BL, Imamura T, Okadome T, Cox GN, Yamashita H, ten Dijke P, Heldin C-H, Miyazono K (1995) Cloning and characterization of a human type II receptor for bone morphogenetic proteins. *Proc Natl Acad Sci USA* 92: 7632–7636

16  Wang T, Li B-Y, Danielson PD, Shah PC, Rockwell S, Lechleider RJ, Martin J, Manganaro T, Donahoe PK (1996) The immunophilin FKBP12 functions as a common inhibitor of the TGFβ family type I receptors. *Cell* 86: 435–444

17  Chen YG, Liu F, Massagué J (1997) Mechanism of TGFβ receptor inhibition by FKBP12. *EMBO J* 16: 3866–3876

18  Huse M, Chen YG, Massagué J, Kuriyan J (1999) Crystal structure of the cytoplasmic domain of the type I TGF β receptor in complex with FKBP12. *Cell* 96: 425–436

19  Luo J, Lodish HF (1997) Positive and negative regulation of type III TGF-β receptor signal transduction by autophosphorylation on multiple serine residues. *EMBO J* 16: 1970–1981

20  Lawler S, Feng XH, Chen RH, Maruoka EM, Turck CW, Griswold-Prenner I, Derynck R (1997) The type II transforming growth factor-β receptor autophosphorylates not only on serine and threonine but also on tyrosine residues. *J Biol Chem* 272: 14850–14859

21  Souchelnytskyi S, ten Dijke P, Miyazono K, Heldin C-H (1996) Phosphorylation of

Ser165 in TGF-β type I receptor modulates TGF-β1-induced cellular responses. *EMBO J* 15: 6231–6240

22    Raftery LA, Twombly V, Wharton K, Gelbart WM (1995) Genetic screens to identify elements of the decapentaplegic signaling pathway in *Drosophila*. *Genetics* 139: 241–254

23    Sekelsky JJ, Newfeld SJ, Raftery LA, Chartoff EH, Gelbart WM (1995) Genetic characterization and cloning of *Mothers against dpp*, a gene required for decapentaplegic function in *Drosophila melanogaster*. *Genetics* 139: 1347–1358

24    Savage C, Das P, Finelli AL, Townsend SR, Sun C-Y, Baird SE, Padgett RW (1996) *Caenorhabditis elegans* genes *sma-2*, *sma-3*, and *sma-4* define a conserved family of transforming growth factor β pathway components. *Proc Natl Acad Sci USA* 93: 790–794

25    Kretzschmar M, Liu F, Hata A, Doody J, Massagué J (1997) The TGF-β family mediator Smad1 is phosphorylated directly and activated functionally by the BMP receptor kinase. *Genes Dev* 11: 984–995

26    Abdollah S, Macías-Silva M, Tsukazaki T, Hayashi H, Attisano L, Wrana JL (1997) TβRI phosphorylation of Smad2 on Ser[465] and Ser[467] is required for Smad2-Smad4 complex formation and signaling. *J Biol Chem* 272: 27678–27685

27    Souchelnytskyi S, Tamaki K, Engström U, Wernstedt C, ten Dijke P, Heldin C-H (1997) Phosphorylation of Ser[465] and Ser[467] in the C terminus of Smad2 mediates interaction with Smad4 and is required for transforming growth factor-β signaling. *J Biol Chem* 272: 28107–28115

28    Chen YG, Massagué J (1999) Smad1 recognition and activation by the ALK1 group of transforming growth factor-β family receptors. *J Biol Chem* 274: 3672–3677

29    Masuyama N, Hanafusa H, Kusakabe M, Shibuya H, Nishida E (1999) Identification of two Smad4 proteins in *Xenopus*. Their common and distinct properties. *J Biol Chem* 274: 12163–12170

30    LeSuer JA, Graff JM (1999) Spemann organizer activity of Smad10. *Development* 126: 137–146

31    Liu F, Hata A, Baker JC, Doody J, Cárcamo J, Harland RM, Massagué J (1996) A human Mad protein acting as a BMP-regulated transcriptional activator. *Nature* 381: 620–623

32    Hata A, Lo RS, Wotton D, Lagna G, Massagué J (1997) Mutations increasing autoinhibition inactivate tumour suppressors Smad2 and Smad4. *Nature* 388: 82–87

33    Shi Y, Hata A, Lo RS, Massagué J, Pavletich NP (1997) A structural basis for mutational inactivation of the tumour suppressor Smad4. *Nature* 388: 87–93

34    Kawabata M, Inoue H, Hanyu A, Imamura T, Miyazono K (1998) Smad proteins exist as monomers *in vivo* and undergo homo- and hetero-oligomerization upon activation by serine/threonine kinase receptors. *EMBO J* 17: 4056–4065

35    Zawel L, Dai JL, Buckhaults P, Zhou S, Kinzler KW, Vogelstein B, Kern SE (1998) Human Smad3 and Smad4 are sequence-specific transcription activators. Mol. *Cell* 1: 611–617

36   Kim J, Johnson K, Chen HJ, Carroll S, Laughon A (1997) *Drosophila* Mad binds to DNA and directly mediates activation of *vestigial* by Decapentaplegic. *Nature* 388: 304–308

37   Shi YG, Wang YF, Jayaraman L, Yang HJ, Massagué J, Pavletich NP (1998) Crystal structure of a Smad MH1 domain bound to DNA: insights on DNA binding in TGF-β signaling. *Cell* 94: 585–594

38   Shioda T, Lechleider RJ, Dunwoodie SL, Li H, Yahata T, de Caestecker MP, Fenner MH, Roberts AB, Isselbacher KJ (1998) Transcriptional activating activity of Smad4: roles of SMAD hetero-oligomerization and enhancement by an associating transactivator. *Proc Natl Acad Sci USA* 95: 9785–9790

39   de Caestecker MP, Hemmati P, Larisch-Bloch S, Ajmera R, Roberts AB, Lechleider RJ (1997) Characterization of functional domains within Smad4/DPC4. *J Biol Chem* 272: 13690–13696

40   Tsukazaki T, Chiang TA, Davison AF, Attisano L, Wrana JL (1998) SARA, a FYVE domain protein that recruits Smad2 to the TGFβ receptor. *Cell* 95: 779–791

41   Feng X-H, Derynck R (1997) A kinase subdomain of transforming growth factor-β (TGF-β) type I receptor determines the TGF-β intracellular signaling specificity. *EMBO J* 16: 3912–3923

42   Chen YG, Hata A, Lo RS, Wotton D, Shi Y, Pavletich N, Massagué J (1998) Determinants of specificity in TGF-β signal transduction. *Genes Dev* 12: 2144–2152

43   Armes NA, Neal KA, Smith JC (1999) A short loop on the ALK-2 and ALK-4 activin receptors regulates signaling specificity but cannot account for all their effects on early *Xenopus* development. *J Biol Chem* 274: 7929–7935

44   Persson U, Izumi H, Souchelnytskyi S, Itoh S, Grimsby S, Engström U, Heldin C-H, Funa K, ten Dijke P (1998) The L45 loop in type I receptors for TGF-β family members is a critical determinant in specifying Smad isoform activation. *FEBS Lett* 434: 83–87

45   Lo RS, Chen YG, Shi Y, Pavletich NP, Massagué J (1998) The L3 loop: a structural motif determining specific interactions between SMAD proteins and TGF-β receptors. *EMBO J* 17: 996–1005

46   Hocevar BA, Brown TL, Howe PH (1999) TGF-β induces fibronectin synthesis through a c-Jun N-terminal kinase-dependent, Smad4-independent pathway. *EMBO J* 18: 1345–1356

47   Nakao A, Imamura T, Souchelnytskyi S, Kawabata M, Ishisaki A, Oeda E, Tamaki K, Hanai J-i, Heldin C-H, Miyazono K et al (1997) TGF-β receptor-mediated signalling through Smad2, Smad3 and Smad4. *EMBO J* 16: 5353–5362

48   Liu F, Pouponnot C, Massagué J (1997) Dual role of the Smad4/DPC4 tumor suppressor in TGFβ-inducible transcriptional complexes. *Genes Dev* 11: 3157–3167

49   Zhang Y, Musci T, Derynck R (1997) The tumor suppressor Smad4/DPC4 as a central mediator of Smad function. *Curr Biol* 7: 270–276

50   Xu X, Yin Z, Hudson JB, Ferguson EL, Frasch M (1998) Smad proteins act in combination with synergistic and antagonistic regulators to target Dpp responses to the *Drosophila* mesoderm. *Genes Dev* 12: 2354–2370

51    Nguyen HT, Xu X (1998) *Drosophila mef2* expression during mesoderm development is controlled by a complex array of cis-acting regulatory modules. *Dev Biol* 204: 550–566

52    Labbé E, Silvestri C, Hoodless PA, Wrana JL, Attisano L (1998) Smad2 and Smad3 positively and negatively regulate TGFβ-dependent transcription through the forkhead DNA-binding protein FAST2. *Mol Cell* 2: 109–120

53    Vindevoghel L, Kon A, Lechleider RJ, Uitto J, Roberts AB, Mauviel A (1998) Smad-dependent transcriptional activation of human type VII collagen gene (COL7A1) promoter by transforming growth factor-β. *J Biol Chem* 273: 13053–13057

54    Yingling JM, Datto MB, Wong C, Frederick JP, Liberati NT, Wang XF (1997) Tumor suppressor Smad4 is a transforming growth factor β-inducible DNA binding protein. *Mol Cell Biol* 17: 7019–7028

55    Zhang Y, Feng XH, Derynck R (1998) Smad3 and Smad4 cooperate with c-Jun/c-Fos to mediate TGF-β-induced transcription. *Nature* 394: 909–913

56    Dennler S, Itoh S, Vivien D, ten Dijke P, Huet S, Gauthier J-M (1998) Direct binding of Smad3 and Smad4 to critical TGFβ-inducible elements in the promoter of human plasminogen activator inhibitor-type 1 gene. *EMBO J* 17: 3091–3100

57    Song CZ, Siok TE, Gelehrter TD (1998) Smad4/DPC4 and Smad3 mediate transforming growth factor-β (TGF-β) signaling through direct binding to a novel TGF-β-responsive element in the human plasminogen activator inhibitor-1 promoter. *J Biol Chem* 273: 29287–29290

58    Stroschein SL, Wang W, Luo K (1999) Cooperative binding of Smad proteins to two adjacent DNA elements in the plasminogen activator inhibitor-1 promoter mediates transforming growth factor β-induced Smad-dependent transcriptional activation. *J Biol Chem* 274: 9431–9441

59    Jonk LJC, Itoh S, Heldin C-H, ten Dijke P, Kruijer W (1998) Identification and functional characterization of a Smad binding element (SBE) in the *JunB* promoter that acts as a transforming growth factor-β, activin, and bone morphogenetic protein-inducible enhancer. *J Biol Chem* 273: 21145–21152

60    Wong C, Rougier-Chapman EM, Frederick JP, Datto MB, Liberati NT, Li J-M, Wang X-F (1999) Smad3/Smad4 and AP-1 complexes synergize in transcriptional activation of the c-Jun promoter by transforming growth factor-β. *Mol Cell Biol* 19: 1821–1830

61    Vindevoghel L, Lechleider RJ, Kon A, de Caestecker MP, Uitto J, Roberts AB, Mauviel A (1998) SMAD3/4-dependent transcriptional activation of the human type VII collagen gene (COL7A1) promoter by transforming growth factor β. *Proc Natl Acad Sci USA* 95: 14769–14774

62    Hunt KK, Fleming JB, Abramian A, Zhang L, Evans DB, Chiao PJ (1998) Overexpression of the tumor suppressor gene *Smad4/DPC4* induces *p21^{wafl}* expression and growth inhibition in human carcinoma cells. *Cancer Res* 58: 5656–5661

63    Thatcher JD, Haun C, Okkema PG (1999) The DAF-3 Smad binds DNA and represses gene expression in the *Caenorhabditis elegans* pharynx. *Development* 126: 97–107

64    Dennler S, Huet S, Gauthier JM (1999) A short amino-acid sequence in MH1 domain

is responsible for functional differences between Smad2 and Smad3. *Oncogene* 18: 1643–1648

65 Yagi K, Goto D, Hamamoto T, Takenoshita S, Kato M, Miyazono K (1999) Alternatively spliced variant of Smad2 lacking exon 3. Comparison with wild-type Smad2 and Smad3. *J Biol Chem* 274: 703–709

66 Derynck R, Zhang Y, Feng X-H (1998) Smads: Transcriptional activators of TGF-β responses. *Cell* 95: 737–740

67 Chen X, Rubock MJ, Whitman M (1996) A transcriptional partner for MAD proteins in TGF-β signalling. *Nature* 383: 691–696

68 Chen X, Weisberg E, Fridmacher V, Watanabe M, Naco G, Whitman M (1997) Smad4 and FAST-1 in the assembly of activin-responsive factor. *Nature* 389: 85–89

69 Zhou S, Zawel L, Lengauer C, Kinzler KW, Vogelstein B (1998) Characterization of human *FAST-1*, a TGFβ and activin signal transducer. *Mol Cell* 2: 121–127

70 Liu B, Dou C-L, Prabhu L, Lai E (1999) FAST-2 is a mammalian winged-helix protein which mediates transforming growth factor β signals. *Mol Cell Biol* 19: 424–430

71 Candia AF, Watabe T, Hawley SHB, Onichtchouk D, Zhang Y, Derynck R, Niehrs C, Cho KWY (1997) Cellular interpretation of multiple TGF-β signals: intracellular antagonism between activin/BVg1 and BMP-2/4 signaling mediated by Smads. *Development* 124: 4467–4480

72 Kaufmann E, Paul H, Friedle H, Metz A, Scheucher M, Clement JH, Knöchel W (1996) Antagonistic actions of activin A and BMP-2/4 control dorsal lip-specific activation of the early response gene *XFD-1'* in *Xenopus laevis* embryos. *EMBO J* 15: 6739–6749

73 Howell M, Hill CS (1997) XSmad2 directly activates the activin-inducible, dorsal mesoderm gene *XFKH1* in *Xenopus* embryos. *EMBO J* 16: 7411–7421

74 Liberati NT, Datto MB, Frederick JP, Shen X, Wong C, Rougier-Chapman EM, Wang X-F (1999) Smads bind directly to the Jun family of AP-1 transcription factors. *Proc Natl Acad Sci USA* 96: 4844–4849

75 Hua XX, Liu XD, Ansari DO, Lodish HF (1998) Synergistic cooperation of TFE3 and Smad proteins in TGF-β-induced transcription of the plasminogen activator inhibitor-1 gene. *Genes Dev* 12: 3084–3095

76 Yanagisawa J, Yanagi Y, Masuhiro Y, Suzawa M, Watanabe M, Kashiwagi K, Toriyabe T, Kawabata M, Miyazono K, Kato S (1999) Convergence of transforming growth factor-β and vitamin D signaling pathways on SMAD transcriptional coactivators. *Science* 283: 1317–1321

77 Roberts AB, Sporn MB (1992) Mechanistic interrelationships between two superfamilies: The steroid/retinoid receptors and transforming growth factor-β. *Cancer Surveys* 14: 205–220

78 Li J-M, Nichols MA, Chandrasekharan S, Xiong Y, Wang X-F (1995) Transforming growth factor β activates the promoter of cyclin-dependent kinase inhibitor p15[INK4B] through an Sp1 consensus site. *J Biol Chem* 270: 26750–26753

79 Datto MB, Yu Y, Wang X-F (1995) Functional analysis of the transforming growth fac-

tor β responsive elements in the WAF1/Cip1/p21 promoter. *J Biol Chem* 270: 28623–28628

80  Datto MB, Li Y, Panus JF, Howe DJ, Xiong Y, Wang XF (1995) Transforming growth factor-β induces the cyclin-dependent kinase inhibitor p21 through a p53-independent mechanism. *Proc Natl Acad Sci USA* 92: 5545–5549

81  Kim Y, Ratziu V, Choi SG, Lalazar A, Theiss G, Dang Q, Kim SJ, Friedman SL (1998) Transcriptional activation of transforming growth factor β1 and its receptors by the Kruppel-like factor Zf9/core promoter-binding protein and Sp1 – Potential mechanisms for autocrine fibrogenesis in response to injury. *J Biol Chem* 273: 33750–33758

82  Greenwel P, Inagaki Y, Hu W, Walsh M, Ramirez F (1997) Sp1 is required for the early response of α2(I) collagen to transforming growth factor-β1. *J Biol Chem* 272: 19738–19745

83  Ammanamanchi S, Kim SJ, Sun LZ, Brattain MG (1998) Induction of transforming growth factor-β receptor type II expression in estrogen receptor-positive breast cancer cells through SP1 activation by 5-aza-2'-deoxycytidine. *J Biol Chem* 273: 16527–16534

84  Li JM, Datto MB, Shen X, Hu PPC, Yu Y, Wang XF (1998) Sp1, but not Sp3, functions to mediate promoter activation by TGF-β through canonical Sp1 binding sites. *Nucleic Acids Res* 26: 2449–2456

85  Moustakas A, Kardassis D (1998) Regulation of the human p21/WAF1/Cip1 promoter in hepatic cells by functional interactions between Sp1 and Smad family members. *Proc Natl Acad Sci USA* 95: 6733–6738

86  Kon A, Vindevoghel L, Kouba DJ, Fujimura Y, Uitto J, Mauviel A (1999) Cooperation between SMAD and NF-kappaB in growth factor regulated type VII collagen gene expression. *Oncogene* 18: 1837–1844

87  Alevizopoulos A, Dusserre Y, Rüegg U, Mermod N (1997) Regulation of the transforming growth factor β-responsive transcription factor CTF-1 by calcineurin and calcium/calmodulin-dependent protein kinase IV. *J Biol Chem* 272: 23597–23605

88  Eresh S, Riese J, Jackson DB, Bohmann D, Bienz M (1997) A CREB-binding site as a target for *decapentaplegic* signalling during *Drosophila* endoderm induction. *EMBO J* 16: 2014–2022

89  Tang SJ, Hoodless PA, Lu Z, Breitman ML, McInnes RR, Wrana JL, Buchwald M (1998) The *Tlx-2* homeobox gene is a downstream target of BMP signalling and is required for mouse mesoderm development. *Development* 125: 1877–1887

90  Hollnagel A, Oehlmann V, Heymer J, Ruther U, Nordheim A (1999) *Id* genes are direct targets of bone morphogenetic protein induction in embryonic stem cells. *J Biol Chem* 274: 19838–19845

91  Kurokawa M, Mitani K, Irie K, Matsuyama T, Takahashi T, Chiba S, Yazaki Y, Matsumoto K, Hirai H (1998) The oncoprotein Evi-1 represses TGF-β signalling by inhibiting Smad3. *Nature* 394: 92–96

92  Verschueren K, Remacle JE, Collart C, Kraft H, Baker BS, Tylzanowski P, Nelles L, Wuytens G, Su M-T, Bodmer R et al (1999) SIP1, a novel zinc finger/homeodomain

repressor, interacts with Smad proteins and binds to 5'-CACCT sequences in candidate target genes. *J Biol Chem* 274: 20489–20498

93   Shi X, Yang X, Chen D, Chang Z, Cao X (1999) Smad1 interacts with homeobox DNA-binding proteins in bone morphogenetic protein signaling. *J Biol Chem* 274: 13711–13717

94   Feng XH, Zhang Y, Wu RY, Derynck R (1998) The tumor suppressor Smad4/DPC4 and transcriptional adaptor CBP/p300 are coactivators for Smad3 in TGF-β-induced transcriptional activation. *Genes Dev* 12: 2153–2163

95   Janknecht R, Wells NJ, Hunter T (1998) TGF-β-stimulated cooperation of smad proteins with the coactivators CBP/p300. *Genes Dev* 12: 2114–2119

96   Topper JN, DiChiara MR, Brown JD, Williams AJ, Falb D, Collins T, Gimbrone MA Jr (1998) CREB binding protein is a required coactivator for Smad-dependent, transforming growth factor-β transcriptional responses in endothelial cells. *Proc Natl Acad Sci USA* 95: 9506–9511

97   Pouponnot C, Jayaraman L, Massagué J (1998) Physical and functional interaction of SMADs and p300/CBP. *J Biol Chem* 273: 22865–22868

98   Nishihara A, Hanai J-i, Okamoto N, Yanagisawa J, Kato S, Miyazono K, Kawabata M (1998) Role of p300, a transcriptional coactivator, in signalling of TGF-β. *Genes Cells* 3: 613–623

99   Shen X, Hu PP, Liberati NT, Datto MB, Frederick JP, Wang XF (1998) TGF-β-induced phosphorylation of Smad3 regulates its interaction with coactivator p300/CREB-binding protein. *Mol Biol Cell* 9: 3309–3319

100  Janknecht R, Hunter T (1996) Transcriptional control: Versatile molecular glue. *Curr Biol* 6: 951–954

101  Wotton D, Lo RS, Lee S, Massagué J (1999) A Smad transcriptional corepressor. *Cell* 97: 29–39

102  Jazwinska A, Kirov N, Wieschaus E, Roth S, Chrsitine R (1999) The *Drosophila* gene *brinker* reveals a novel mechanism of Dpp target gene regulation. *Cell* 96: 563–573

103  Campbell G, Tomlinson A (1999) Transducing the Dpp morphogen gradient in the wing of *Drosophila*: regulation of Dpp targets by *brinker*. *Cell* 96: 553–562

104  Minami M, Kinoshita N, Kamoshida Y, Tanimoto H, Tabata T (1999) *brinker* is a target of Dpp in *Drosophila* that negatively regulates Dpp-dependent genes. *Nature* 398: 242–246

105  Topper JN, Cai J, Qiu Y, Anderson KR, Xu Y-Y, Deeds JD, Feeley R, Gimeno CJ, Woolf EA, Tayber O et al (1997) Vascular *MADs*: Two novel *MAD*-related genes selectively inducible by flow in human vascular endothelium. *Proc Natl Acad Sci USA* 94: 9314–9319

106  Hayashi H, Abdollah S, Qiu Y, Cai J, Xu YY, Grinnell BW, Richardson MA, Topper JN, Gimbrone MAJ, Wrana JL et al (1997) The MAD-related protein Smad7 associates with the TGFβ receptor and functions as an antagonist of TGFβ signaling. *Cell* 89: 1165–1173

107 Imamura T, Takase M, Nishihara A, Oeda E, Hanai J, Kawabata M, Miyazono K (1997) Smad6 inhibits signalling by the TGF-β superfamily. *Nature* 389: 622–626

108 Nakayama T, Snyder MA, Grewal SS, Tsuneizumi K, Tabata T, Christian JL (1998) *Xenopus* Smad8 acts downstream of BMP-4 to modulate its activity during vertebrate embryonic patterning. *Development* 125: 857–867

109 Tsuneizumi K, Nakayama T, Kamoshida Y, Kornberg TB, Christian JL, Tabata T (1997) *Daughters against dpp* modulates *dpp* organizing activity in *Drosophila* wing development. *Nature* 389: 627–631

110 Souchelnytskyi S, Nakayama T, Nakao A, Morén A, Heldin C-H, Christian JL, ten Dijke P (1998) Physical and functional interaction of murine and *Xenopus* Smad7 with bone morphogenetic protein receptors and transforming growth factor-β receptors. *J Biol Chem* 273: 25364–25370

111 Inoue H, Imamura T, Ishidou Y, Takase M, Udagawa Y, Oka Y, Tsuneizumi K, Tabata T, Miyazono K, Kawabata M (1998) Interplay of signal mediators of *decapentaplegic* (Dpp): Molecular characterization of *mothers against dpp, medea*, and *daughters against dpp*. *Mol Biol Cell* 9: 2145–2156

112 Lebrun JJ, Takabe K, Chen Y, Vale W (1999) Roles of pathway-specific and inhibitory Smads in activin receptor signaling. *Mol Endocrinol* 13: 15–23

113 Itoh S, Landström M, Hermansson A, Itoh F, Heldin C-H, Heldin N-E, ten Dijke P (1998) Transforming growth factor β1 induces nuclear export of inhibitory Smad7. *J Biol Chem* 273: 29195–29201

114 Ishisaki A, Yamato K, Nakao A, Nonaka K, Ohguchi M, ten Dijke P, Nishihara T (1998) Smad7 is an activin-inducible inhibitor of activin-induced growth arrest and apoptosis in mouse B cells. *J Biol Chem* 273: 24293–24296

115 Ishisaki A, Yamato K, Hashimoto S, Nakao A, Tamaki K, Nonaka K, ten Dijke P, Sugino H, Nishihara T (1999) Differential inhibition of Smad6 and Smad7 on bone morphogenetic protein- and activin-mediated growth arrest and apoptosis in B cells. *J Biol Chem* 274: 13637–13642

116 Bhushan A, Chen Y, Vale W (1998) Smad7 inhibits mesoderm formation and promotes neural cell fate in *Xenopus* embryos. *Dev Biol* 200: 260–268

117 Casellas R, Brivanlou AH (1998) Xenopus Smad7 inhibits both the activin and BMP pathways and acts as a neural inducer. *Dev Biol* 198: 1–12

118 Afrakhte M, Morén A, Jossan S, Itoh S, Sampath K, Westermark B, Heldin C-H, Heldin N-E, ten Dijke P (1998) Induction of inhibitory Smad6 and Smad7 mRNA by TGF-β family members. *Biochem Biophys Res Commun* 249: 505–511

119 Takase M, Imamura T, Sampath TK, Takeda K, Ichijo H, Miyazono K, Kawabata M (1998) Induction of Smad6 mRNA by bone morphogenetic proteins. *Biochem Biophys Res Commun* 244: 26–29

120 Ulloa L, Doody J, Massagué J (1999) Inhibition of transforming growth factor-β/SMAD signalling by the interferon-gamma/STAT pathway. *Nature* 397: 710–713

121 Kleeff J, Maruyama H, Friess H, Büchler MW, Falb D, Korc M (1999) Smad6 suppresses

TGF-β-induced growth inhibition in COLO-357 pancreatic cancer cells and is overexpressed in pancreatic cancer. *Biochem Biophys Res Commun* 255: 268–273

122 Kretzschmar M, Doody J, Massagué J (1997) Opposing BMP and EGF signalling pathways converge on the TGF-β family mediator Smad1. *Nature* 389: 618–622

123 Kretzschmar M, Doody J, Timokhina I, Massagué J (1999) A mechanism of repression of TGFβ/Smad signaling by oncogenic Ras. *Genes Dev* 13: 804–816

124 Yue J, Hartsough MT, Frey RS, Frielle T, Mulder KM (1999) Cloning and expression of a rat Smad1: Regulation by TGFβ and modulation by the Ras/MEK pathway. *J Cell Physiol* 178: 387–396

125 De Caestecker MP, Parks WT, Frank CJ, Castagnino P, Bottaro DP, Roberts AB, Lechleider RJ (1998) Smad2 transduces common signals from receptor serine-threonine and tyrosine kinases. *Genes Dev* 12: 1587–1592

126 Yamaguchi K, Shirakabe K, Shibuya H, Irie K, Oishi I, Ueno N, Taniguchi T, Nishida E, Matsumoto K (1995) Identification of a member of the MAPKKK family as a potential mediator of TGF-β signal transduction. *Science* 270: 2008–2011

127 Shibuya H, Yamaguchi K, Shirakabe K, Tonegawa A, Gotoh Y, Ueno N, Irie K, Nishida E, Matsumoto K (1996) TAB1: An activator of the TAK1 MAPKKK in TGF-β signal transduction. *Science* 272: 1179–1182

128 Shibuya H, Iwata H, Masuyama N, Gotoh Y, Yamaguchi K, Irie K, Matsumoto K, Nishida E, Ueno N (1998) Role of TAK1 and TAB1 in BMP signaling in early *Xenopus* development. *EMBO J* 17: 1019–1028

129 Yamaguchi K, Nagai S-i, Ninomiya-Tsuji J, Nishita M, Tamai K, Irie K, Ueno N, Nishida E, Shibuya H, Matsumoto K (1999) XIAP, a cellular member of the inhibitor of apoptosis protein family, links the receptors to TAB1-TAK1 in the BMP signaling pathway. *EMBO J* 18: 179–187

130 Kurozumi K, Nishita M, Yamaguchi K, Fujita T, Ueno N, Shibuya H (1998) BRAM1, a BMP receptor-associated molecule involved in BMP signalling. *Genes Cells* 3: 257–264

131 Shirakabe K, Yamaguchi K, Shibuya H, Irie K, Matsuda S, Moriguchi T, Gotoh Y, Matsumoto K, Nishida E (1997) TAK1 mediates the ceramide signaling to stress-activated protein kinase/c-Jun N-terminal kinase. *J Biol Chem* 272: 8141–8144

132 Atfi A, Djelloul S, Chastre E, Davis R, Gespach C (1997) Evidence for a role of Rho-like GTPases and stress-activated protein kinase/c-Jun N-terminal kinase (SAPK/JNK) in transforming growth factor β-mediated signaling. *J Biol Chem* 272: 1429–1432

133 Frey RS, Mulder KM (1997) Involvement of extracellular signal-regulated kinase 2 and stress-activated protein kinase Jun N-terminal kinase activation by transforming growth factor β in the negative growth control of breast cancer cells. *Cancer Res* 57: 628–633

134 Atfi A, Buisine M, Mazars A, Gespach C (1997) Induction of apoptosis by DPC4, a transcriptional factor regulated by transforming growth factor-β through stress-activated protein kinase/c-Jun N-terminal kinase (SAPK/JNK) signaling pathway. *J Biol Chem* 272: 24731–24734

135 Sano Y, Harada J, Tashiro S, Gotoh-Mandeville R, Maekawa T, Ishii S (1999) ATF-2 is

a common nuclear target of Smad and TAK1 pathways in transforming growth factor-β signaling. *J Biol Chem* 274: 8949–8957

136  Brown JD, DiChiara MR, Anderson KR, Gimbrone MA Jr, Topper JN (1999) MEKK-1, a component of the stress (stress-activated protein kinase/c-Jun N-terminal kinase) pathway, can selectively activate Smad2-mediated transcriptional activation in endothelial cells. *J Biol Chem* 274: 8797–8805

137  Hartsough MT, Frey RS, Zipfel PA, Buard A, Cook SJ, McCormick F, Mulder KM (1996) Altered transforming growth factor β signaling in epithelial cells when Ras activation is blocked. *J Biol Chem* 271: 22368–22375

138  Mucsi I, Skorecki KL, Goldberg HJ (1996) Extracellular signal-regulated kinase and the small GTP-binding protein, Rac, contribute to the effects of transforming growth factor-β1 on gene expression. *J Biol Chem* 271: 16567–16572

139  Yue J, Frey RS, Mulder KM (1999) Cross-talk between the Smad1 and Ras/MEK signaling pathways for TGFβ. *Oncogene* 18: 2033–2037

140  Cui W, Fowlis DJ, Bryson S, Duffie E, Ireland H, Balmain A, Akhurst RJ (1996) TGFβ1 inhibits the formation of benign skin tumors, but enhances progression to invasive spindle carcinomas in transgenic mice. *Cell* 86: 531–542

141  Matzuk MM, Finegold MJ, Su J-GJ, Hsueh AJW, Bradley A (1992) α-Inhibin is a tumour-suppressor gene with gonadal specificity in mice. *Nature* 360: 313–319

142  Markowitz S, Wang J, Myeroff L, Parsons R, Sun L, Lutterbaugh J, Fan RS, Zborowska E, Kinzler KW, Vogelstein B et al (1995) Inactivation of the type II TGF-β receptor in colon cancer cells with microsatellite instability. *Science* 268: 1336–1338

143  Kim IY, Ahn HJ, Zelner DJ, Shaw JW, Sensibar JA, Kim JH, Kato M, Lee C (1996) Genetic change in transforming growth factor β (TGF-β) receptor type I gene correlates with insensitivity to TGF-β1 in human prostate cancer cells. *Cancer Res* 56: 44–48

144  DeCoteau JF, Knaus PI, Yankelev H, Reis MD, Lowsky R, Lodish HF, Kadin ME (1997) Loss of functional cell surface transforming growth factor β (TGF-β) type 1 receptor correlates with insensitivity to TGF-β in chronic lymphocytic leukemia. *Proc Natl Acad Sci USA* 94: 5877–5881

145  Goggins M, Shekher M, Turnacioglu K, Yeo CJ, Hruban RH, Kern SE (1998) Genetic alterations of the transforming growth factor β receptor genes in pancreatic and biliary adenocarcinomas. *Cancer Res* 58: 5329–5332

146  Chen TP, Carter D, Garrigue-Antar L, Reiss M (1998) Transforming growth factor-β type I receptor kinase mutant associated with metastatic breast cancer. *Cancer Res* 58: 4805–4810

147  Hahn SA, Schutte M, Hoque ATMS, Moskaluk CA, da Costa LT, Rozenblum E, Weinstein CL, Fischer A, Yeo CJ, Hruban RH et al (1996) *DPC4*, a candidate tumor suppressor gene at human chromosome 18q21.1. *Science* 271: 350–353

148  Hahn SA, Bartsch D, Schroers A, Galehdari H, Becker M, Ramaswamy A, Schwarte-Waldhoff I, Maschek H, Schmiegel W (1998) Mutations of the *DPC4/Smad4* gene in biliary tract carcinoma. *Cancer Res* 58: 1124–1126

149  Thiagalingam S, Lengauer C, Leach FS, Schutte M, Hahn SA, Overhauser J, Willson

JKV, Markowitz S, Hamilton SR, Kern SE et al (1996) Evaluation of candidate tumour suppressor genes on chromosome 18 in colorectal cancers. *Nature Genetics* 13: 343–346

150 Riggins RG, Kinzler KW, Vogelstein B, Thiagalingam S (1997) Frequency of *Smad* gene mutations in human cancers. *Cancer Res* 57: 2578–2580

151 Eppert K, Scherer SW, Ozcelik H, Pirone R, Hoodless P, Kim H, Tsui L-C, Bapat B, Gallinger S, Andrulis IL et al (1996) MADR2 maps to 18q21 and encodes a TGFβ-regulated MAD-related protein that is functionally mutated in colorectal carcinoma. *Cell* 86: 543–552

152 Riggins GJ, Thiagalingam S, Rozenblum E, Weinstein CL, Kern SE, Hamilton SR, Willson JKV, Markowitz SD, Kinzler KW, Vogelstein B (1996) *Mad*-related genes in the human. Nature Genetics 13: 347–349

153 Sirard C, de la Pompa JL, Elia A, Itie A, Mirtsos C, Cheung A, Hahn S, Wakeham A, Schwartz L, Kern SE et al (1998) The tumor suppressor gene *Smad4/Dpc4* is required for gastrulation and later for anterior development of the mouse embryo. *Genes Dev* 12: 107–119

154 Yang X, Li CL, Xu XL, Deng CX (1998) The tumor suppressor SMAD4/DPC4 is essential for epiblast proliferation and mesoderm induction in mice. *Proc Natl Acad Sci USA* 95: 3667–3672

155 Waldrip WR, Bikoff EK, Hoodless PA, Wrana JL, Robertson EJ (1998) Smad2 signaling in extraembryonic tissues determines anterior-posterior polarity of the early mouse embryo. *Cell* 92: 797–808

156 Datto MB, Frederick JP, Pan L, Borton AJ, Zhuang Y, Wang X-F (1999) Targeted disruption of Smad3 reveals an essential role in transforming growth factor β-mediated signal transduction. *Mol Cell Biol* 19: 2495–2504

157 Zhu Y, Richardson JA, Parada LF, Graff JM (1998) Smad3 mutant mice develop metastatic colorectal cancer. *Cell* 94: 703–714

158 Yang X, Letterio JJ, Lechleider RJ, Chen L, Hayman R, Gu H, Roberts AB, Deng CX (1999) Targeted disruption of SMAD3 results in impaired mucosal immunity and diminished T cell responsiveness to TGF-β. *EMBO J* 18: 1280–1291

# The transforming growth factor family and the endothelium

*Jennifer R. Gamble, Pu Xia and Mathew A. Vadas*

Division of Immunology, Hanson Centre for Cancer Research, Institute of Medical & Veterinary Science and The University of Adelaide, Frome Road, Adelaide 5000, South Australia

## Transforming growth factor (TGF) and the endothelium

The initial data that transforming growth factors could influence the growth and behaviour of endothelial cells in culture suggested that these factors may have a key role in the regulation of blood vessels [1–6]. Subsequently, TGF was also shown to regulate the smooth muscle cell component of the vessel wall [7–11] and to influence the composition of the extracellular matrix [12–16]. Thirteen years on, the mechanisms underlying this regulation of the blood vessel and in particular the endothelium are far from clear. It is now apparent that the overall effect of the TGFs is time- and site-dependent thus demonstrating the complex nature of these molecules in endothelial cell biology. This chapter will discuss some of the better recognised and understood effects of TGF (and primarily TGF-β) on the endothelium. The complexity of these effects demonstrates the difficulty in considering (at present) the TGF receptor : ligand system as a target for clinical therapy.

## TGF in endothelial cell differentiation

TGF-β isoforms and their receptors are expressed in the early stages of mouse and human embryogenesis [17–22] suggesting they play a critical role in developmental processes. This has been confirmed, at least for TGF-$β_1$, by the use of the gene targetting technology.

## TGF-$β_1$ gene deletion and differentiation

50% of homozygous null mice for TGF-β and 25% of heterozygous mice for TGF-$β_1$ die at around 10.5 dpc. These mice show major defects in vasculogenesis and in the development of the haematopoietic system [23].

In the absence of the TGF-$\beta_1$ gene, the differentiation of mesoderm into endothelial cells appears to proceed normally. TGF-$\beta$ –/– embryos have no specific abnormalities. However, the defect in the vascular system is principally in the yolk sac, affecting vasculogenesis and haematopoiesis. In wild type mice, the two endothelial monolayers associated with the mesothelial and endodermal lining are in close apposition. In contrast, in the TGF-$\beta$ –/– yolk sac, these two endothelial cell layers are partially detached, cell contacts are incomplete and a distended vessel forms. In some mice, blood cell leakage into the yolk sac cavity was observed. Although the mechanism for the loss of junctional integrity in the knock-out mice is unknown at present, *in vitro* observations have demonstrated that TGF-$\beta_1$ regulates expression of the gap junctional proteins connexin 43 and connexin 37, which are important in cell-cell communication [24]. Furthermore, TGF-$\beta$-treated endothelial cells (ECs) undergoing angiogenesis-like reorganisation *in vitro* demonstrate tight junction formation and organisation of basal lamina-like material on the albuminal plasma membrane [25] suggesting TGF-$\beta$ regulation of junctional complexes. However, some studies also demonstrate that TGF-$\beta_1$ is able to disrupt cell junctions highlighting the multi-functional nature of this factor [26, 27]. The requirement for TGF-$\beta$ signalling in vessel organisation in the yolk sac has been confirmed by somatic chimeras from embryonic stem (ES) cells transfected with kinase-deficient TGF-$\beta$RII mutants [28].

Molecular analysis of the endothelial cells in TGF-$\beta$ –/– mice using the Flk-1 cDNA probe, the receptor for the angiogenic factor, vascular endothelial cell growth factor (VEGF), showed a reduction in the number of endothelial cells expressing Flk-1 in the yolk sacs compared to TGF +/+ mice [23]. Interestingly, however, TGF-$\beta$1 down-regulates Flk-1 expression at least in mature endothelial cells [29]. The Flk-1 knock-out mice confirm the essential role for this receptor in vasculogenesis producing a phenotype deficient in mature ECs [30–32] since their migration and expansion does not occur.

The rescue of the TGF-$\beta_1$ –/– mice to term was originally thought to be mediated through maternal transfer of TGF-$\beta_1$. However, transfer of TGF-$\beta_1$ –/– embryos into TGF-$\beta_1$ –/– mothers still allowed some embryos to develop to term, suggesting factors other than TGF-$\beta_1$ are involved in this rescue [23, 33]. The phenotype of TGF –/– mice is indistinguishable from that obtained in mice where the TGF-$\beta$ receptor II is deleted (TGF-$\beta$RII –/–) [34]. However, 100% of the TGF-$\beta$RII –/– mice are embryonic lethal compared to the 50% for TGF-$\beta_1$ –/– mice demonstrating that signalling through TGF-$\beta$RII is essential for vasculogenesis (and haematopoiesis) in the yolk sac. The phenotype of these mice also shows that the putative factor that is able to rescue the TGF-$\beta_1$ –/– embryos belongs to the TGF supergene family [34]. Since TGF-$\beta_3$ null mice are viable, although exhibiting abnormal lung development and cleft palate, it suggests this factor is not TGF-$\beta_3$ [35, 36].

The development of *in vitro* assays that mimic aspects of differentiation [37–40] have confirmed that TGF-$\beta_1$ directly stimulates vasculogenesis [41]. Zhang et al.

have shown that embryonic stem cells transfected with the cDNA for TGF-$\beta_1$ differentiate *in vitro* into cystic embryonic bodies with tubular structure outgrowth. These tubes are of endothelial cell origin as judged by morphological and histological criteria. Furthermore, no haematopoiesis was seen suggesting TGF-$\beta_1$ promoted vasculogenesis but is not sufficient for haematopoietic differentiation [41]. Indeed, TGF-$\beta_1$ is known to be a potent inhibitor of early aspects of haematopoiesis [42].

## Endoglin gene deletion and differentiation

The essential nature of TGF-$\beta$ signalling in vascular development has recently been extended to encompass endoglin. Li et al. [43] have shown that mice deficient in endoglin, one of the transmembrane proteins that binds TGF-$\beta$ and which is expressed in endothelial cells, die from defective vascular development. Ultra-structural analysis showed that ECs formed the primary capillary network, but that endothelial remodelling did not take place. Furthermore, there was a general absence of supporting cells, such as pericytes or vascular smooth muscle cells around the capillary network. The phenotype of these mice suggested that endothelial cell expression of endoglin is required for vascular smooth muscle cell development and that these peri-endothelial cells are essential for endothelial cell organisation.

## TGF and angiogenesis

The process of angiogenesis involves a number of steps including EC activation resulting in migration, proliferation, reorganisation and finally vessel stabilisation. From *in vitro* studies, it is likely that TGF-$\beta$ can affect all stages and thus has both angiogenic and anti-angiogenic properties. Its angiogenic role, however, is unlikely to be direct, mediated instead through its effects on bystander cells and associated with local inflammatory reactions [44]. Inflammatory cells such as neutrophils, T cells, fibroblasts and monocytes, associated with these lesions and initially recruited there by chemotactic properties of TGF-$\beta$ [45–50] release angiogenic factors such as basic fibroblast growth factor (bFGF) and VEGF [44, 48, 49, 51, 52] which thus stimulate angiogenesis. An excellent review by Pepper [53] discusses at length the background behind this conclusion and the discrepancies between the *in vivo* and *in vitro* data.

The case against a direct angiogenic role for TGF-$\beta$1 is strengthened by gene therapy data where over-expression of TGF-$\beta$ in the vessel wall does not result in an angiogenic response [54, 55]. Indeed most of the TGF-$\beta$ was expressed in smooth muscle cells and resulted in extracellular matrix deposition, and hyperplasia. Further, transgenic animals for TGF-$\beta$ do not show signs of enhanced angiogenesis [55–57].

## EC migration and TGF-β

TGF-β can both promote and inhibit EC movement.

For a cell to move, it must alter its interaction with both the extracellular matrix (ECM) and with neighbouring cells. TGF-β down-regulates the $\beta_1$ integrins and perhaps specifically $\alpha_5\beta_1$, which is involved in EC attachment to the ECM [58] and which also has been localised to regions of cell:cell contact [59]. This loss of cell-cell and cell-matrix contact is likely to promote cell migration. Interestingly, TGF-β can also upregulate $\alpha_5\beta_1$ and synergizes with FGF in this regard [60], thus suggesting TGF-β may regulate both the initial (induction; cell proliferation and migration) and late (stabilisation; inhibition of proliferation and migration) phases of angiogenesis.

The integrin $\alpha_v\beta_3$ is considered a hallmark of an angiogenic vessel since it is absent on resting ECs but is rapidly induced on migrating ECs [61, 62]. Indeed, antibodies to $\alpha_v\beta_3$, peptide antagonists or a naturally occurring fragment of the matrix metalloproteinase MMP-2 (which binds $\alpha_v\beta_3$) are able to block many angiogenic-dependent pathologies [63–65]. In addition, $\alpha_v$ null mice are embryonic lethal due to vascular defects [66]. TGF-β upregulates $\alpha_v\beta_3$ at both the protein and mRNA levels [67] suggesting it potentiates the angiogenic state.

## TGF-β and invasion

In agreement with cell migration studies, TGF-β can exert a dual role on EC invasion.

The enzyme system consisting of urokinase plasminogen activator (uPA) and urokinase plasminogen activator inhibitor (PAI) is involved in the migration and matrix remodelling of ECs. The uPA receptor (uPAR) can function as an adhesion receptor for vitronectin and can co-localise with focal contacts, at the leading edge of migrating cells, and regulates the function of the $\beta_1$ integrins [68–70]. TGF-$\beta_1$ can act on both systems, stimulating the release of both uPA and PAI [71, 72] and regulating the expression of $\beta_1$ integrins [58, 60]. TGF-β also regulates some of the matrix metalloproteinases, MMPs, which are involved in EC invasion [73, 74], and their inhibitors, the tissue inhibitors of metalloproteinases (TIMPs) [74].

## TGF-β and EC proliferation

*In vitro* data using ECs plated as 2 dimensional (2D) monolayers demonstrated that TGF-β inhibited EC proliferation [1]. However, EC proliferation is a critical component of angiogenesis. This potential contradiction may suggest two points. Firstly, it is possible that the 2D cultures more accurately reflect wounding of ECs in large vessels as is seen in balloon angioplasty where application of TGF-β inhibits proliferation. Cells plated in 2D cultures and those plated within a gel (3 dimensional matrix) show that TGF-β inhibits ECs in 2D but promotes proliferation of the cells in the 3D cultures [75]. Furthermore, the effects of TGF on uPA production also differ between 2D and 3D cultures [76, 77]. Secondly, the contradictions may suggest that the effect of TGF-β on inhibiting the proliferation of ECs and thus angiogenesis, takes place predominantly in the stabilisation stage. Indeed, the stabilisation phase is associated with smooth muscle cell (SMC) or pericyte contact with the endothelium and cocultures of SMC and ECs generate active TGF-β [78]. TGF-$\beta_1$ also induces SMC differentiation [79]. In diabetic retinopathy, one of the initial changes associated with induction of angiogenesis vessels is a loss of pericyte contact [80].

## TGF-β and EC reorganisation

In addition to effects on proliferation, migration and adhesion, TGF-β is also involved in the reorganisation of ECs into a classical vessel-like structure. This reorganisation presumably reflects the maturation of the blood vessel into a patent vessel.

Work, principally from the Madri laboratory, showed that although cell proliferation is not altered by TGF-$\beta_1$ when cells are plated into 3D matrices, they migrate together, form lumen and undergo cell-cell interactions [25, 81, 82] as denoted by the relocalisation of the tight junction protein, ZO-1. This TGF-$\beta_1$-stimulated remodelling is mediated through nitric oxide (NO) [83]. NO also regulates VEGF-mediated EC functions [84] and induces apoptosis, a requirement for vascular remodelling [85, 86]. The apoptosis associated with this remodelling is regulated by TGF-β [83, 85, 87].

Analysis of the effect of TGFs on the VEGF system further supports the concept that it can act both as an angiogenesis promoter and inhibitor. *In vitro* TGF-$\beta_1$ and TGF-α induced the expression of the major angiogenic factor, VEGF, in many cell types [52, 88, 89]. However, TGF-β is also able to inhibit VEGF-induced angiogenesis [90] and inhibits the expression of Flk-1 on endothelial cells [29]. This is in contrast to the embryonic studies that show a requirement for TGF in Flk-1 induction and its essential role in VEGF induced embryonic vasculogenesis and angiogenesis [23]. Thus, it is possible that angiogenesis in the embryo and in the adult are, in many respects, fundamentally different events and that the activity of TGF reflects these differences. In support of this concept, Lee et al. [91] have recently shown that the surface glycoprotein Thy-1 is expressed on adult but not embryonic angiogenic endothelium.

## TGF-β and inflammation

The principal feature of an inflammatory response is the activation of ECs to render them pro-adhesive and pro-thrombotic. Many of the factors which induce this alteration are well described such as tumour necrosis factor (TNF) [92], interleukin-1 (IL-1) [93], shear stress [94], lipopolysaccharide (LPS) [95] and ionising radiation [96]. However, we initially reasoned that negative regulators, factors which hinder this pro-inflammatory state or which initiate the resolution of the inflammatory state, must also act on the endothelium. This hypothesis led to the description that TGF-β acts as such a negative regulator, inhibiting the adhesion and subsequent transmigration of neutrophils and T lymphocytes [97–99]. This control is brought about by the inhibition of adhesion molecules on the EC surface and chemotactic factors produced by the endothelium which are essential for neutrophil egress, namely E-selectin and interleukin-8 (IL-8) [99, 100]. This role for TGF-β has been substantiated and extended in a number of different *in vitro* systems, including models for the CNS [101–105] for the lung [106], for high endothelial venules [107, 108] and for the micro-vasculature [104, 105]. Rhodes et al. [109] have demonstrated that endogenous endothelial derived TGF-$β_1$ is also anti-adhesive.

Coculture of ECs and SMC inhibits the induction of E-selectin on the endothelial cells and vascular cell adhesion molecule-1 (VCAM-1) on the SMC, a process postulated to be mediated through the active TGF-β made as a result of the interaction of these two cell types [78, 110]. More recently, TGF-β has been shown to decrease the expression of the TNF receptor subunit, p75, suggesting an additional anti-inflammatory mechanism [111]. Interestingly, shear stress, as well as inducing adhesion molecule expression on ECs [94], also induces TGF-β transcription, protein expression and activation. This regulation of TGF-β is mediated through endothelial $K^+$ channels [112]. However, all is not simple. The effect of TGF-β on adhesion molecule expression is selective, as we originally showed, it inhibits E-selectin but not VCAM [100, 106]. Furthermore, the inhibitory effects can depend on time of treatment, on the pro-inflammatory stimulant used, or the growth conditions of the cells [97, 100, 113], and on the interaction with other cell types [114].

## TGF-β gene deletion and inflammation

The *in vitro* data on the anti-adhesive role for TGF-β in inflammation is supported by the TGF-$β_1$ knock-out mice. Approximately 50% are embryonic lethal. However, the remainder of the mice are born healthy but rapidly develop a wasting syndrome and die soon thereafter. The essential feature of the wasting syndrome is multifocal inflammatory infiltrates seen in all vital organs [115, 116]. Increased expression of adhesion molecules on leukocytes from the TGF-β –/– mice resulted in enhanced adhesion to extracellular matrix and to the endothelium [117]. Administration of fibronectin peptides blocked TGF-β –/– leukocyte adhesion both to Fn and to endothelial cells *in vitro* and blocked leukocyte infiltration into the tissues of TGF-β –/– mice [117]. Thus, $β_1$ integrins, at the very least appear to be important players in leukocyte attachment. Increases in expression of $α_4β_1$ (VLA-4), the ligand for the endothelial adhesion molecule VCAM-1, and for Fn were also seen in the leukocytes of TGF-β −/− mice. The phenotype of the TGF-β −/− mice suggest two important points. Firstly, that TGF-$\beta_1$ not only is essential to resolve inflammation, but also is an integral player in maintaining the basal, anti-inflammatory nature of the endothelium. Secondly, the results show that other TGF-β isoforms cannot substitute for TGF-$\beta_1$ in this regard.

The initial attempts to regulate the adhesive nature of the endothelium by TGF are encouraging. In myocardial ischemia and reperfusion, the essential feature of which is neutrophil accumulation as a result of endothelial dysfunction, TGF-β treatment exerts a significant cardioprotective effect [118]. In experimental autoimmune disease in mice, TGF-$\beta_1$ also exerts a significant protective effect, reducing the number of infiltrating T lymphocytes that bind to the endothelium and egress from the blood into the CNS [103].

## TGF in endothelial cell associated disease

Changes in TGF and its receptors have been documented in a large number of diseases associated with endothelial perturbations including rheumatoid arthritis [119], intracranial saccular aneurysms [120] and diabetic retinopathy [121]. The diseases discussed here are those where the link between TGF and endothelial cell function is more widely understood.

### Cancer

The role of TGF-β in cancer is clearly complex, not only because of the multifactorial progression to tumourgenesis but also, at least for solid tumours, because of the involvement of the vascular system in tumour growth. TGF-β is likely to be inhibitory during the early phases of tumour growth since it inhibits tumour cell proliferation and inhibits Flk-1 expression [29] and VEGF-induced angiogenesis [90]. However, during the later phases, loss of cell growth control by TGF may influence both the tumour and the vascular compartments. What is now clear is that the vascular bed is a prime target for tumour control.

The expansion of the initial avascular tumour bed is critically dependent on the ability of the tumour cells to stimulate the endogenous vascular compartment. However, it is important to point out that tumour angiogenesis is a complex phenomenon influenced by the angiogenic factors secreted by the tumour cells and the host vascular system, and driven by such factors as the hypoxic environment (reviewed in [122, 123]). In addition, it is now apparent that there are a number of "endogenous" inhibitors of angiogenesis which function to limit vascular expansion. These include angiostatin, a cleavage product of plasminogen [124], and endostatin, a cleavage product of collagen VIII [125].

High levels of TGF-β are found in many tumours, such as prostate, where loss of TGF-RII expression is also seen and which correlates with poor prognosis [126–128]. These changes are likely to lead to loss of cell growth control for the tumour cells. However, TGF-β also inhibits angiostatin production by inhibiting the plasminogen/plasmin system which generates the active molecule [129]. Thus, high TGF-β levels may act on the vascular system to remove these natural anti-angiogenic control mechanisms. In addition, as previously discussed under angiogenesis, TGF-β regulates VEGF expression, EC attachment and the activity of invasion promoting enzyme systems. Indeed, high levels of uPA are correlated with blood vessel invasion in colorectal cancer [130].

*Endoglin*

Endoglin (CD105) is a homodimeric transmembrane protein that binds TGF-$\beta_1$ and TGF-$\beta_3$. It is highly expressed on macrophages, stromal cells and endothelial cells [89, 131–133]. Over-expression of endoglin is able to modulate the cellular responses to TGF-β and thus is postulated to act as a regulator of TGF-β signalling rather than as a direct signalling molecule [134, 135]. In myoblasts and the monocytic line U937, the over-expression of endoglin results in the abrogation of TGF-β inhibition of cell proliferation [134] and enhanced production in response to TGF-$\beta_1$ of plasminogen activator inhibitor-1, a gene involved in the early phase of angiogenesis and which, like TGF-β, inhibits angiostatin production [129]. Over-expression of endoglin in endothelial cells may result in the same loss of function of TGF-$\beta_1$ control.

Endoglin and one of its ligands, TGF-$\beta_3$, is significantly elevated in the plasma of patients with breast cancer with node metastasis compared to patients who show absence of node involvement. No correlation with TGF-$\beta_1$ was observed [128]. In another study of breast cancer, a positive correlation was seen between microvessel density and TGF-$\beta_2$, TGF-RI and RII expression [127]. In childhood brain tumours [136] and in malignant melanomas [137], there was an elevated expression of endoglin on the endothelial cells. The blood vessels associated with these highly vascularised tumours are characterised by a large perivascular space and the absence of contact between the blood vessels and the adjacent parenchyma, reminiscent of the contact-mediating role of TGF-β in vasculogenesis [136].

Endoglin is thus considered a proliferation-associated antigen since it is strongly expressed on tumour-associated vasculature [138] but to lower levels on normal adult endothelium and in non-cycling ECs grown in culture. Antibody and immunotoxin to endoglin inhibited cell proliferation and also inhibited urokinase-type plasminogen activator [139–141]. Thus it is conceivable that endoglin may be a therapeutic target for tumour-associated vasculature.

## Adhesion

The homing of tumour cells to specific organs and therefore initiation of potential metastatic clones requires their interaction with the endothelium and egress into the tissues. The effect of TGF on EC-tumour cell adhesion is variable depending on the system. It can enhance the interaction through effects on both cell types [142] or through regulation of integrin expression on the tumour cell [143]. However, TGF-β can also inhibit tumour cell adhesion through regulation of adhesion molecules on the micro-endothelium [144, 145].

## Hereditary hemorrhagic telangiectasia (HHT)

HHT is an autosomal dominant disorder showing localised angiodysplasia and anteriovenous malformations in the brain, lung and liver [146–148]. Germline mutations in endoglin are responsible for HHT-1 and mutations in ALK-1, a TGF-βRI serine threonine kinase receptor with an unknown ligand, results in HHT-2 [146, 149]. The essentially null phenotype that arises from these mutations results in reduced protein and mRNA levels of endoglin and ALK-1 [149]. The localised nature of this disease is intriguing and suggests other vascular bed-specific events are also operating. However, the reduced endoglin seen in HHT-1 together with the elevated levels of endoglin identified in endothelial cells associated with certain solid tumours suggests the importance of endoglin (and presumably ALK-1) in the regulation of endothelial cell function.

## Psoriasis

Although the exact pathogenesis of psoriasis is not known, the disease is characterised by a large inflammatory infiltrate in the psoriatic lesions. *in vitro* dermal endothelium from patients with psoriasis fail to respond to the negative regulation of TGF-$\beta_1$ [104, 150]. Thus the ECs remain adhesive for CD4[+] T cells and CD45RO[+] helper/inducer cells [151] and TGF-β isoforms do not down-regulate E-selectin expression. The defect in responsiveness of the endothelium may, in part, be explained by a reduction in the function of TGF-β receptors. Both a decrease in the number of high affinity receptors for TGF-$\beta_1$ and a decrease in the signal transduction pathway mediated through a decrease in the auto-phosphorylation of the TGF-β type II receptor [151] have been noted. Alteration in endoglin levels associated with changes in the inflammatory infiltrate in the psoriatic plaque have also been found [152]. Further, increased levels of VEGF are found [153, 154] which may be responsible for the increased vascular permeability. As discussed previously, TGF-β and TGF-α both upregulate VEGF expression [52, 88, 89].

## Wounding

There are at least two types of wound healing; that which occurs as a result of an incisional wound where fibroblast and keratinocyte responses are paramount and secondly, wound healing as a result of direct vessel damage as is seen in balloon angioplasty. Only the latter will be considered here.

The wound edge after balloon angioplasty is characterised by proliferating, migrating endothelial cells with platelet aggregation. TGF-β isoforms and receptors are upregulated at the wound edge [155–158] suggesting their involvement in damage and repair of the vessel. However, as for so many other pathologies, the TGF-β effect is likely to be time- and site-dependent. TGF-β regulates expression of specific integrins on ECs which are involved in EC-ECM interactions [58, 60]. Thus, TGF-β may promote migration of ECs by inhibiting adhesion with the ECM. However, the EC proliferative response is inhibited by the addition of exogenous TGF-β [1]. TGF-β together with platelet-derived growth factor (PDGF), both released from aggregating platelets, leads to an increase in VEGF production from SMC, suggesting a platelet-mediated stimulatory effect on endothelial cell regeneration [159]. Also associated with the regenerating endothelium is an upregulation of endothelial derived nitric oxide synthase (eNOS) [160], the enzyme responsible for production of endothelial-derived NO. NO regulates neutrophil-endothelial interactions [161–163]. Anti-TGF-β neutralising antibody inhibited the eNOS [160], suggesting that TGF-β may be essential for inhibiting the inflammatory infiltrate at wound sites. Interestingly, in a rat model of balloon angioplasty [164], injection of TGF-3R:Fc chimera protein, which should neutralise available TGF-β, had little effect on re-endothelialisation of the wounded aorta but inhibited the induction of alpha SMC actin expression in the advertitia. This supports the *in vitro* data showing that TGF-β inhibits SMC differentiation and proliferation [9, 10, 165]. We have shown previously that TGF-β inhibits the TNF- and IL-1-induced adhesion molecule expression on SMC [110] which may be important in regulating the immobilisation and activation of inflammatory cells in the general area of vessel injury.

## TGF and endothelial cell signalling

It is not understood why the EC should display contrasting responses to TGF. However, it is apparent that these responses are concentration dependent [90], that the cells' environment can regulate the expression of the TGF receptors [77] and that TGF modulates the cellular response to itself and to other growth factors [4, 166, 167].

The intracellular signalling pathways that mediate the diverse endothelial cell responses to the TGF family of factors are even less well understood although the identification of the family of Smad proteins that translocate to the nucleus and thereby exert their functions should aid our investigations into this area. Most

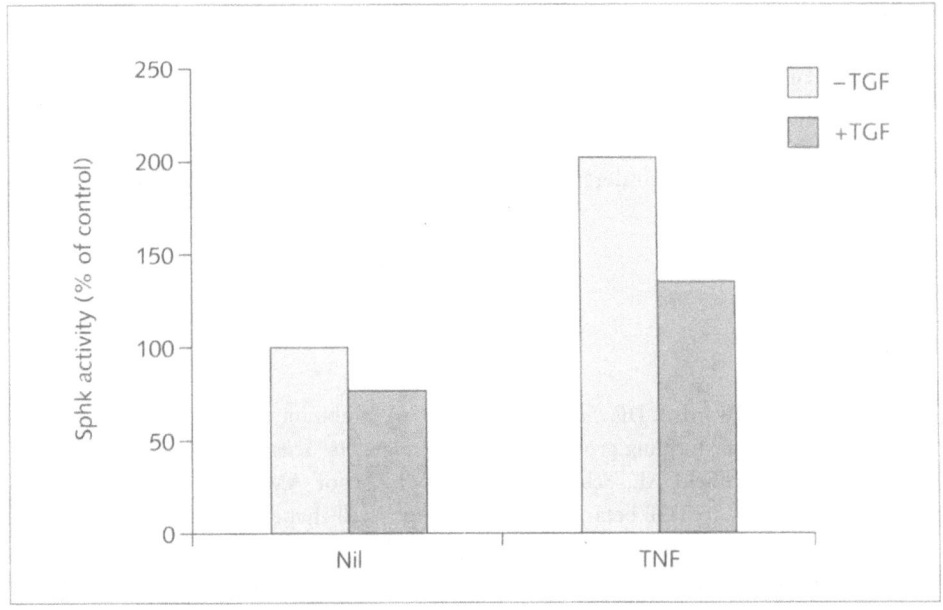

*Figure 1*
*TGF-β inhibited SphK activation in endothelial cells.*
*The primary endothelial cells were treated with or without TNF (1 ng/ml) for 10 min in the presence or absence of TGF-β (0.2 ng/ml). The SphK activity in vivo was then measured in the permeabilized cells. Data represent the mean of the two experiments.*

recently, it has been shown that H-Ras is involved in the transcription effects of TGF-β but not the anti-proliferative effects [168]. Data from our laboratory would suggest that the enzyme sphingosine kinase (SphK) is a potential target. SphK is a unique lipid kinase responsible for the formation of sphingosine-1-phosphate that serves as an intracellular and/or extracellular mediator to regulate a variety of cellular functions such as calcium mobilisation, cell motility, survival and proliferation [169– 171]. Stimulation of ECs with cytokines such as TNF-β and IL-1 and growth factors resulted in a rapid and transient activation of SphK and generation of sphingosine-1-phosphate. We have shown recently that the SphK pathway is critically involved in EC adhesion molecule expression, and in EC survival and activation [167, 172]. The finding that TGF-β inhibited the activation of SphK (Fig. 1; Xia et al., unpublished observations) suggests a novel signalling pathway responsible for TGF-β anti-inflammatory and anti-proliferative effects in ECs. The pathway linking SphK, the TGF receptors and their associated downstream Smads is yet to be determined.

## Conclusion

The effects of the TGF family of proteins on the endothelium is complex. Our quest to understand the biological processes initiated by the binding of TGF to the endothelial cells will be greatly facilitated by the identification of the signalling pathways involved and by an understanding of the impact of cell phenotype on the function of these pathways.

## References

1    Heimark RL, Twardzik DR, Schwartz SM (1986) Inhibition of endothelial regeneration by type-beta transforming growth factor from platelets. *Science* 233: 1078–1080

2    Sutton AB, Canfield AE, Schor SL, Grant ME, Schor AM (1991) The response of endothelial cells to TGF beta-1 is dependent upon cell shape proliferative state and the nature of the substratum. *J Cell Sci* 99: ( Pt 4) 777–787

3    Roberts AB, Sporn MB (1989) Regulation of endothelial cell growth, architecture, and matrix synthesis by TGF-beta. *Am Rev Respir Dis* 140: 1126–1128

4    Takehara K, LeRoy EC, Grotendorst GR (1987) TGF-beta inhibition of endothelial cell proliferation: alteration of EGF binding and EGF-induced growth-regulatory (competence) gene expression. *Cell* 49: 415–422

5    Madri JA, Pratt BM, Tucker AM (1988) Phenotypic modulation of endothelial cells by transforming growth factor-beta depends upon the composition and organization of the extracellular matrix. *J Cell Biol* 106: 1375–1384

6    Muller G, Behrens J, Nussbaumer U, Bohlen P, Birchmeier W (1987) Inhibitory action of transforming growth factor beta on endothelial cells. *Proc Natl Acad Sci USA* 84: 5600–5604

7    Wight TN, Potter-Perigo S, Aulinskas T (1989) Proteoglycans and vascular cell proliferation. *Am Rev Respir Dis* 140: 1132–1135

8    Goodman LV, Majack RA (1989) Vascular smooth muscle cells express distinct transforming growth factor-beta receptor phenotypes as a function of cell density in culture. *J Biol Chem* 264: 5241–5244

9    Owens GK, Geisterfer AA, Yang YW, Komoriya A (1988) Transforming growth factor-beta-induced growth inhibition and cellular hypertrophy in cultured vascular smooth muscle cells. *J Cell Biol* 107: 771–780

10   Majack RA (1987) Beta-type transforming growth factor specifies organizational behavior in vascular smooth muscle cell cultures. *J Cell Biol* 105: 465–471

11   Majack RA, Majesky MW, Goodman LV (1990) Role of PDGF-A expression in the control of vascular smooth muscle cell growth by transforming growth factor-beta. *J Cell Biol* 111: 239–247

12   Chen JK, Hoshi H, McKeehan WL (1987) Transforming growth factor type beta specif-

ically stimulates synthesis of proteoglycan in human adult arterial smooth muscle cells. *Proc Natl Acad Sci USA* 84: 5287–5291

13 Rifkin DB, Moscatelli D, Bizik J, Quarto N, Blei F, Dennis P, Flaumenhaft R, Mignatti P (1990) Growth factor control of extracellular proteolysis. *Cell Differ Dev* 32: 313–318

14 Laiho M, Saksela O, Andreasen PA, Keski-Oja J (1986) Enhanced production and extracellular deposition of the endothelial-type plasminogen activator inhibitor in cultured human lung fibroblasts by transforming growth factor-beta. *J Cell Biol* 103: 2403–2410

15 Ma C, Chegini N (1999) Regulation of matrix metalloproteinases (MMPs) and their tissue inhibitors in human myometrial smooth muscle cells by TGF-beta1. *Mol Hum Reprod* 5: 950–954

16 Ignotz RA, Massague J (1987) Cell adhesion protein receptors as targets for transforming growth factor-beta action. *Cell* 51: 189–197

17 Roelen BA, van Rooijen MA, Mummery CL (1997) Expression of ALK-1, a type 1 serine/threonine kinase receptor, coincides with sites of vasculogenesis and angiogenesis in early mouse development. *Dev Dyn* 209: 418–430

18 Gerhart J (1999) 1998 warkany lecture: signaling pathways in development (In Process Citation). *Teratology* 60: 226–239

19 Mishina Y, Crombie R, Bradley A, Behringer RR (1999) Multiple roles for activin-like kinase-2 signaling during mouse embryogenesis. *Dev Biol* 213: 314–326

20 Saadeh PB, Mehrara BJ, Steinbrech DS, Dudziak ME, Greenwald JA, Luchs JS, Spector JA, Ueno H, Gittes GK, Longaker MT (1999) Transforming growth factor-beta1 modulates the expression of vascular endothelial growth factor by osteoblasts. *Am J Physiol* 277: C628–C637

21 Capdevila J, Belmonte JC (1999) Extracellular modulation of the Hedgehog, Wnt and TGF-beta signalling pathways during embryonic development. *Curr Opin Genet Dev* 9: 427–433

22 Raftery LA, Sutherland DJ (1999) TGF-beta family signal transduction in *Drosophila* development: from Mad to Smads. *Dev Biol* 210: 251–268

23 Dickson MC, Martin JS, Cousins FM, Kulkarni AB, Karlsson S, Akhurst RJ (1995) Defective haematopoiesis and vasculogenesis in transforming growth factor-beta 1 knock out mice. *Development* 121: 1845–1854

24 Larson DM, Wrobleski MJ, Sagar GD, Westphale EM, Beyer EC (1997) Differential regulation of connexin43 and connexin37 in endothelial cells by cell density, growth, and TGF-beta1. *Am J Physiol* 272: C405–C415

25 Merwin JR, Anderson JM, Kocher O, Van Itallie CM, Madri JA (1990) Transforming growth factor beta 1 modulates extracellular matrix organization and cell-cell junctional complex formation during *in vitro* angiogenesis. *J Cell Physiol* 142: 117–128

26 Hurst V IV, Goldberg PL, Minnear FL, Heimark RL, Vincent PA (1999) Rearrangement of adherens junctions by transforming growth factor-beta1: role of contraction. *Am J Physiol* 276: L582–L595

27 Petroll WM, Jester, JV, Barry-Lane PA, Cavanagh HD (1996) Effects of basic FGF and

TGF beta 1 on F-actin and ZO-1 organization during cat endothelial wound healing. *Cornea* 15: 525–532

28    Goumans MJ, Zwijsen A, van Rooijen MA, Huylebroeck, Roelen BA, Mummery CL (1999) Transforming growth factor-beta signalling in extraembryonic mesoderm is required for yolk sac vasculogenesis in mice. *Development* 126: 3473–3483

29    Mandriota SJ, Menoud PA, Pepper MS (1996) Transforming growth factor beta 1 down-regulates vascular endothelial growth factor receptor 2/flk-1 expression in vascular endothelial cells. *J Biol Chem* 271: 11500–11505

30    Shalaby F, Ho J, Stanford WL, Fischer KD, Schuh AC, Schwartz L, Bernstein A, Rossant J (1997) A requirement for Flk1 in primitive and definitive hematopoiesis and vasculogenesis. *Cell* 89: 981–990

31    Schuh AC, Faloon P, Hu QL, Bhimani M, Choi K (1999) *In vitro* hematopoietic and endothelial potential of flk-1(–/–) embryonic stem cells and embryos. *Proc Natl Acad Sci USA* 96: 2159–2164

32    Shalaby F, Rossant J, Yamaguchi TP, Gertsenstein M, Wu XF, Breitman ML, Schuh AC (1995) Failure of blood-island formation and vasculogenesis in Flk-1-deficient mice. *Nature* 376: 62–66

33    Letterio JJ, Geiser AG, Kulkarni AB, Roche NS, Sporn MB, Roberts AB (1994) Maternal rescue of transforming growth factor-beta 1 null mice. *Science* 264: 1936–1938

34    Oshima M, Oshima H, Taketo MM (1996) TGF-beta receptor type II deficiency results in defects of yolk sac hematopoiesis and vasculogenesis. *Dev Biol* 179: 297–302

35    Proetzel G, Pawlowski SA, Wiles MV, Yin M, Boivin GP, Howles PN, Ding J, Ferguson MW, Doetschman T (1995) Transforming growth factor-beta 3 is required for secondary palate fusion. *Nat Genet* 11: 409–414

36    Kaartinen V, Voncken JW, Shuler C, Warburton D, Bu D, Heisterkamp N, Groffen J (1995) Abnormal lung development and cleft palate in mice lacking TGF-beta 3 indicates defects of epithelial-mesenchymal interaction. *Nat Genet* 11: 415–421

37    Suda Y, Suzuki M, Ikawa Y, Aizawa S (1987) Mouse embryonic stem cells exhibit indefinite proliferative potential. *J Cell Physiol* 133: 197–201

38    Wiles MV, Keller G (1991) Multiple hematopoietic lineages develop from embryonic stem (ES) cells in culture. *Development* 111: 259–267

39    Wang R, Clark R, Bautch VL (1992) Embryonic stem cell-derived cystic embryoid bodies form vascular channels: an *in vitro* model of blood vessel development. *Development* 114: 303–316

40    Vittet D, Prandini MH, Berthier R, Schweitzer A, Martin-Sisteron H, Uzan G, Dejana E (1996) Embryonic stem cells differentiate *in vitro* to endothelial cells through successive maturation steps. *Blood* 88: 3424–3431

41    Zhang XJ, Tsung HC, Caen JP, Li XL, Yao Z, Han ZC (1998) Vasculogenesis from embryonic bodies of murine embryonic stem cells transfected by Tgf-beta1 gene. *Endothelium* 6: 95–106

42    Keller JR, Mantel C, Sing GK, Ellingsworth LR, Ruscetti SK, Ruscetti FW (1988) Transforming growth factor beta 1 selectively regulates early murine hematopoietic progeni-

tors and inhibits the growth of IL-3-dependent myeloid leukemia cell lines. *J Exp Med* 168: 737–750

43  Li DY, Sorensen LK, Brooke BS, Urness LD, Davis EC, Taylor DG, Boak BB, Wendel DP (1999) Defective angiogenesis in mice lacking endoglin. *Science* 284: 1534–1537

44  Wiseman DM, Polverini PJ, Kamp DW, Leibovich SJ (1988) Transforming growth factor-beta (TGF beta) is chemotactic for human monocytes and induces their expression of angiogenic activity. *Biochem Biophys Res Commun* 157: 793–800

45  Brandes ME, Mai UE, Ohura K, Wahl SM (1991) Type I transforming growth factor-beta receptors on neutrophils mediate chemotaxis to transforming growth factor-beta. *J Immunol* 147: 1600–1606

46  Wahl SM, McCartney-Francis N, Mergenhagen SE (1989) Inflammatory and immuno-modulatory roles of TGF-beta. *Immunol Today* 10: 258–261

47  Assoian RK, Fleurdelys BE, Stevenson HC, Miller PJ, Madtes DK, Raines EW, Ross R, Sporn MB (1987) Expression and secretion of type beta transforming growth factor by activated human macrophages. *Proc Natl Acad Sci USA* 84: 6020–6024

48  Wahl SM, Hunt DA, Wakefield LM, McCartney-Francis N, Wahl LM, Roberts AB, Sporn MB (1987) Transforming growth factor type beta induces monocyte chemotaxis and growth factor production. *Proc Natl Acad Sci USA* 84: 5788–5792

49  McCartney-Francis N, Mizel D, Wong H, Wahl L, Wahl S (1990) TGF-beta regulates production of growth factors and TGF-beta by human peripheral blood monocytes. *Growth Factors* 4: 27–35

50  Reibman J, Meixler S, Lee TC, Gold LI, Cronstein BN, Haines KA, Kolasinski SL, Weissmann G (1991) Transforming growth factor beta 1, a potent chemoattractant for human neutrophils, bypasses classic signal-transduction pathways. *Proc Natl Acad Sci USA* 88: 6805–6809

51  Berse B, Hunt JA, Diegel RJ, Morganelli P, Yeo K, Brown F, Fava RA (1999) Hypoxia augments cytokine (transforming growth factor-beta (TGF-beta) and IL-1)-induced vascular endothelial growth factor secretion by human synovial fibroblasts. *Clin Exp Immunol* 115: 176–182

52  Pertovaara L, Kaipainen A, Mustonen T, Orpana A., Ferrara N, Saksela O, Alitalo K (1994) Vascular endothelial growth factor is induced in response to transforming growth factor-beta in fibroblastic and epithelial cells. *J Biol Chem* 269: 6271–6274

53  Pepper MS (1997) Transforming growth factor-beta: vasculogenesis, angiogenesis, and vessel wall integrity. *Cytokine Growth Factor Rev* 8: 21–43

54  Nabel EG, Shum L, Pompili VJ, Yang ZY, San H, Shu HB, Liptay S, Gold L, Gordon D, Derynck R (1993) Direct transfer of transforming growth factor beta 1 gene into arteries stimulates fibrocellular hyperplasia. *Proc Natl Acad Sci USA* 90: 10759–10763

55  Schulick AH, Taylor AJ, Zuo W, Qiu CB, Dong G, Woodward RN, Agah R, Roberts AB, Virmani R, Dichek DA (1998) Overexpression of transforming growth factor beta1 in arterial endothelium causes hyperplasia, apoptosis, and cartilaginous metaplasia. *Proc Natl Acad Sci USA* 95: 6983–6988

56  Koh GY, Kim SJ, Klug MG, Park K, Soonpaa MH, Field LJ (1995) Targeted expression

of transforming growth factor-beta 1 in intracardiac grafts promotes vascular endothelial cell DNA synthesis. *J Clin Invest* 95: 114–121

57    Cui W, Fowlis DJ, Bryson S, Duffie E, Ireland H, Balmain A, Akhurst RJ (1996) TGF-beta1 inhibits the formation of benign skin tumors, but enhances progression to invasive spindle carcinomas in transgenic mice. *Cell* 86: 531–542

58    Frank R, Adelmann-Grill BC, Herrmann K, Haustein UF, Petri JB, Heckmann M (1996) Transforming growth factor-beta controls cell-matrix interaction of microvascular dermal endothelial cells by downregulation of integrin expression. *J Invest Dermatol* 106: 36–41

59    Bradley JR, Pober JS (1996) Prolonged cytokine exposure causes a dynamic redistribution of endothelial cell adhesion molecules to intercellular junctions. *Lab Invest* 75: 463–472

60    Collo G, Pepper MS (1999) Endothelial cell integrin alpha5beta1 expression is modulated by cytokines and during migration *in vitro*. *J Cell Sci* 112 (Pt 4): 569–578

61    Brooks PC, Clark RA, Cheresh DA (1994) Requirement of vascular integrin alpha v beta 3 for angiogenesis. *Science* 264: 569–571

62    Brooks PC, Montgomery AM, Rosenfeld M, Reisfeld RA, Hu T, Klier G, Cheresh DA (1994) Integrin alpha v beta 3 antagonists promote tumor regression by inducing apoptosis of angiogenic blood vessels. *Cell* 79: 1157–1164

63    Brooks PC, Stromblad S, Klemke R, Visscher D, Sarkar FH, Cheresh DA (1995) Anti-integrin alpha v beta 3 blocks human breast cancer growth and angiogenesis in human skin (see comments). *J Clin Invest* 96: 1815–1822

64    Drake CJ, Cheresh DA, Little CD (1995) An antagonist of integrin alpha v beta 3 prevents maturation of blood vessels during embryonic neovascularization. *J Cell Sci* 108 (Pt 7): 2655–2661

65    Brooks PC, Silletti S, von Schalscha TL, Friedlander M, Cheresh DA (1998) Disruption of angiogenesis by PEX, a noncatalytic metalloproteinase fragment with integrin binding activity. *Cell* 92: 391–400

66    Bader BL, Rayburn H, Crowley D, Hynes RO (1998) Extensive vasculogenesis, angiogenesis, and organogenesis precede lethality in mice lacking all alpha v integrins. *Cell* 95: 507–519

67    Basson CT, Kocher O, Basson MD, Asis A, Madri JA (1992) Differential modulation of vascular cell integrin and extracellular matrix expression *in vitro* by TGF-beta 1 correlates with reciprocal effects on cell migration. *J Cell Physiol* 153: 118–128

68    Wei Y, Lukashev M, Simon DI, Bodary SC, Rosenberg S, Doyle MV, Chapman HA (1996) Regulation of integrin function by the urokinase receptor. *Science* 273: 1551–1555

69    Waltz DA, Natkin LR, Fujita RM, Wei Y, Chapman HA (1997) Plasmin and plasminogen activator inhibitor type 1 promote cellular motility by regulating the interaction between the urokinase receptor and vitronectin. *J Clin Invest* 100: 58–67

70    Chapman HA (1997) Plasminogen activators, integrins, and the coordinated regulation of cell adhesion and migration. *Curr Opin Cell Biol* 9: 714–724

71    Sandberg T, Casslen B, Gustavsson B, Benraad TJ (1998) Human endothelial cell migration is stimulated by urokinase plasminogen activator:plasminogen activator inhibitor 1 complex released from endometrial stromal cells stimulated with transforming growth factor beta1; possible mechanism for paracrine stimulation of endometrial angiogenesis. *Biol Reprod* 59: 759–767

72    Pepper MS, Belin D, Montesano R, Orci L, Vassalli JD (1990) Transforming growth factor-beta 1 modulates basic fibroblast growth factor-induced proteolytic and angiogenic properties of endothelial cells *in vitro*. *J Cell Biol* 111: 743–755

73    Puyraimond A, Weitzman JB, Babiole E, Menashi S (1999) Examining the relationship between the gelatinolytic balance and the invasive capacity of endothelial cells. *J Cell Sci* 112 (Pt 9): 1283–1290

74    Ito K, Ryuto M, Ushiro S, Ono M, Sugenoya A, Kuraoka A, Shibata Y, Kuwano M (1995) Expression of tissue-type plasminogen activator and its inhibitor couples with development of capillary network by human microvascular endothelial cells on Matrigel. *J Cell Physiol* 162: 213–224

75    Iruela-Arispe ML, Sage EH (1993) Endothelial cells exhibiting angiogenesis *in vitro* proliferate in response to TGF-beta 1. *J Cell Biochem* 52: 414–430

76    Zimrin AB, Maciag T (1996) Progress towards a unifying hypothesis for angiogenesis (editorial). *J Clin Invest* 97: 1359

77    Sankar S, Mahooti-Brooks N, Bensen L., McCarthy TL, Centrella M, Madri JA (1996) Modulation of transforming growth factor beta receptor levels on microvascular endothelial cells during *in vitro* angiogenesis. *J Clin Invest* 97: 1436–1446

78    Antonelli-Orlidge A, Saunders KB, Smith SR, D'Amore PA (1989) An activated form of transforming growth factor beta is produced by cocultures of endothelial cells and pericytes. *Proc Natl Acad Sci USA* 86: 4544–4548

79    Hirschi KK, Rohovsky SA, D'Amore PA (1998) PDGF, TGF-beta, and heterotypic cell-cell interactions mediate endothelial cell-induced recruitment of 10T1/2 cells and their differentiation to a smooth muscle fate (published erratum appears in *J Cell Biol* (1998) Jun 1; 141 (5): 1287). *J Cell Biol* 141: 805–814

80    Speiser P, Gittelsohn AM, Patz A (1968) Studies on diabetic retinopathy. 3. Influence of diabetes on intramural pericytes. *Arch Ophthalmol* 80: 332–337

81    Madri JA, Bell L, Merwin JR (1992) Modulation of vascular cell behavior by transforming growth factors beta. *Mol Repro Dev* 32: 121–126

82    Merwin JR, Roberts A, Kondaiah P, Tucker A, Madri J (1991) Vascular cell responses to TGF-beta 3 mimic those of TGF-beta 1 *in vitro*. *Growth Factors* 5: 149–158

83    Papapetropoulos A, Desai KM, Rudic RD, Mayer B, Zhang R, Ruiz-Torres MP, Garcia-Cardena G, Madri JA, Sessa WC (1997) Nitric oxide synthase inhibitors attenuate transforming-growth-factor-beta 1-stimulated capillary organization *in vitro*. *Am J Pathol* 150: 1835–1844

84    Papapetropoulos A, Garcia-Cardena G, Madri JA, Sessa WC (1997) Nitric oxide production contributes to the angiogenic properties of vascular endothelial growth factor in human endothelial cells. *J Clin Invest* 100: 3131–3139

85 Pollman MJ, Naumovski L, Gibbons GH (1999) Endothelial cell apoptosis in capillary network remodeling. *J Cell Physiol* 178: 359–370

86 Meyer GT, Matthias LJ, Noack L, Vadas MA, Gamble JR (1997) Lumen formation during angiogenesis *in vitro* involves phagocytic activity, formation and secretion of vacuoles, cell death, and capillary tube remodelling by different populations of endothelial cells. *Anat Rec* 249: 327–340

87 Choi ME, Ballermann BJ (1995) Inhibition of capillary morphogenesis and associated apoptosis by dominant negative mutant transforming growth factor-beta receptors. *J Biol Chem* 270: 21144–21150

88 Bottomley MJ, Webb NJ, Watson CJ, Holt PJ, Freemont AJ, Brenchley PE (1999) Peripheral blood mononuclear cells from patients with rheumatoid arthritis spontaneously secrete vascular endothelial growth factor (VEGF): specific up-regulation by tumour necrosis factor-alpha (TNF-alpha) in synovial fluid. *Clin Exp Immunol* 117: 171–176

89 Gougos A, Letarte M (1988) Identification of a human endothelial cell antigen with monoclonal antibody 44G4 produced against a pre-B leukemic cell line. *J Immunol* 141: 1925–1933

90 Pepper MS, Vassalli JD, Orci L, Montesano R (1993) Biphasic effect of transforming growth factor-beta 1 on *in vitro* angiogenesis. *Exp Cell Res* 204: 356–363

91 Lee WS, Jain MK, Arkonac BM, Zhang D, Shaw SY, Kashiki S, Maemura K, Lee SL, Hollenberg NK, Lee ME et al (1998) Thy-1, a novel marker for angiogenesis upregulated by inflammatory cytokines (see comments). *Circ Res* 82: 845–851

92 Gamble JR, Harlan JM, Klebanoff SJ, Vadas MA (1985) Stimulation of the adherence of neutrophils to umbilical vein endothelium by human recombinant tumor necrosis factor. *Proc Natl Acad Sci USA* 82: 8667–8671

93 Bevilacqua MP, Pober JS, Wheeler ME, Cotran RS, Gimbrone MA Jr (1985) Interleukin 1 acts on cultured human vascular endothelium to increase the adhesion of polymorphonuclear leukocytes, monocytes, and related leukocyte cell lines. *J Clin Invest* 76: 2003–2011

94 Morigi M, Zoja C, Figliuzzi M, Foppolo M, Micheletti G, Bontempelli M, Saronni M, Remuzzi G, Remuzzi A (1995) Fluid shear stress modulates surface expression of adhesion molecules by endothelial cells. *Blood* 85: 1696–1703

95 Doherty DE, Zagarella L, Henson PM, Worthen GS (1989) Lipopolysaccharide stimulates monocyte adherence by effects on both the monocyte and the endothelial cell. *J Immunol* 143: 3673–3679

96 Hallahan D, Clark ET, Kuchibhotla J, Gewertz BL, Collins T (1995) E-selectin gene induction by ionizing radiation is independent of cytokine induction. *Biochem Biophys Res Commun* 217: 784–795

97 Gamble JR, Vadas MA (1988) Endothelial adhesiveness for blood neutrophils is inhibited by transforming growth factor-beta. *Science* 242: 97–99

98 Gamble JR, Vadas MA (1991) Endothelial cell adhesiveness for human T lymphocytes is inhibited by transforming growth factor-beta 1. *J Immunol* 146: 1149–1154

99  Smith WB, Noack L, Khew-Goodall Y, Isenmann S, Vadas, MA, Gamble JR (1996) Transforming growth factor-beta 1 inhibits the production of IL-8 and the transmigration of neutrophils through activated endothelium. *J Immunol* 157: 360–368

100 Gamble JR, Khew-Goodall Y, Vadas MA (1993) Transforming Growth Factor-beta Inhibits E-Selectin Expression on Human Endothelial Cells. *J Immunology* 150: 4494–4503

101 Dore-Duffy P, Balabanov R, Washington R, Swanborg RH (1994) Transforming growth factor beta 1 inhibits cytokine-induced CNS endothelial cell activation. *Mol Chem Neuropathol* 22: 161–175

102 McCarron RM, Wang L, Racke MK, McFarlin DE, Spatz M (1993) Cytokine-regulated adhesion between encephalitogenic T lymphocytes and cerebrovascular endothelial cells. *J Neuroimmunol* 43: 23–30

103 Fabry Z, Topham DJ, Fee D, Herlein J, Carlino JA, Hart MN, Sriram S (1995) TGF-beta 2 decreases migration of lymphocytes *in vitro* and homing of cells into the central nervous system *in vivo*. *J Immunol* 155: 325–332

104 Cai JP, Falanga V, Chin YH (1991) Transforming growth factor-beta regulates the adhesive interactions between mononuclear cells and microvascular endothelium. *J Invest Dermatol* 97: 169–174

105 Bereta J, Bereta M, Cohen S, Cohen MC (1993) Regulation of VCAM-1 expression and involvement in cell adhesion to murine microvascular endothelium. *Cell Immunol* 147: 313–330

106 Suzuki Y, Tanigaki T, Heimer D, Wang W, Ross WG, Murphy GA, Sakai A., Sussman HH, Vu TH, Raffin TA (1994) TGF-beta 1 causes increased endothelial ICAM-1 expression and lung injury. *J Appl Physiol* 77: 1281–1287

107 Chin YH, Cai, JP, Xu XM (1992) Transforming growth factor-beta 1 and IL-4 regulate the adhesiveness of Peyer's patch high endothelial venule cells for lymphocytes. *J Immunol* 148: 1106–1112

108 Chin YH, Ye MW, Cai JP, Xu XM (1996) Differential regulation of tissue-specific lymph node high endothelial venule cell adhesion molecules by tumour necrosis factor and transforming growth factor-beta 1. *Immunology* 87: 559–565

109 Rhodes JM, Engelmyer E, Tilberg AF, Gifford RR (1995) Transforming growth factor-beta 1 serves as an autocrine inhibitor of human endothelial cell/lymphocyte adhesion. *J Surg Res* 59: 719–724

110 Gamble JR, Bradley S, Noack L, Vadas MA (1995) TGF-beta and endothelial cells inhibit VCAM-1 expression on human vascular smooth muscle cells. *Arterioscler Thromb Vasc Biol* 15: 949–955

111 Weiss JM, Cuff CA, Berman JW (1999) TGF-beta downmodulates cytokine-induced monocyte chemoattractant protein (MCP)-1 expression in human endothelial cells. A putative role for TGF-beta in the modulation of TNF receptor expression. *Endothelium* 6: 291–302

112 Ohno M, Cooke JP, Dzau VJ, Gibbons GH (1995) Fluid shear stress induces endothe-

lial transforming growth factor beta-1 transcription and production. Modulation by potassium channel blockade. *J Clin Invest* 95: 1363–1369

113 Kang YH, Brummel SE, Lee CH (1996) Differential effects of transforming growth factor-beta 1 on lipopolysaccharide induction of endothelial adhesion molecules. *Shock* 6: 118–125

114 Weiss JM, Downie SA, Lyman WD, Berman JW (1998) Astrocyte-derived monocyte-chemoattractant protein-1 directs the transmigration of leukocytes across a model of the human blood-brain barrier. *J Immunol* 161: 6896–6903

115 Fawcett J, Buckley C, Holness CL, Bird IN, Spragg JH, Saunders J, Harris A, Simmons DL (1995) Mapping the homotypic binding sites in CD31 and the role of CD31 adhesion in the formation of interendothelial cell contacts. *J Cell Biol* 128: 1229–1241

116 Kulkarni AB, Huh CG, Becker D, Geiser A, Lyght M, Flanders KC, Roberts AB, Sporn MB, Ward JM, Karlsson S (1993) Transforming growth factor beta 1 null mutation in mice causes excessive inflammatory response and early death. *Proc Natl Acad Sci USA* 90: 770–774

117 Hines KL, Kulkarni AB, McCarthy JB, Tian H, Ward JM, Christ M, McCartney-Francis NL, Furcht LT, Karlsson S, Wahl SM (1994) Synthetic fibronectin peptides interrupt inflammatory cell infiltration in transforming growth factor beta 1 knockout mice. *Proc Natl Acad Sci USA* 91: 5187–5191

118 Lefer AM, Ma XL, Weyrich AS, Scalia R (1993) Mechanism of the cardioprotective effect of transforming growth factor beta 1 in feline myocardial ischemia and reperfusion. *Proc Natl Acad Sci USA* 90: 1018–1022

119 Szekanecz Z, Haines GK, Harlow LA, Shah MR, Fong TW, Fu R, Lin SJ, Rayan G, Koch AE (1995) Increased synovial expression of transforming growth factor (TGF)-beta receptor endoglin and TGF-beta 1 in rheumatoid arthritis: possible interactions in the pathogenesis of the disease. *Clin Immunol Immunopathol* 76: 187–194

120 Takenaka K, Sakai H, Yamakawa H, Yoshimura S, Kumagai M, Yamakawa H, Nakashima S, Nozawa Y, Sakai N (1999) Polymorphism of the endoglin gene in patients with intracranial saccular aneurysms. *J Neurosurg* 90: 935–938

121 Pascal MM, Forrester JV, Knott RM (1999) Glucose-mediated regulation of transforming growth factor-beta (TGF-beta) and TGF-beta receptors in human retinal endothelial cells. *Curr Eye Res* 19: 162–170

122 Hanahan D, Folkman J (1996) Patterns and emerging mechanisms of the angiogenic switch during tumorigenesis. *Cell* 86: 353–364

123 Holash J, Maisonpierre PC, Compton D, Boland P, Alexander CR, Zagzag D, Yancopoulos GD, Wiegand SJ (1999) Vessel cooption, regression, and growth in tumors mediated by angiopoietins and VEGF. *Science* 284: 1994–1998

124 O'Reilly MS, Holmgren L, Shing Y, Chen C, Rosenthal RA, Moses M, Lane WS, Cao Y, Sage EH, Folkman J (1994) Angiostatin: a novel angiogenesis inhibitor that mediates the suppression of metastases by a Lewis lung carcinoma (see comments). *Cell* 79: 315–328

125 O'Reilly MS, Boehm T, Shing Y, Fukai N, Vasios G, Lane WS, Flynn E, Birkhead JR,

Olsen BR, Folkman J (1997) Endostatin: an endogenous inhibitor of angiogenesis and tumor growth. *Cell* 88: 277–285

126  Wikstrom P, Stattin P, Franck-Lissbrant I, Damber JE, Bergh A (1998) Transforming growth factor beta1 is associated with angiogenesis, metastasis, and poor clinical outcome in prostate cancer. *Prostate* 37: 19–29

127  de Jong JS, van Diest PJ, van der Valk P, Baak JP (1998) Expression of growth factors, growth-inhibiting factors, and their receptors in invasive breast cancer. II: Correlations with proliferation and angiogenesis. *J Pathol* 184: 53–57

128  Li C, Wang J, Wilson PB, Kumar P, Levine E, Hunter RD, Kumar S (1998) Role of transforming growth factor beta3 in lymphatic metastasis in breast cancer. *Int J Cancer* 79: 455–459

129  O'Mahony CA, Albo D, Tuszynski GP, Berger DH (1998) Transforming growth factor-beta 1 inhibits generation of angiostatin by human pancreatic cancer cells. *Surgery* 124: 388–393

130  Nakata S, Ito K, Fujimori M, Shingu K, Kajikawa S, Adachi W, Matsuyama I, Tsuchiya S, Kuwano M, Amano J (1998) Involvement of vascular endothelial growth factor and urokinase-type plasminogen activator receptor in microvessel invasion in human colorectal cancers. *Int J Cancer* 79: 179–186

131  Lastres P, Bellon T, Cabanas C, Sanchez-Madrid F, Acevedo A, Gougos A, Letarte M, Bernabeu C (1992) Regulated expression on human macrophages of endoglin, an Arg-Gly-Asp-containing surface antigen. *Eur J Immunol.* 22: 393–397

132  St Jacques S, Cymerman U, Pece N, Letarte M (1994) Molecular characterization and in situ localization of murine endoglin reveal that it is a transforming growth factor-beta binding protein of endothelial and stromal cells. *Endocrinology* 134: 2645–2657

133  O'Connell PJ, McKenzie A, Fisicaro N, Rockman SP, Pearse MJ, d'Apice AJ (1992) Endoglin: a 180-kD endothelial cell and macrophage restricted differentiation molecule. *Clin Exp Immunol* 90: 154–159

134  Lastres P, Letamendia A, Zhang H, Rius C, Almendro N, Raab U, Lopez LA, Langa C, Fabra A, Letarte M, Bernabeu C (1996) Endoglin modulates cellular responses to TGF-beta 1. *J Cell Biol* 133: 1109–1121

135  Letamendia A, Lastres P, Botella LM, Raab U, Langa C, Velasco B, Attisano L, Bernabeu C (1998) Role of endoglin in cellular responses to transforming growth factor-beta. A comparative study with betaglycan. *J Biol Chem* 273: 33011–33019

136  Bodey B, Bodey B Jr, Siegel SE, Kaiser HE (1998) Upregulation of endoglin (CD105) expression during childhood brain tumor-related angiogenesis. Anti-angiogenic therapy. Anticancer Res 18: 1485–1500

137  Bodey B, Bodey B Jr, Siegel SE, Kaiser HE (1998) Immunocytochemical detection of endoglin is indicative of angiogenesis in malignant melanoma. *Anticancer Res* 18: 2701–2710

138  Miller DW, Graulich W, Karges B, Stahl S, Ernst M, Ramaswamy A, Sedlacek HH, Muller R, Adamkiewicz J (1999) Elevated expression of endoglin, a component of the

TGF-beta-receptor complex, correlates with proliferation of tumor endothelial cells. *Int J Cancer* 81: 568–572

139 Matsuno F, Haruta Y, Kondo M, Tsai H, Barcos M, Seon BK (1999) Induction of lasting complete regression of preformed distinct solid tumors by targeting the tumor vasculature using two new anti-endoglin monoclonal antibodies. *Clin Cancer Res 5*: 371–382

140 Maier JA, Delia D, Thorpe PE, Gasparini G (1997) *In vitro* inhibition of endothelial cell growth by the antiangiogenic drug AGM-1470 (TNP-470) and the anti-endoglin antibody TEC-11. *Anticancer Drugs* 8: 238–244

141 Burrows FJ, Derbyshire EJ, Tazzari PL, Amlot P, Gazdar AF, King SW, Letarte M, Vitetta ES, Thorpe PE (1995) Up-regulation of endoglin on vascular endothelial cells in human solid tumors: implications for diagnosis and therapy. *Clin Cancer Res 1*: 1623–1634

142 Teti A, De Giorgi A, Spinella MT, Migliaccio S, Canipari R, Onetti MA, Faraggiana T (1997) Transforming growth factor-beta enhances adhesion of melanoma cells to the endothelium *in vitro*. *Int J Cancer* 72: 1013–1020

143 Loganadane LD, Vassy J, Legrand C, Fauvel-Lafeve F (1999) Transforming growth factor-beta 1 increases the adhesion of MDA-MB-231 mammary adenocarcinoma cells to the microvascular subendothelium. *Cell Adhes Commun* 7: 57–71

144 Chen TC, Hinton DR, Yong VW, Hofman FM (1997) TGF-B2 and soluble p55 TNFR modulate VCAM-1 expression in glioma cells and brain derived endothelial cells. *J Neuroimmunol* 73: 155–161

145 Bereta J, Bereta M, Coffman FD, Cohen S, Cohen MC (1992) Inhibition of basal and tumor necrosis factor-enhanced binding of murine tumor cells to murine endothelium by transforming growth factor-beta 1. *J Immunol* 148: 2932–2940.

146 Marchuk DA (1998) Genetic abnormalities in hereditary hemorrhagic telangiectasia. *Curr Opin Hematol 5*: 332–338

147 Fernandez-Ruiz E, St Jacques S, Bellon T, Letarte M, Bernabeu C (1993) Assignment of the human endoglin gene (END) to 9q34→qter. *Cytogenet Cell Genet* 64: 204–207

148 McAllister KA, Grogg KM, Johnson DW, Gallione CJ, Baldwin MA, Jackson CE, Helmbold EA, Markel DS, McKinnon WC, Murrell J (1994) Endoglin, a TGF-beta binding protein of endothelial cells, is the gene for hereditary haemorrhagic telangiectasia type 1. *Nat Genet* 8: 345–351

149 Lux A, Attisano L, Marchuk DA (1999) Assignment of transforming growth factor beta1 and beta3 and a third new ligand to the type I receptor ALK-1. *J Biol Chem* 274: 9984–9992

150 Cai JP, Falanga V, Taylor JR, Chin YH (1992) Transforming growth factor-beta differentially regulates the adhesiveness of normal and psoriatic dermal microvascular endothelial cells for peripheral blood mononuclear cells. *J Invest Dermatol* 98: 405–409

151 Cai JP, Falanga V, Taylor JR, Chin YH (1996) Transforming growth factor-beta receptor binding and function are decreased in psoriatic dermal endothelium. *J Invest Dermatol* 106: 225–231

152 van de Kerkhof PC, Rulo HF, van Pelt JP, Vlijmen-Willems IM, De Jong EM (1998) Expression of endoglin in the transition between psoriatic uninvolved and involved skin. *Acta Derm Venereol* 78: 19–21

153 Detmar M (1996) Molecular regulation of angiogenesis in the skin (editorial). *J Invest Dermatol* 106: 207–208

154 Detmar M, Brown LF, Claffey KP, Yeo KT, Kocher O, Jackman RW, Berse B, Dvorak HF (1994) Overexpression of vascular permeability factor/vascular endothelial growth factor and its receptors in psoriasis. *J Exp Med* 180: 1141–1146

155 Rotatori DS, Kerr NC, Raphael B, McLaughlin BJ, Shimizu R, Stern GA, Schultz GS (1994) Elevation of transforming growth factor alpha in cat aqueous tumor after corneal endothelial injury. *Invest Ophthalmol Vis Sci* 35: 143–149

156 Ward MR, Agrotis A, Kanellakis P, Dilley R, Jennings G, Bobik A (1997) Inhibition of protein tyrosine kinases attenuates increases in expression of transforming growth factor-beta isoforms and their receptors following arterial injury. *Arterioscler Thromb Vasc Biol* 17: 2461–2470

157 Yang L, Qiu CX, Ludlow A, Ferguson MW, Brunner G (1999) Active transforming growth factor-beta in wound repair: determination using a new assay. *Am J Pathol* 154: 105–111

158 Frank S, Madlener M, Werner S (1996) Transforming growth factors beta1, beta2, and beta3 and their receptors are differentially regulated during normal and impaired wound healing. *J Biol Chem* 271: 10188–10193

159 Kronemann N, Bouloumi A, Bassus S, Kirchmaier CM, Busse R, Schini-Kerth VB (1999) Aggregating human platelets stimulate expression of vascular endothelial growth factor in cultured vascular smooth muscle cells through a synergistic effect of transforming growth factor-beta(1) and platelet-derived growth factor(AB). *Circulation* 100: 855–860

160 Poppa V, Miyashiro JK, Corson MA, Berk BC (1998) Endothelial NO synthase is increased in regenerating endothelium after denuding injury of the rat aorta. *Arterioscler Thromb Vasc Biol* 18: 1312–1321

161 Cockrell A, Laroux FS, Jourd'heuil D, Kawachi S, Gray L, Van der HH, Grisham MB (1999) Role of inducible nitric oxide synthase in leukocyte extravasation *in vivo*. *Biochem Biophys Res Commun* 257: 684–686

162 Lefer DJ, Jones SP, Girod WG, Baines A, Grisham MB, Cockrell AS, Huang PL, Scalia R (1999) Leukocyte-endothelial cell interactions in nitric oxide synthase-deficient mice. *Am J Physiol* 276: H1943–H1950

163 Fowler AA III, Fisher BJ, Sweeney LB, Wallace TJ, Natarajan R, Ghosh SS, Ghosh S (1999) Nitric oxide regulates interleukin-8 gene expression in activated endothelium by inhibiting NF-kappaB binding to DNA: effects on endothelial function. *Biochem Cell Biol* 77: 201–208

164 Smith JD, Bryant SR, Couper LL, Vary CP, Gotwals PJ, Koteliansky VE, Lindner V (1999) Soluble transforming growth factor-beta type II receptor inhibits negative remodeling, fibroblast transdifferentiation, and intimal lesion formation but not endothelial growth. *Circ Res* 84: 1212–1222

165 Hirschi KK, Rohovsky SA, D'Amore PA (1998) PDGF, TGF-beta, and heterotypic cell-cell interactions mediate endothelial cell-induced recruitment of 10T1/2 cells and their differentiation to a smooth muscle fate [published erratum appears in *J Cell Biol* (1998) Jun 1; 141 (5): 1287). *J Cell Biol* 141: 805–814

166 Sankar S, Mahooti-Brooks N, Centrella M, McCarthy TL, Madri JA (1995) Expression of transforming growth factor type III receptor in vascular endothelial cells increases their responsiveness to transforming growth factor beta 2. *J Biol Chem* 270: 13567–13572

167 Fafeur V, Terman BI, Blum J, Bohlen P (1990) Basic FGF treatment of endothelial cells down-regulates the 85-KDa TGF beta receptor subtype and decreases the growth inhibitory response to TGF-beta 1. *Growth Factors* 3: 237–245

168 Yamamoto H, Atsuchi N, Tanaka H, Ogawa W, Abe M, Takeshita A, Ueno H (1999) Separate roles for H-Ras and Rac in signaling by transforming growth factor (TGF)-beta. H-Ras is essential for activation of MAP kinase, partially required for transcriptional activation by TGF-beta, but not required for signaling of growth suppression by TGF-beta. *Eur J Biochem* 264: 110–119

169 Spiegel S, Merrill AH Jr (1996) Sphingolipid metabolism and cell growth regulation. *FASEB J* 10: 1388–1397

170 Olivera A, Spiegel S (1993) Sphingosine-1-phosphate as second messenger in cell proliferation induced by PDGF and FCS mitogens. *Nature* 365: 557–560

171 Olivera A, Kohama T, Edsall L, Nava V, Cuvillier O, Poulton S, Spiegel S. (1999) Sphingosine kinase expression increases intracellular sphingosine-1-phosphate and promotes cell growth and survival (In Process Citation). *J Cell Biol* 147: 545–558

172 Xia P, Gamble JR, Rye KA, Wang L, Hii CS, Cockerill P, Khew-Goodall Y, Bert AG, Barter PJ, Vadas MA (1998) Tumor necrosis factor-alpha induces adhesion molecule expression through the sphingosine kinase pathway. *Proc Natl Acad Sci USA* 95: 14196–14201

# TGF-β and macrophages in the rise and fall of inflammation

Nancy L. McCartney-Francis and Sharon M. Wahl

Oral Infection and Immunity Branch, National Institute of Dental and Craniofacial Research, National Institutes of Health, 30 Convent Drive, Building 30, Bethesda, MD 20892-4352, USA

## Introduction

Macrophages represent one of the most influential classes of cells within the body that functions not only in host defense against infectious agents and tumor cells, but also in immune events ranging from antigen processing and presentation to production of mediators that regulate immune and inflammatory responses [1, 2]. One such mediator that plays a prominent role in inducing responses in and regulating responses by cells of monocyte/macrophage lineage is transforming growth factor-beta (TGF-β) [3, 4]. Known for its diverse functions in numerous biological processes encompassing embryogenesis to tumorigenesis, TGF-β's most divergent properties are observed in immune reactions [3, 5, 6]. Induced and potentiated by, as well as suppressed by TGF-β, inflammatory responses rise and then fall, culminating in tissue repair and resolution of inflammation. However, imbalance between the pro-inflammatory properties and immunosuppressive activities of TGF-β can result in chronic states of inflammation and fibrosis. These imbalances are most graphic in the TGF-$\beta_1$ knockout mice, which die of a multifocal inflammatory response and multisystem failure [7, 8], and the TGF-$\beta_1$ overexpressing mice which exhibit tissue fibrosis and kidney failure [9]. Furthermore, dysregulation of immune homeostasis by aberrant expression of, or response to, TGF-β is associated with infectious diseases and autoimmunity [5, 6, 10]. Understanding of these opposing activities of TGF-β is vital to the design of therapeutic interventions for such life-threatening diseases.

## The rise of inflammation: initiation by TGF-β

### Mononuclear cell recruitment and activation

The inflammatory process is a complex cascade of events that involves recruitment and migration of cells into a site of injury, infection or antigen deposition, followed

TGF-β and Related Cytokines in Inflammation, edited by Samuel N. Breit and Sharon M. Wahl
© 2001 Birkhäuser Verlag Basel/Switzerland

by activation, proliferation and differentiation of cells within the lesion, modulation of integrin expression, and synthesis of inflammatory mediators and proteases to rid the host of the inciting agent [11]. Resolution of the response involves apoptosis and matrix deposition. One of the first steps in the initiation of this inflammatory sequence involves aggregation and degranulation of platelets with the release of a myriad of inflammatory mediators including TGF-β from the α-granules. Whereas several of these mediators activate the plasma protease systems which contribute to the acute inflammatory response (vasodilation, vascular permeability, neutrophil recruitment and activation) [12], TGF-β functions in the early inflammatory response as a potent chemoattractant for monocytes/macrophages as well as lymphocytes, neutrophils, and fibroblasts. Femtomolar concentrations of TGF-β are effective in inducing the migration of mononuclear cells *in vitro* [13, 14] and identification of TGF-β within sites of acute inflammation suggests an important role in the initial stages of inflammation. TGF-β is also released from connective tissue reservoirs and from the recruited inflammatory cells. Furthermore, local injection of TGF-β into the skin or joint cavity results in a rampant influx of leukocytes [15–17]. Thus, the establishment of a concentration-dependent chemotactic gradient of TGF-β radiating from the inflammatory site promotes the migration of leukocytes from the vasculature into the tissue.

Recruitment of leukocytes into a site of injury or infection depends not only on chemotactic signals but also on cellular and matrix interactions [18, 19]. During the sequence of events leading to the migration of cells into the tissue, leukocytes first encounter and bind to activated endothelial cells. Cell adhesion to other cells and to extracellular matrix is mediated by membrane adhesion molecules including selectins and integrins. In addition to providing a chemotactic gradient, TGF-β and other stimuli promote emigration of leukocytes into tissues by inducing the expression of specific α and $\beta_1$ integrin subunits [20, 21]. Picomolar concentrations of TGF-β upregulate monocyte expression of $\alpha_5\beta_1$, the functional receptor for fibronectin, and $\alpha_3\beta_1$, the ligand for laminin and type IV collagen. Increased integrin expression is accompanied by enhanced monocyte binding to endothelium and extracellular matrix, thus facilitating the targeting and retention of circulating cells to sites of injury or infection. The importance of adhesive events in the initiation of inflammation is evident by the therapeutic efficacy of synthetic fibronectin peptide antagonists in delayed wound healing, chronic inflammation, and autoimmune disease [22–25].

In addition to modulation of adhesion molecule expression, monocytes, in response to TGF-β, express increased levels of the 92 kDa and 72 kDa gelatinase/type IV collagenases [20]. Degradation of the basement membrane, of which collagen IV is a major component, facilitates the migration of cells from the circulation into and through the tissues. Moreover, at the site of tissue injury, proteolytic degradation and clearance of damaged matrix is essential to eventual resolution and repair. Coordinated regulation of these pathways, chemotaxis, adhesion, and enzymatic degradation of the extracellular matrix by TGF-β, as well as other inflammatory mediators, some of which are induced by TGF-β, contributes to the initiation and amplification of the cellular inflammatory response.

One important component in the initiation of inflammation is the activation of the cytokine cascade which modulates cell function and mobilizes host defense mechanisms. Upregulation of pro-inflammatory cytokines including interleukin-1β (IL-1β) [13], tumor necrosis factor α (TNF-α) [26], and IL-6 [27] in nonactivated monocytes and monocyte-derived macrophages by TGF-β serves to potentiate the inflammatory cascade by acting on endothelial cells, fibroblasts and lymphocytes to promote angiogenesis, matrix synthesis, and lymphocyte activation and proliferation (reviewed in [5]). In turn, these activated cells synthesize and secrete TGF-β [26, 28–31]. In a paracrine and autocrine manner, this TGF-β further augments cytokine and mediator production in surrounding cells and, importantly, can also upregulate its own expression, acting through transcription factor activator protein-1 (AP-1) to activate transcription of TGF-β [32], and thus intensify the inflammatory response.

As part of its early pro-inflammatory profile, TGF-β may modulate expression of the Fcγ receptor III (FcγRIII, CD16), a molecule that binds the Fc portion of immunoglobulin and is found on the surface of natural killer cells, a small subpopulation of peripheral blood monocytes, and differentiated, mature macrophages. By rapidly upregulating FcγRIII on the surface of newly recruited monocytes, TGF-β contributes to phagocytosis and clearance of IgG-opsonized particles and immune complexes together with increased respiratory burst activity and superoxide generation [33]. Once activated, however, macrophages downregulate respiratory burst activity in response to TGF-β as part of the resolution phase (see below). Phagocytosis also occurs when TGF-β promotes macrophage recognition of phosphatidylserine, which is expressed on the outer membrane leaflet of apoptotic cells [34]. This process triggers the release of additional TGF-β, likely a key mechanism for suppression rather than exacerbation of inflammation during clearance of apoptotic cells.

## Regulation of TGF-β expression and signaling

Whereas the pro-inflammatory activities of TGF-β and the ensuing acute inflammatory cascade serve to maximize the host's ability to rapidly respond to infection or injury and initiate repair, and excess TGF-β generated in response to infection can dampen this host response, it is obvious that these events must be under tight regulatory control to prevent persistent and pathogenic inflammation and fibrosis. Expression of TGF-β in macrophages and other cell types is regulated at both transcriptional and translational levels [35]. Although the three mammalian isoforms of TGF-β (TGF-$\beta_1$, -$\beta_2$, -$\beta_3$) are encoded by unique genes, they share 70–80% amino acid identity and conserved structural features, bind to the same family of receptors, and induce overlapping responses (reviewed in [36]). However, differences within the promoters and 5' and 3' untranslated regions likely account for isoform-specific expression patterns [35]. TGF-$\beta_1$ is the most abundant isoform expressed by monocytes/macrophages. Unlike TGF-$\beta_2$ and TGF-$\beta_3$, the TGF-$\beta_1$ promoter lacks TATA and CAAT boxes and contains AP-1 and Erg-1 response elements [37]. TGF-$\beta_1$ transcription is differentially affected by growth factors; for example, nerve growth factor acts through the Erg-1 site [38] and TGF-$\beta_1$ autoinduction occurs through the AP-1 binding site [32]. TGF-$\beta_1$ transcription is also influenced by viral infection through the Erg-1 binding site by transactivator proteins of hepatitis B virus and cytomegalovirus [39, 40] and through the AP-1 site by HTLV-1 transactivating protein Tax [41]. Oncogenes *src* and *abl* activate TGF-$\beta$ through Erg-1 and AP-1, whereas *ras*, *jun*, and *fos* activate only through AP-1 [37]. These multiple regulatory sites in the TGF-$\beta_1$ promoter, which are absent in the TGF-$\beta_2$ and TGF-$\beta_3$ promoters, may account for the selective overexpression of TGF-$\beta_1$ in inflammatory and infectious situations. TGF-$\beta_2$ and TGF-$\beta_3$ promoters, in contrast, contain cAMP-response elements, suggesting that transcription is under hormonal and developmental control [35]. Both TGF-$\beta_1$ and TGF-$\beta_3$ are regulated by Sp-1 transcription factor and, whereas the retinoblastoma gene product (Rb) induces TGF-$\beta_2$ through the ATF-2 transcription factor, Rb may negatively influence TGF-$\beta_1$ expression through inhibition of the *fos* gene.

TGF-$\beta$ responsive promoters also contain cis- and trans-acting elements that mediate transcriptional effects of TGF-$\beta$. Of significance is the association of these transactivating factors with the TGF-$\beta$ signal transducers, Smads (mammalian homologue of *Drosophila Mad; Mad* = mothers against decapentaplegic), which deliver specific TGF-$\beta$ signals from the cytoplasm to the nucleus of target cells (see below). In addition, TGF-$\beta$ transcriptional repression is controlled through inhibitory response elements. For example, binding of a Fos protein complex to the transin/stromelysin promoter confers an inhibitory signal [42]. Inhibitory elements are also found in promoters of urokinase, elastase, collagenase, and *c-myc*, all genes sensitive to down-regulation by TGF-$\beta$ [35]. Thus, the transcriptional activation of TGF-$\beta$ and the target gene response to TGF-$\beta$ contribute to the outcome of inflammation, wound healing and tissue remodeling.

Another absolutely critical level of regulation occurs through the conformation of the TGF-$\beta$ molecule itself. Although secreted by virtually all cells of the body, TGF-$\beta$ is synthesized as a large inactive precursor molecule which is unable to bind to its signaling receptors. Since TGF-$\beta$ receptors are ubiquitously expressed, the secretion of a biologically inactive molecule requiring proteolytic activation avoids unnecessary signal transduction and system overload. The precursor molecule is cleaved by proteolysis through the action of endopeptidases such as furin to yield the mature 112 amino acid, 25 kDa TGF-$\beta$ molecule [43]. TGF-$\beta$ is secreted as a complex of the 25 kDa disulfide-linked homodimer of mature TGF-$\beta$, a noncovalently associated 75 kDa latency associated protein (LAP) representing the precursor cleavage product and, in most cases, a covalently bound 135 kDa latent TGF-β binding protein (LTBP). LAP, which contains mannose-6-phosphate residues, may facilitate binding of the secreted latent complex to the cell surface *via* mannose-6-phosphate /insulin growth factor II receptors. TGF-β itself rapidly enhances monocyte insulin-like growth factor II receptor mRNA (Wild et al., unpublished observations) which likely promotes this process. LAP of TGF-$\beta_1$ and -$\beta_3$ isoforms also contains arginine-glycine-aspartic acid (RGD) residues which, at least in the case of LAP-TGF-$\beta_1$, can bind $\alpha_v\beta_1$ integrin [44], a TGF-β-inducible binding protein (Wild et al., unpublished observations). This association fosters cell attachment and migration as well as signaling events [44]. In contrast to LAP, LTBP functions as an anchoring protein to localize TGF-β to extracellular matrix, providing a readily accessible reservoir of TGF-β for activation by plasmin and thrombospondin.

Activation of TGF-β probably occurs through multiple, not well-delineated mechanisms including, but not limited to, proteolytic processing by plasmin, exposure to low dose radiation, low pH, and reactive oxygen species [45]. Nitric oxide (NO)-induced nitrosylation and inactivation of LAP may also play a role [46]. Recent evidence implicates mannose-6-phosphate receptor binding, integrin binding, and interaction with thrombospondin-1 in the TGF-β activation process [45]. For example, activation of latent TGF-β secreted by murine alveolar macrophages in bleomycin-induced pulmonary fibrosis was shown to be dependent upon plasmin, but activation also required binding of latent TGF-β to the macrophage cell surface *via* thrombospondin-1 and its receptor CD36 [47, 48], as reviewed in [45]. In activated mouse peritoneal cells, plasmin activation of TGF-β involved coordinated actions with mannose-6-phosphate receptor, transglutaminase, and the urokinase receptor [49, 50]. By confocal analysis of IFN-γ + lipopolysaccharide (LPS)-stimulated macrophages, activation of TGF-β by a cell membrane-bound protease was accompanied by loss of LAP immunoreactivity and gain of TGF-β epitopes which colocalized with betaglycan (TβRIII) [51], also suggesting that activation occurs on the cell surface. Activation of latent TGF-β may also occur through cytoskeletal associated-integrin $\alpha_v\beta_6$ in epithelial cells which induce conformational changes in the latent complex such that mature TGF-β can bind to nearby TGF-β receptors to initiate signaling [52]. Despite the overwhelming *in vitro* evidence for involvement of plasmin, plasminogen-deficient mice share no pathological features with the TGF-$\beta_1$ knockout mice [53], implicating redundant proteolytic processes. On the other hand, thrombospondin-1 knockout mice display similar features as TGF-$\beta_1$ knockout mice but the symptomology is not as severe [54].

Although TGF-β is rapidly synthesized, secreted, and/or activated, mechanisms are in place to rapidly inactivate or sequester this highly active polypeptide (reviewed in [55]). Secreted TGF-β is rapidly scavenged by $\alpha_2$-macroglobulin and cleared from the circulation. Within the tissues, binding to biglycan, decorin, elastin, or fibromodulin renders TGF-β inactive and sequesters the molecule in the extracellular matrix. Binding of α-fetoprotein to TGF-$\beta_2$ occurs without loss of activity

[56], whereas binding to thrombospondin-1 can either activate or prevent activation of TGF-β, depending on the region of the thrombospondin-1 molecule which binds to latent TGF-β [57]. Matrix-bound latent TGF-β provides a reservoir of latent TGF-β. Proteolytic cleavage to release latent TGF-β represents an extracellular mechanism for regulation of its activation.

Once activated, the biological effects of the mature TGF-β are elicited through receptor binding and signaling (Fig. 1) [58]. Freshly isolated circulating monocytes express type I (50–60 kDa, TβRI) and type II (75–85 kDa, TβRII) transmembrane TGF-β receptors and are exquisitely sensitive to TGF-β stimulation. As shown for other cells, receptor binding of TGF-β and the ensuing signaling cascade results in modulation of targeted genes including cytokines, integrins, and proteases, as well as TGF-β gene expression. TGF-β receptor-mediated signaling is initiated by binding to TβRII, a constitutively-active serine-threonine kinase [58]. Recruitment of the TβRI into the signaling complex is followed by the sequential phosphorylation of TβRI and downstream signaling elements which include the nuclear transcriptional factors Smad 2 and Smad 3 [59]. The Smad molecules are localized to the TβRI in the membrane by an adaptor molecule SARA (Smad anchor for receptor activation), which subsequently allows for efficient TβR1-mediated phosphorylation of Smad 2 and 3 [60]. The phosphorylated pathway-specific Smad proteins then dissociate from the receptor complex and hetero-oligomerize with the common mediator Smad 4 and translocate to the nucleus, where they act as transcriptional activators of TGF-β-regulated genes. Although *in vitro* studies have shown some similar, interchangeable functions of Smad 2 and Smad 3, Smad 3 is uniquely able to bind directly to DNA *via* the Mad homology domain (MH1) to transactivate TGF-β-responsive genes such as plasminogen activator inhibitor-1 (PAI) [61–63], type VII collagen [64], and JunB [65]. Furthermore, mice bearing null mutations of the Smad 3 or Smad 2 gene display distinct phenotypes, with Smad 2 null mice dying *in utero* [66] and Smad 3 null mice surviving into adulthood [67–69]. In functional studies, Smad 3 deficient monocytes fail to chemotax to TGF-β, but not other stimuli, and autocrine induction of TGF-β$_1$ is impaired, implicating Smad 3 in TGF-β-mediated macrophage activation [21]. Importantly, these studies have provided the first evidence that independent TGF-β signaling events may be mediated by individual Smads, thus offering potential insight into selective functional regulation for therapeutic benefit.

Whereas Smad-mediated gene activation occurs through direct binding of the Smad complex to DNA or interaction with specific DNA-binding proteins, such as Fast1, association with transcriptional coactivators such as CBP (Creb binding protein) and its functional homolog p300 [70] and MSG1 (melanocyte-specific gene-1) [71] or transcriptional corepressors such as the homeodomain protein TGIF (5'TG3' interacting factor) [72] also influences transcription of TGF-β-regulated genes. Smad-mediated transcription is blocked by binding of adenoviral transforming protein E1A to CBP/p300 [73] or by interaction of the nuclear zinc finger pro-

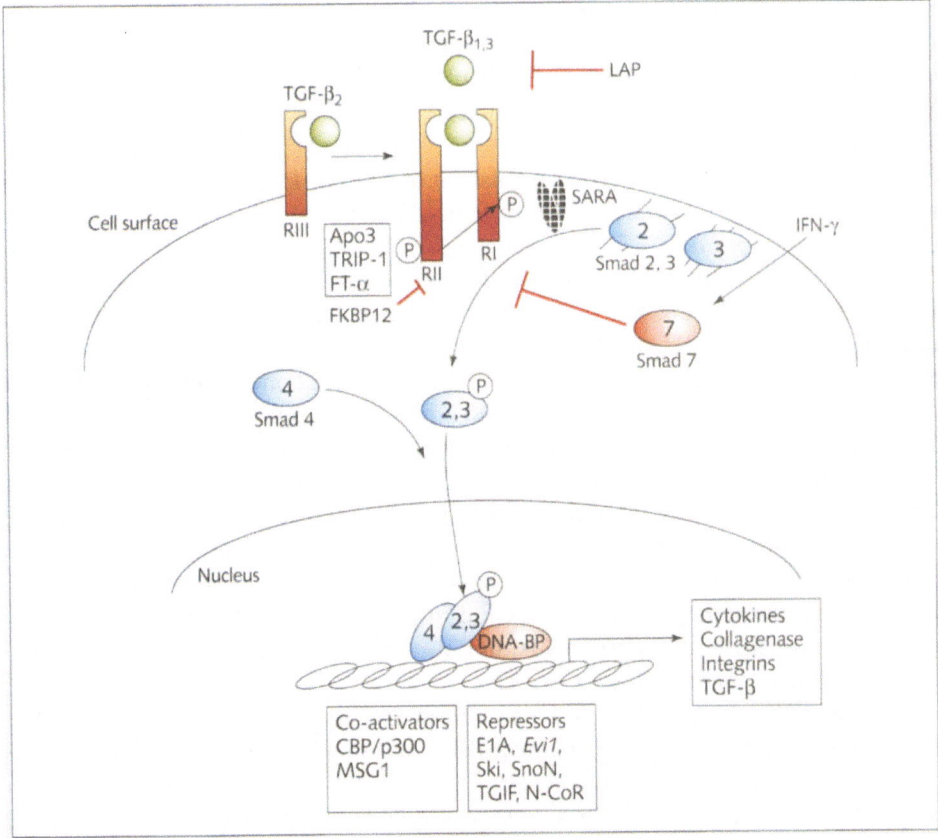

*Figure 1*

*Regulation of TGF-β signaling and signaling crosstalk*

*Signaling is initiated by binding of TGF-β to TβRII, followed by recruitment and phosphorylation of TβRI. Unphosphorylated transcription factors Smad 2 or Smad 3 are sequestered in the cytoplasm through association with microtubules. Recruitment of the Smads to TβRI in the plasma membrane is mediated by SARA (Smad anchor for receptor activation). Upon subsequent phosphorylation and activation of Smad 2 or Smad 3, the receptor-SARA-Smad complex dissociates and the phosphorylated Smad proteins are then hetero-oligomerized with Smad 4 and translocated to the nucleus, where they activate transcription of TGF-β-regulated genes by either direct binding to DNA response elements or to DNA binding cofactors. Induced by IFN-γ, inhibitor Smad 7 interacts with activated TβRI, thus antagonizing the receptor-mediated phosphorylation of Smad 2 and Smad 3. Association of the Smad signaling complex with coactivators CBP/p300 and MSG1 or corepressors TGIF, N-CoR, Ski, SnoN, Evi1, and E1a also influence transcription of TGF-β-regulated genes. Degradation and clearance of phosphorylated Smad 2 from the nucleus following TGF-β stimulation occurs through the ubiquitin-dependent proteasome pathway, thus terminating its signaling capacity.*

tein Evi-1 with Smad 3 [74]. Nuclear oncoproteins Ski and SnoN bind to Smad proteins and, through the recruitment and complexing with corepressor N-CoR, prevent Smad-mediated transcriptional activation of TGF-β-responsive genes [75, 76]. Whereas expression of Ski is not affected by TGF-β, SnoN is rapidly induced by TGF-β and interacts with Smad 2 and Smad 4 to repress signaling, suggesting a role for SnoN in the negative feedback regulation of TGF-β signaling. In contrast to the interaction of Smad 2 and Smad 4 with SnoN, Smad 3 rapidly degrades SnoN, thus enabling transcription of TGF-β target genes.

Two inhibitory Smad proteins, Smad 6 and Smad 7, act as anti-Smads and, by binding to the TβRI, prevent the receptor-mediated phosphorylation of Smad 2/3, thus interrupting the signaling cascade [77, 78]. Smad 6 inhibits phosphorylation of Smad 2 but not Smad 3 and may preferentially inhibit bone morphogenic protein (BMP) signaling. On the other hand, Smad 7 inhibits phosphorylation of both Smad 2 and Smad 3, and it has been suggested that Smad 7 has a higher selectivity for TGF-β signaling [79], even though both Smad 6 and Smad 7 are rapidly induced by TGF-β [80]. The therapeutic potential of Smad 7 interruption of TGF-β signaling was recently demonstrated in a mouse model of bleomycin-induced lung fibrosis [81]. Gene transfer of Smad 7, but not Smad 6, prevented lung fibrosis, documenting not only the pathogenic role of TGF-β in tissue fibrosis and the biological differences between the two anti-Smads, but also the ability to selectively target specific TGF-β-dependent pathways.

Recent studies have suggested a Smad-dependent link between the TGF-β signaling pathway and IFN-γ signaling pathway [82]. IFN-γ, which signals through the Jak-Stat pathway, was found to induce expression of the inhibitory Smad 7 molecule. These data are consistent with the known antagonistic relationship between IFN-γ and TGF-β [83–87]. TGF-β, in turn, is inhibitory to IFN-γ-regulated genes, including inducible nitric oxide synthase (iNOS), an important macrophage product for host defense [88]. In the absence of TGF-β$_1$, unchecked IFN-γ-induced IRF-1 and Stat-1 expression results in persistent NO production, a potential contributor to the early demise of the TGF-β$_1$ null mice (McCartney-Francis et al., unpublished observations).

The contribution of TGF-β to recruitment and activation of monocytes and macrophages at a site of injury or infection facilitates the accumulation of cells to clear the inciting agent, enabling resolution of the inflammatory response and the initiation of tissue repair.

## The fall of inflammation: resolution by TGF-β

### Anti-inflammatory and immunosuppressive effects of TGF-β

Inflammation is a dynamic process involving pro-inflammatory activities of cellular migration, adhesion, and activation and matrix synthesis countered by the immunosuppressive activities of cytokines, inflammatory mediator down-modulation, and inhibition of lymphocyte proliferation, with the ultimate goal of the entire process being elimination of the inciting agent, resolution of inflammation, and tissue repair (Fig. 2) [89]. TGF-β plays an important part in each of these processes, and the state of cellular differentiation which underlies TGF-β receptor expression in large part determines the outcome of the TGF-β response. Whereas resting monocytes express an optimal number (about 400 high affinity type I/II TGF-β receptors) of receptors [90], upon activation and differentiation, receptor expression is reduced and the macrophages become relatively insensitive to the pro-inflammatory signals triggered by TGF-β in immature populations [5]. In activated macrophages, TGF-β, at higher concentrations, becomes a potent immunosuppressive agent and macrophage deactivator, as evidenced by TGF-β-mediated inhibition of hydrogen peroxide and NO release, cytotoxic activity, TNF-α and IL-1β production, and expression of prostaglandin synthase-2 by murine macrophages [91-96]. The macrophage response to TGF-β is influenced by the cytokine milieu that the cell is exposed to [86, 97], the context in which the cytokine is presented [98, 99], and the temporal nature of cytokine exposure, as well as the state of differentiation and receptor expression. Priming of macrophages with TGF-β prior to exposure to particulate stimuli [100], lipopolysaccharide (LPS) [86], or IFN-γ [97] prevented the generation of inflammatory cytokines and NO. The suppressive effects of TGF-β could be reversed by prior exposure to IFN-γ, providing evidence that TGF-$\beta_1$ and IFN-γ deliver antagonistic signals [82].

This inverse relationship is reflected in TGF-$\beta_1$ transgenic mouse models. TGF-$\beta_1$-deficient mice develop clinical symptoms of an autoimmune Sjogren's-like syndrome characterized by increased IFN-γ expression, circulating autoantibodies, leukocyte infiltration, and elevated MHC class I and II antigens [24]. Dysregulated macrophage function in these mice is highlighted by increased RNA expression of inflammatory cytokines TNF-α, IL-1β, and IL-6 [8, 24] and inducible nitric oxide synthase and by elevated circulating levels of nitrite/nitrate [101] (McCartney-Francis et al., unpublished observations). Whereas TGF-β is a potent deactivator of IFN-γ-induced NO in macrophages [88], NO production is reduced in TGF-$\beta_1$ overexpressing transgenic mice (TGF-$\beta_1$/albumin) following induction of septic shock [102].

As part of the resolution process, lymphocytes, which express few TGF-β receptors until activated, become increasingly sensitive to the immunosuppressive properties of TGF-β. Since lymphocyte proliferation involves the pro-inflammatory cytokine IL-1, a product of TGF-β-stimulated monocytes, as is the IL-1 receptor antagonist, TGF-β inhibition of activated macrophages reduces pro-inflammatory IL-1 levels [103, 104]. Inhibition of proliferation by TGF-β also occurs more directly through induction of cyclin dependent kinase (CDK) inhibitors p21$^{CIP1/WAF1}$ and p15$^{INK4B}$ which block the activities of cyclin/cdk complexes, arresting the cell cycle in G1 phase [105]. Additional TGF-β-dependent mechanisms of T cell suppression

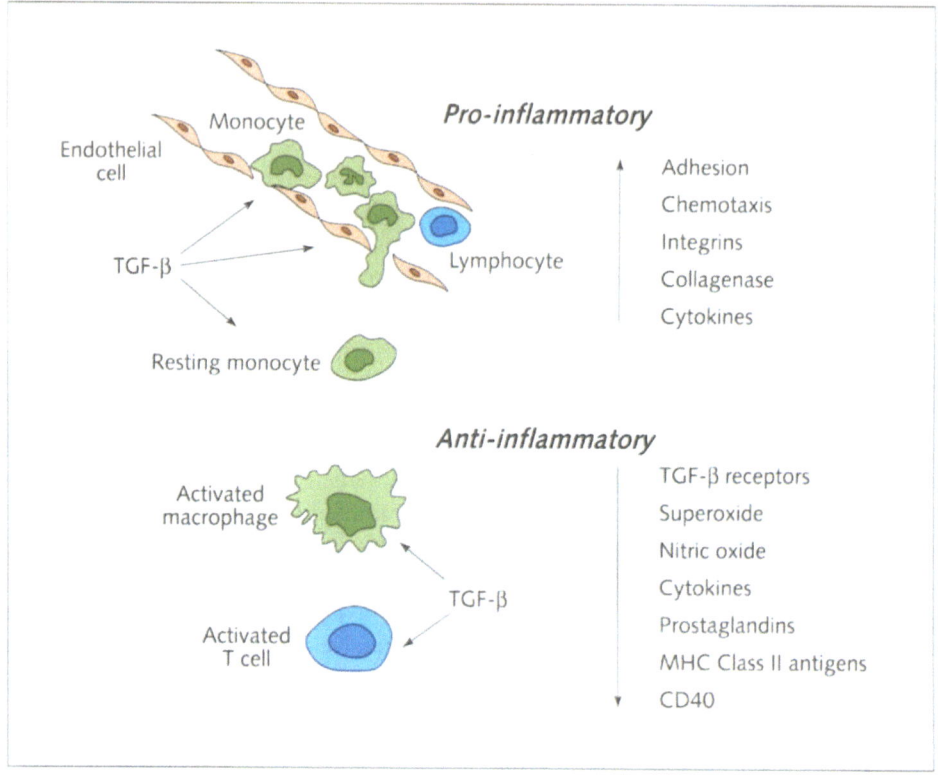

Figure 2

*The rise and fall of inflammation: regulation by TGF-β*

*Bacterial infection or traumatic insult causes platelet degranulation and release of TGF-β into the tissue. A potent chemotactic factor, TGF-β recruits cells from the circulation into the tissue. TGF-β-induced integrin expression enhances monocyte adhesion and retention to endothelium and matrix and upregulation of collagenases facilitates migration of cells into and through the tissue. Activation of the pro-inflammatory cytokine cascade in newly recruited or non-activated inflammatory cells by increased concentrations of TGF-β potentiates the response by promoting angiogenesis, matrix synthesis, and lymphocyte activation and proliferation. Autocrine production of TGF-β further intensifies the inflammatory response. TGF-β-dependent activation is transient, likely due to TGF-β-increased SnoN expression, which participates in negative feedback regulation of TGF-β signaling. Consequently, once activation and differentiation of monocytes occurs, not only is TGF-β receptor expression reduced, but macrophages become insensitive to the pro-inflammatory signals, and TGF-β becomes a macrophage deactivator (inhibition of superoxide, nitric oxide, cytokine, and prostaglandin production). Meanwhile, receptor expression is upregulated on activated T cells and these cells become sensitive to the immunosuppressive properties of TGF-β.*

may involve effects on antigen presentation, since TGF-β down-regulates expression of major histocompatibility complex (MHC) class II on macrophages and B cells. In the absence of TGF-β, as in the TGF-$\beta_1$ null mice, expression of proliferating cell nuclear antigen (PCNA) and cdk (p34$^{cdc2}$) in inflamed tissues is elevated, indicative of uncontrolled proliferation [24, 106].

TGF-β may also contribute to resolution by shifting the cytokine profile towards an anti-inflammatory milieu. Depending on the environment, TGF-β may foster presentation of antigen by macrophages to elicit a Th2 (IL-4) as opposed to a Th1 (IFN-γ, IL-2) response. This has been shown to be the situation for TGF-$\beta_2$ [107], which may be especially important in immunoprivileged sites such as the eye, brain and fetal/placental unit, as well as for TGF-$\beta_1$, evident in diabetic mice [108]. The mechanism of this altered T cell response which is driven by autoregulation of endogenous TGF-β, may lie in reduced macrophage capacity to produce IL-12. Deficient IL-12 production results in failure of T cells to produce IFN-γ [109]. In addition, in the presence of TGF-β, CD40 expression is diminished thus reducing the costimulatory signal for responding T cells. TGF-β also inhibits B cell proliferation, Ig production, and membrane Ig expression and, as evident in the TGF-$\beta_1$ null mouse, B cell function and antibody dysregulation contribute to the lethal phenotype [110].

Apoptosis or programmed cell death is an important process for controlling accumulation of cells in inflammatory lesions. Unstimulated monocytes in the absence of serum undergo apoptosis which can be prevented by the inflammatory cytokines IL-1β, TNF-α, granulocyte macrophage colony stimulating factor (GM-CSF), and IFN-γ [111], whereas chemotactic factors, including TGF-β, are independently incapable of rescuing monocytes from apoptosis. Thus, if monocytes are recruited to a site of inflammation in which resolution and/or insufficient pro-inflammatory cytokines are present, these cells will undergo apoptosis and be cleared, and not perpetuate the response. However, macrophages induced to undergo apoptosis by serum deprivation could be rescued by TGF-β by a mechanism believed to involve TβRII- and mitogen-activated protein kinase-mediated signaling pathways [112]. In epithelial cells, expression of TGF-β signaling molecule Smad 3, but not Smad 2, has been implicated in the apoptotic process since Smad 3 mRNA expression is downregulated by TGF-β concomitantly with prevention of apoptosis [113]. Whether a similar situation occurs in macrophages is unknown.

The critical process of resolution of inflammation and tissue remodeling includes phagocytosis of apoptotic cells by tissue macrophages, thus allowing for the removal of cellular debris while preventing the release of toxic and potentially immunogenic intracellular molecules ([114], reviewed in [115]). TGF-β may contribute to the anti-inflammatory consequences of apoptotic cell clearance which is an active process, involving receptor recognition and cytokine modulation. Binding and phagocytosis of apoptotic cells by macrophages induces the expression of TGF-$\beta_1$, prostaglandin E$_2$, and platelet-activating factor and the subsequent inhibition of pro-inflammatory cytokine production, including IL-1$\beta$, IL-8, and TNF-$\alpha$, as well as IL-10, GM-CSF, leukotriene C$_4$ and thromboxane B2 [116]. Restoration of cytokine production by treatment with anti-TGF-$\beta$ antibody supports an autocrine/paracrine inhibitory mechanism involving TGF-$\beta$ [116].

## Wound healing, macrophages, and TGF-$\beta$

In addition to clearance of the inciting agent(s), phagocytosis of dead and dying cells and other debris, and elaboration of cytotoxic mediators to enhance killing of pathogens, macrophages play a central role in tissue repair. The ability to rapidly close a wound is crucial to protection of the host from bacterial invasion and to ultimately restore the integrity of the tissue. Wound healing studies have demonstrated that the degree of macrophage infiltration influences the rate and quality of healing in terms of scarring and the macrophage profile is remarkably affected by the relative levels of TGF-$\beta$ isoform expression (reviewed in [117]). Reduced infiltration and paucity of TGF-$\beta_1$ and -$\beta_2$ correlates with scar-free healing of fetal wounds [118, 119]. In contrast, sustained levels of TGF-$\beta_1$ contribute to scarring in adult wounds and reduction of inflammation through neutralizing antibody or antisense oligonucleotides to TGF-$\beta_1$ and -$\beta_2$ or through exogenous TGF-$\beta_3$ minimizes scarring [120]. Recent studies in TGF-$\beta_1$-overexpressing mice (TGF-$\beta_1$ under the control of the albumin promoter) that express elevated circulating levels of TGF-$\beta_1$ demonstrated reduced scarring of cutaneous wounds associated with reduced levels of TGF-$\beta_1$ within the wound site and increased TGF-$\beta_3$ protein and T$\beta$RII [121]. These studies parallel recent findings in another model of inflammation in which increased circulating levels of TGF-$\beta$ *via* gene therapy decrease leukocyte infiltration and fibrosis. This decrease occurred in part by reduced chemokine synthesis and likely also through loss of the TGF-$\beta$ chemotactic gradient otherwise emanating from the inflammatory lesions [122, 123].

In the TGF-$\beta_1$ null mice, the absence of TGF-$\beta_1$ has multiple effects on the healing process. Full-thickness skin wounds in TGF-$\beta_1$ null mice were characterized by decreased granulation tissue, collagen deposition, vascularity, and epithelialization, but extensive inflammatory cell infiltration, consistent with the rampant accumulation of leukocytes in multiple other tissues in these mice [124]. As expected, TGF-$\beta_1$ was absent, but TGF-$\beta_3$ was elevated in the wounds of the TGF-$\beta_1$ null mice and scarring was minimal [125]. Suppression of inflammation with rapamycin resulted in normal wound healing in TGF-$\beta_1$ null mice [126]. Interestingly, the TGF-$\beta_1$ deficient mice lack epidermal Langerhans cells [127]. The lack of Langerhans cells appears to be an independent consequence of the absence of TGF-$\beta$ since it precedes the appearance of inflammatory lesions in these mice and is not corrected by immunosuppressive therapy (rapamycin or SCID, nude, RAG2 background) [3]. However, dendritic cells could be expanded from the bone marrow of the TGF-$\beta_1$

null mice in medium containing fetal calf serum and GM-CSF, and upon transplantation into lethally-irradiated wild type mice repopulate the recipient skin [128], supporting the critical role of TGF-β in dendritic cell development [129]. TGF-$\beta_1$ transgenic mice, both knockouts and overexpressors, as well as newly-engineered gene-switch bigenic mice, in which TGF-$\beta_1$ can be focally induced in the epidermis at different expression levels and developmental stages, will be useful tools for studying the role of TGF-β in wound healing [130].

In total, the data suggest that TGF-β's potent leukocyte recruitment activity, in the absence of infection, may not necessarily be in the best interests of the host. Minimizing the inflammatory cell accumulation appears to favor healing with less scar formation, although this has to be balanced with the potential risk of infectious complications since we do not exist in a germ-free environment. In this regard, Smad 3 null mice in which TGF-β signaling is interrupted, display accelerated cutaneous wound healing with an increased rate of re-epithelialization and significantly reduced monocyte infiltration [21]. Application of topical TGF-β to the wounds did not increase monocyte recruitment nor affect re-epithelialization, documenting the requirement for Smad 3 in these cellular responses, but did increase matrix deposition, defining Smad 3-dependent and independent events in healing. Parallel *in vitro* studies using macrophages from Smad 3 null mice confirmed that an intact TGF-β/Smad 3 signaling pathway is required for TGF-β-mediated monocyte recruitment, although these cells respond normally to other stimuli. Furthermore, primary Smad 3 null keratinocytes displayed a reduced sensitivity to TGF-β-mediated growth inhibition, whereas fibroblast matrix synthesis was not jeopardized. Thus, it appears that the TGF-β/Smad 3 signaling pathway contributes to a delay in wound healing and that targeting of Smad 3 might be considered a beneficial approach to accelerate or facilitate impaired wound healing.

## Microbial subversion of the host response: role of TGF-β

Although TGF-β is important in the initial recruitment and activation of phagocytic cells to sites of infection, infectious organisms have the capacity to commandeer this peptide for their own benefit. Microorganisms can mediate host suppression and avoid immune surveillance by taking advantage of the TGF-β inhibitory pathway. Infection of macrophages by intracellular parasites such as *Trypanosoma cruzi* [131] results in TGF-β-mediated immune suppression, a clever parasite device to promote parasite replication and exacerbate infection (reviewed in [132]). Successful parasitic infection depends on its ability to subvert the host immune response and particularly the cytokine repertoire. Since IFN-γ plays a central role in the intracellular inhibition of parasite replication through iNOS and NO [133], parasites must disarm this molecule. Host TGF-β, produced during acute parasitic infection, may increase host susceptibility by inhibition of IL-12, a potent inducer of IFN-γ

[134], and IFN-γ-induced iNOS [133], thus allowing unrestricted growth of the parasites. Similar mechanisms for TGF-β-mediated suppression of innate immune responses controlling infection with *Leishmania major* in mice have also been observed [135, 136]. Interestingly, elevated TGF-β and reduced IFN-γ are also found in mice deficient for the iNOS gene which correlates with enhanced dissemination of the parasites [137].

Treatment of leishmania-resistant mice with TGF-β changes the immune response from a Th1 pattern (increased IFN-γ) to a dominant Th2 response (increased IL-10), resulting in increased susceptibility to disease [138, 139]. Whereas treatment of a resistant mouse strain with TGF-β increases parasitemia, neutralization of TGF-β with anti-TGF-β in leishmania-sensitive mice reduces parasitic growth and affords protection [138, 140]. TGF-β not only increases disease susceptibility in murine leishmaniasis, but production of active TGF-β by leishmania-infected human macrophages also promotes parasitic infection [141]. Infection with another macrophage parasite, *Toxoplasma gondii*, demonstrates a parallel pattern with increased release of TGF-β [142]. T. gondii also reduces macrophage TNF receptors, which may be a downstream effect of elevated TGF-β [142]. Active TGF-β released by mycobacterial-infected monocyte/macrophages facilitates intracellular mycobacterial replication while blocking macrophage effector functions [143, 144]. Furthermore, neutralization of TGF-β by antibody, decorin, or LAP resulted in reduction of bacterial growth [143, 144]. In contrast to this pattern of microbial induction of TGF-β which in turn suppresses host defense, recent evidence suggests that TGF-β inhibits malarial infections [145]. Severity of murine malarial infection is reportedly inversely proportional to TGF-β production [145]. Why some infectious organisms thrive in a TGF-β-rich environment and others are inhibited is totally unclear, but deciphering these pathways is critical to development of therapeutic approaches.

## Therapeutic modulation of TGF-β

Because of the clinical relevance of TGF-β in the regulation of inflammation, host defense and wound repair, the ability to therapeutically target TGF-β to modulate disease processes is of great interest. As is evident by its multifunctional actions, in some circumstances, elevating TGF-β levels may be beneficial whereas in others, inhibiting TGF-β may be the goal. Animal studies have documented the efficacy of systemically delivered TGF-β in suppressing arthritis [146], wound healing [121], and reducing the incidence and severity of experimental allergic encephalomyelitis [147–149]. Whereas locally-delivered TGF-β exacerbates arthritis [16], intra-articular injection of TGF-β antibody effectively suppresses joint inflammation [150]. More recently, gene transfer of TGF-β cDNA into skeletal muscle with elevated circulating TGF-β levels has been effective in the treatment of experimental arthritis

[123], fibrosis [122], diabetes [151], systemic lupus erythematosus [152], and colitis [153]. On the other hand, consistent with the bifunctional actions of this molecule, neutralizing antibodies and TGF-β antagonists, including gene transfer of decorin, have shown efficacy in other diseases, particularly those characterized by fibrosis [154]. Newer techniques are now being devised to better target and neutralize TGF-β; for example, intramuscular injection of a TGF-β-receptor-IgG Fc chimeric cDNA reduces fibrosis in nephritic rats [155]. These and other approaches using genetically-engineered macrophages [156] to modulate the endogenous expression of TGF-β and to directly target the inflammatory site may become effective therapeutic strategies of the future. Importantly, newly-emerging information on the TGF-β signaling promoters (Smad 2, 3, 4), inhibitors (Smad 6, 7), and transcriptional corepressors (Ski, SnoN) provide new opportunities to selectively target TGF-β actions which are not beneficial nor supportive of the desirable outcome of host defense processes.

# References

1   Morrissette N, Gold E, Aderem A (1999) The macrophage – a cell for all seasons. *Trends Cell Biol* 9: 199–201

2   Gordon S (1999) Macrophages and the immune response. In: W Paul (ed): *Fundamentals of immunology*. Lippincott-Raven, Philadelphia, 533–545

3   Letterio JJ, Roberts AB (1998) Regulation of immune responses by TGF-beta. *Annu Rev Immunol* 16: 137–161

4   Ashcroft G (1999) Bidirectional regulation of macrophage function by TGF-β. *Microbes Infect* 1: 1275–1282

5   McCartney-Francis NL, Wahl SM (1994) Transforming growth factor beta: a matter of life and death. *J Leukoc Biol* 55: 401–409

6   McCartney-Francis NL, Frazier-Jessen M, Wahl SM (1998) TGF-beta: a balancing act. *Int Rev Immunol* 16: 553–580

7   Kulkarni AB, Huh CG, Becker D, Geiser A, Lyght M, Flanders KC, Roberts AB, Sporn MB, Ward JM, Karlsson S (1993) Transforming growth factor beta 1 null mutation in mice causes excessive inflammatory response and early death. *Proc Natl Acad Sci USA* 90: 770–774

8   Shull MM, Ormsby I, Kier AB, Pawlowski S, Diebold RJ, Yin M, Allen R, Sidman C, Proetzel G, Calvin D et al (1992) Targeted disruption of the mouse transforming growth factor-beta 1 gene results in multifocal inflammatory disease. *Nature* 359: 693–699

9   Sanderson N, Factor V, Nagy P, Kopp J, Kondaiah P, Wakefield L, Roberts AB, Sporn MB, Thorgeirsson SS (1995) Hepatic expression of mature transforming growth factor beta 1 in transgenic mice results in multiple tissue lesions. *Proc Natl Acad Sci USA* 92: 2572–2576

10   Chen W, Wahl SM (1999) Manipulation of TGF-β in controlling autoimmune and infectious diseases. *Microbes Infect* 1: 1367–1380

11   Wahl SM (1992) Transforming growth factor beta (TGF-beta) in inflammation: a cause and a cure. *J Clin Immunol* 12: 61–74

12   Rosenberg HF, Gallin JI (1999) Inflammation. In: W Paul (ed): *Fundamental immunology*. Lippincott-Raven, Philadelphia, 1051–1066

13   Wahl SM, Hunt DA, Wakefield LM, McCartney-Francis N, Wahl LM, Roberts AB, Sporn MB (1987) Transforming growth factor type beta induces monocyte chemotaxis and growth factor production. *Proc Natl Acad Sci USA* 84: 5788–5792

14   Wiseman DM, Polverini PJ, Kamp DW, Leibovich SJ (1988) Transforming growth factor-beta (TGF beta) is chemotactic for human monocytes and induces their expression of angiogenic activity. *Biochem Biophys Res Commun* 157: 793–800

15   Roberts AB, Sporn MB, Assoian RK, Smith JM, Roche NS, Wakefield LM, Heine UI, Liotta LA, Falanga V, Kehrl JH et al (1986) Transforming growth factor type beta: rapid induction of fibrosis and angiogenesis *in vivo* and stimulation of collagen formation *in vitro*. *Proc Natl Acad Sci USA* 83: 4167–4171

16   Allen JB, Manthey CL, Hand AR, Ohura K, Ellingsworth L, Wahl SM (1990) Rapid onset synovial inflammation and hyperplasia induced by transforming growth factor beta. *J Exp Med* 171: 231–247

17   Fava RA, Olsen NJ, Postlethwaite AE, Broadley KN, Davidson JM, Nanney LB, Lucas C, Townes AS (1991) Transforming growth factor beta 1 (TGF-beta 1) induced neutrophil recruitment to synovial tissues: implications for TGF-beta-driven synovial inflammation and hyperplasia. *J Exp Med* 173: 1121–1132

18   Albelda SM, Smith CW, Ward PA (1994) Adhesion molecules and inflammatory injury. *FASEB J* 8: 504–512

19   Wahl SM, Feldman GM, McCarthy JB (1996) Regulation of leukocyte adhesion and signaling in inflammation and disease. *J Leukoc Biol* 59: 789–796

20   Wahl SM, Allen JB, Weeks BS, Wong HL, Klotman PE (1993) Transforming growth factor beta enhances integrin expression and type IV collagenase secretion in human monocytes. *Proc Natl Acad Sci USA* 90: 4577–4581

21   Ashcroft GS, Yang X, Glick AB, Weinstein M, Letterio JJ, Mizel DE, Anzano M, Greenwell-Wild T, Wahl SM, Deng C et al (1999) Mice lacking SMAD3 show accelerated wound healing and an impaired local inflammatory response. *Nature Cell Biol* 1: 260–266

22   Wahl SM, Allen JB, Hines KL, Imamichi T, Wahl AM, Furcht LT, McCarthy JB (1994) Synthetic fibronectin peptides suppress arthritis in rats by interrupting leukocyte adhesion and recruitment. *J Clin Invest* 94: 655–662

23   Hines KL, Kulkarni AB, McCarthy JB, Tian H, Ward JM, Christ M, McCartney-Francis NL, Furcht LT, Karlsson S, Wahl SM (1994) Synthetic fibronectin peptides interrupt inflammatory cell infiltration in transforming growth factor beta 1 knockout mice. *Proc Natl Acad Sci USA* 91: 5187–5191

24   McCartney-Francis NL, Mizel DE, Redman RS, Frazier-Jessen M, Panek RB, Kulkarni

AB, Ward JM, McCarthy JB, Wahl SM (1996) Autoimmune Sjogren's-like lesions in salivary glands of TGF-beta1-deficient mice are inhibited by adhesion-blocking peptides. *J Immunol* 157: 1306–1312

25  McCartney-Francis NL, Mizel DE, Frazier-Jessen M, Kulkarni AB, McCarthy JB, Wahl SM (1997) Lacrimal gland inflammation is responsible for ocular pathology in TGF-beta 1 null mice. *Am J Pathol* 151: 1281–1288

26  McCartney-Francis N, Mizel D, Wong H, Wahl L, Wahl S (1990) TGF-beta regulates production of growth factors and TGF-beta by human peripheral blood monocytes. Growth Factors 4: 27–35

27  Turner M, Chantry D, Feldmann M (1990) Transforming growth factor beta induces the production of interleukin 6 by human peripheral blood mononuclear cells. *Cytokine* 2: 211–216

28  Assoian RK, Fleurdelys BE, Stevenson HC, Miller PJ, Madtes DK, Raines EW, Ross R, Sporn MB (1987) Expression and secretion of type beta transforming growth factor by activated human macrophages. *Proc Natl Acad Sci USA* 84: 6020–6024

29  Grotendorst GR, Smale G, Pencev D (1989) Production of transforming growth factor beta by human peripheral blood monocytes and neutrophils. *J Cell Physiol* 140: 396–402

30  Kehrl JH, Wakefield LM, Roberts AB, Jakowlew S, Alvarez-Mon M, Derynck R, Sporn MB, Fauci AS (1986) Production of transforming growth factor beta by human T lymphocytes and its potential role in the regulation of T cell growth. *J Exp Med* 163: 1037–1050

31  Lafyatis R, Thompson NL, Remmers EF, Flanders KC, Roche NS, Kim SJ, Case JP, Sporn MB, Roberts AB, Wilder RL (1989) Transforming growth factor-beta production by synovial tissues from rheumatoid patients and streptococcal cell wall arthritic rats. Studies on secretion by synovial fibroblast-like cells and immunohistologic localization. *J Immunol* 143: 1142–1148

32  Kim SJ, Angel P, Lafyatis R, Hattori K, Kim KY, Sporn MB, Karin M, Roberts AB (1990) Autoinduction of transforming growth factor beta 1 is mediated by the AP-1 complex. *Mol Cell Biol* 10: 1492–1497

33  Welch GR, Wong HL, Wahl SM (1990) Selective induction of Fc gamma RIII on human monocytes by transforming growth factor-beta. *J Immunol* 144: 3444–3448

34  Rose DM, Fadok VA, Riches DW, Clay KL, Henson PM (1995) Autocrine/paracrine involvement of platelet-activating factor and transforming growth factor-beta in the induction of phosphatidylserine recognition by murine macrophages. *J Immunol* 155: 5819–5825

35  Roberts AB (1998) Molecular and cell biology of TGF-beta. *Miner Electrolyte Metab* 24: 111–119

36  Massague J, Cheifetz S, Laiho M, Ralph DA, Weis FM, Zentella A (1992) Transforming growth factor-beta. *Cancer Surv* 12: 81–103

37  Kim SJ, Romeo D, Yoo YD, Park K (1994) Transforming growth factor-beta: expression in normal and pathological conditions. *Horm Res* 42: 5–8

38  Kim SJ, Park K, Rudkin BB, Dey BR, Sporn MB, Roberts AB (1994) Nerve growth factor induces transcription of transforming growth factor-beta 1 through a specific promoter element in PC12 cells. *J Biol Chem* 269: 3739–3744

39  Yoo YD, Ueda H, Park K, Flanders KC, Lee YI, Jay G, Kim SJ (1996) Regulation of transforming growth factor-beta 1 expression by the hepatitis B virus (HBV) X transactivator. Role in HBV pathogenesis. *J Clin Invest* 97: 388–395

40  Yoo YD, Chiou CJ, Choi KS, Yi Y, Michelson S, Kim S, Hayward GS, Kim SJ (1996) The IE2 regulatory protein of human cytomegalovirus induces expression of the human transforming growth factor beta1 gene through an Egr-1 binding site. *J Virol* 70: 7062–7070

41  Kim SJ, Kehrl JH, Burton J, Tendler CL, Jeang KT, Danielpour D, Thevenin C, Kim KY, Sporn MB, Roberts AB (1990) Transactivation of the transforming growth factor beta 1 (TGF-beta 1) gene by human T lymphotropic virus type 1 tax: a potential mechanism for the increased production of TGF-beta 1 in adult T cell leukemia. *J Exp Med* 172: 121–129

42  Kerr LD, Miller DB, Matrisian LM (1990) TGF-beta 1 inhibition of transin/stromelysin gene expression is mediated through a Fos binding sequence. *Cell* 61: 267–278

43  Dubois CM, Laprise MH, Blanchette F, Gentry LE, Leduc R (1995) Processing of transforming growth factor beta 1 precursor by human furin convertase. *J Biol Chem* 270: 10618–10624

44  Munger JS, Harpel JG, Giancotti FG, Rifkin DB (1998) Interactions between growth factors and integrins: latent forms of transforming growth factor-beta are ligands for the integrin alphavbeta1. *Mol Biol Cell* 9: 2627–2638

45  Khalil N (1999) TGF-β: From latent to active. *Microbes Infect* 1: 1255–1263

46  Vodovotz Y, Chesler L, Chong H, Kim SJ, Simpson JT, DeGraff W, Cox GW, Roberts AB, Wink DA, Barcellos-Hoff MH (1999) Regulation of transforming growth factor beta1 by nitric oxide. *Cancer Res* 59: 2142–2149

47  Khalil N, Corne S, Whitman C, Yacyshyn H (1996) Plasmin regulates the activation of cell-associated latent TGF-beta 1 secreted by rat alveolar macrophages after *in vivo* bleomycin injury. *Am J Respir Cell Mol Biol* 15: 252–259

48  Yesner LM, Huh HY, Pearce SF, Silverstein RL (1996) Regulation of monocyte CD36 and thrombospondin-1 expression by soluble mediators. *Arterioscler Thromb Vasc Biol* 16: 1019–1025

49  Nunes I, Shapiro RL, Rifkin DB (1995) Characterization of latent TGF-beta activation by murine peritoneal macrophages. *J Immunol* 155: 1450–1459

50  Falcone DJ, McCaffrey TA, Mathew J, McAdam K, Borth W (1995) THP-1 macrophage membrane-bound plasmin activity is up-regulated by transforming growth factor-beta 1 *via* increased expression of urokinase and the urokinase receptor. *J Cell Physiol* 164: 334–343

51  Chong H, Vodovotz Y, Cox GW, Barcellos-Hoff MH (1999) Immunocytochemical localization of latent transforming growth factor-beta1 activation by stimulated macrophages. *J Cell Physiol* 178: 275–283

52  Munger JS, Huang X, Kawakatsu H, Griffiths MJ, Dalton SL, Wu J, Pittet JF, Kaminski N, Garat C, Matthay MA et al (1999) The integrin alpha v beta 6 binds and activates latent TGF beta 1: a mechanism for regulating pulmonary inflammation and fibrosis. *Cell* 96: 319–328

53  Bugge TH, Flick MJ, Daugherty CC, Degen JL (1995) Plasminogen deficiency causes severe thrombosis but is compatible with development and reproduction. *Genes Dev* 9: 794–807

54  Crawford SE, Stellmach V, Murphy-Ullrich JE, Ribeiro SM, Lawler J, Hynes RO, Boivin GP, Bouck N (1998) Thrombospondin-1 is a major activator of TGF-beta1 *in vivo*. *Cell* 93: 1159–1170

55  Miyazono K, Ichijo H, Heldin CH (1993) Transforming growth factor-beta: latent forms, binding proteins and receptors. *Growth Factors* 8: 11–22

56  Altman DJ, Schneider SL, Thompson DA, Cheng HL, Tomasi TB (1990) A transforming growth factor beta 2 (TGF-beta 2)-like immunosuppressive factor in amniotic fluid and localization of TGF-beta 2 mRNA in the pregnant uterus. *J Exp Med* 172: 1391–1401

57  Schultz-Cherry S, Chen H, Mosher DF, Misenheimer TM, Krutzsch HC, Roberts DD, Murphy-Ullrich JE (1995) Regulation of transforming growth factor-beta activation by discrete sequences of thrombospondin 1. *J Biol Chem* 270: 7304–7310

58  Massague J (1998) TGF-beta signal transduction. *Annu Rev Biochem* 67: 753–791

59  Derynck R, Zhang Y, Feng XH (1998) Smads: transcriptional activators of TGF-beta responses. *Cell* 95: 737–740

60  Tsukazaki T, Chiang TA, Davison AF, Attisano L, Wrana JL (1998) SARA, a FYVE domain protein that recruits Smad2 to the TGFbeta receptor. *Cell* 95: 779–791

61  Hua X, Liu X, Ansari DO, Lodish HF (1998) Synergistic cooperation of TFE3 and smad proteins in TGF-beta-induced transcription of the plasminogen activator inhibitor-1 gene. *Genes Dev* 12: 3084–3095

62  Song CZ, Siok TE, Gelehrter TD (1998) Smad4/DPC4 and Smad3 mediate transforming growth factor-beta (TGF-beta) signaling through direct binding to a novel TGF-beta-responsive element in the human plasminogen activator inhibitor-1 promoter. *J Biol Chem* 273: 29287–29290

63  Dennler S, Itoh S, Vivien D, ten Dijke P, Huet S, Gauthier JM (1998) Direct binding of Smad3 and Smad4 to critical TGF beta-inducible elements in the promoter of human plasminogen activator inhibitor-type 1 gene. *EMBO J* 17: 3091–3100

64  Vindevoghel L, Lechleider RJ, Kon A, de Caestecker MP, Uitto J, Roberts AB, Mauviel A (1998) SMAD3/4-dependent transcriptional activation of the human type VII collagen gene (COL7A1) promoter by transforming growth factor beta. *Proc Natl Acad Sci USA* 95: 14769–14774

65  Jonk LJ, Itoh S, Heldin CH, ten Dijke P, Kruijer W (1998) Identification and functional characterization of a Smad binding element (SBE) in the JunB promoter that acts as a transforming growth factor-beta, activin, and bone morphogenetic protein-inducible enhancer. *J Biol Chem* 273: 21145–21152

66  Weinstein M, Yang X, Li C, Xu X, Gotay J, Deng CX (1998) Failure of egg cylinder elongation and mesoderm induction in mouse embryos lacking the tumor suppressor smad2. *Proc Natl Acad Sci USA* 95: 9378–9383

67  Yang X, Letterio JJ, Lechleider RJ, Chen L, Hayman R, Gu H, Roberts AB, Deng C (1999) Targeted disruption of SMAD3 results in impaired mucosal immunity and diminished T cell responsiveness to TGF-beta. *EMBO J* 18: 1280–1291

68  Datto MB, Frederick JP, Pan L, Borton AJ, Zhuang Y, Wang XF (1999) Targeted disruption of Smad3 reveals an essential role in transforming growth factor beta-mediated signal transduction. *Mol Cell Biol* 19: 2495–2504

69  Zhu Y, Richardson JA, Parada LF, Graff JM (1998) Smad3 mutant mice develop metastatic colorectal cancer. *Cell* 94: 703–714

70  Feng XH, Zhang Y, Wu RY, Derynck R (1998) The tumor suppressor Smad4/DPC4 and transcriptional adaptor CBP/p300 are coactivators for smad3 in TGF-beta-induced transcriptional activation. *Genes Dev* 12: 2153–2163

71  Shioda T, Lechleider RJ, Dunwoodie SL, Li H, Yahata T, de Caestecker MP, Fenner MH, Roberts AB, Isselbacher KJ (1998) Transcriptional activating activity of Smad4: roles of SMAD hetero-oligomerization and enhancement by an associating transactivator. *Proc Natl Acad Sci USA* 95: 9785–9790

72  Wotton D, Lo RS, Lee S, Massague J (1999) A Smad transcriptional corepressor. *Cell* 97: 29–39

73  Topper JN, DiChiara MR, Brown JD, Williams AJ, Falb D, Collins T, Gimbrone MA Jr (1998) CREB binding protein is a required coactivator for Smad-dependent, transforming growth factor beta transcriptional responses in endothelial cells [published erratum appears in *Proc Natl Acad Sci USA* (1998) Oct 13; 95 (21): 12735]. *Proc Natl Acad Sci USA* 95: 9506–9511

74  Kurokawa M, Mitani K, Irie K, Matsuyama T, Takahashi T, Chiba S, Yazaki Y, Matsumoto K, Hirai H (1998) The oncoprotein Evi-1 represses TGF-beta signalling by inhibiting Smad3. *Nature* 394: 92–96

75  Luo K, Stroschein SL, Wang W, Chen D, Martens E, Zhou S, Zhou Q (1999) The Ski oncoprotein interacts with the Smad proteins to repress TGFbeta signaling. *Genes Dev* 13: 2196–2206

76  Stroschein S, Wang W, Zhou S, Zhou Q, Luo K (1999) Negative feedback regulation of TGF-β signaling by the SnoN oncoprotein. *Science* 286: 771–774

77  Imamura T, Takase M, Nishihara A, Oeda E, Hanai J, Kawabata M, Miyazono K (1997) Smad6 inhibits signalling by the TGF-beta superfamily. *Nature* 389: 622–626

78  Nakao A, Afrakhte M, Moren A, Nakayama T, Christian JL, Heuchel R, Itoh S, Kawabata M, Heldin NE, Heldin CH et al (1997) Identification of Smad7, a TGFbeta-inducible antagonist of TGF-beta signalling. *Nature* 389: 631–635

79  Zhang Y, Derynck R (1999) Regulation of Smad signalling by protein associations and signalling crosstalk. *Trends Cell Biol* 9: 274–279

80  Afrakhte M, Moren A, Jossan S, Itoh S, Sampath K, Westermark B, Heldin CH, Heldin

NE, ten Dijke P(1998) Induction of inhibitory Smad6 and Smad7 mRNA by TGF-beta family members. *Biochem Biophys Res Commun* 249: 505–511

81 Nakao A, Fujii M, Matsumura R, Kumano K, Saito Y, Miyazono K, Iwamoto I (1999) Transient gene transfer and expression of Smad7 prevents bleomycin-induced lung fibrosis in mice. *J Clin Invest* 104: 5–11

82 Ulloa L, Doody J, Massague J (1999) Inhibition of transforming growth factor-beta/SMAD signalling by the interferon-gamma/STAT pathway. *Nature* 397: 710–713

83 Czarniecki CW, Chiu HH, Wong GH, McCabe SM, Palladino MA (1988) Transforming growth factor-beta 1 modulates the expression of class II histocompatibility antigens on human cells. *J Immunol* 140: 4217–4223

84 Bauvois B, Rouillard D, Sanceau J, Wietzerbin J (1992) IFN-gamma and transforming growth factor-beta 1 differently regulate fibronectin and laminin receptors of human differentiating monocytic cells. *J Immunol* 148: 3912–3919

85 Schmitt E, Hoehn P, Huels C, Goedert S, Palm N, Rude E, Germann T (1994) T helper type 1 development of naive CD4+ T cells requires the coordinate action of interleukin-12 and interferon-gamma and is inhibited by transforming growth factor-beta. *Eur J Immunol* 24: 793–798

86 Hausmann EH, Hao SY, Pace JL, Parmely MJ (1994) Transforming growth factor beta 1 and gamma interferon provide opposing signals to lipopolysaccharide-activated mouse macrophages. *Infect Immun* 62: 3625–3632

87 Strober W, Kelsall B, Fuss I, Marth T, Ludviksson B, Ehrhardt R, Neurath M (1997) Reciprocal IFN-gamma and TGF-beta responses regulate the occurrence of mucosal inflammation. *Immunol Today* 18: 61–64

88 Vodovotz Y, Bogdan C, Paik J, Xie QW, Nathan C (1993) Mechanisms of suppression of macrophage nitric oxide release by transforming growth factor beta. *J Exp Med* 178: 605–613

89 Wahl S (1999) Transforming growth factor-β (TGF-β) in the resolution and repair of inflammation. In: J Gallin, R Snyderman (eds): *Inflammation: Basic principles and clinical correlates.* Lippincott Williams and Wilkins, Philadelphia, 883–892

90 Brandes ME, Wakefield LM, Wahl SM (1991) Modulation of monocyte type I transforming growth factor-beta receptors by inflammatory stimuli. *J Biol Chem* 266: 19697–19703

91 Tsunawaki S, Sporn M, Ding A, Nathan C (1988) Deactivation of macrophages by transforming growth factor-beta. *Nature* 334: 260–262

92 Ding A, Nathan CF, Graycar J, Derynck R, Stuehr DJ, Srimal S (1990) Macrophage deactivating factor and transforming growth factors-beta 1, -beta 2 and -beta 3 inhibit induction of macrophage nitrogen oxide synthesis by IFN-gamma. *J Immunol* 145: 940–944

93 Nelson BJ, Ralph P, Green SJ, Nacy CA (1991) Differential susceptibility of activated macrophage cytotoxic effector reactions to the suppressive effects of transforming growth factor-beta 1. *J Immunol* 146: 1849–1857

94 Espevik T, Figari IS, Shalaby MR, Lackides GA, Lewis GD, Shepard HM, Palladino MA

Jr (1987) Inhibition of cytokine production by cyclosporin A and transforming growth factor beta. *J Exp Med* 166: 571–576

95  Bogdan C, Paik J, Vodovotz Y, Nathan C (1992) Contrasting mechanisms for suppression of macrophage cytokine release by transforming growth factor-beta and interleukin-10. *J Biol Chem* 267: 23301–23308

96  Reddy ST, Gilbert RS, Xie W, Luner S, Herschman HR (1994) TGF-beta 1 inhibits both endotoxin-induced prostaglandin synthesis and expression of the TIS10/prostaglandin synthase 2 gene in murine macrophages. *J Leukoc Biol* 55: 192–200

97  Erwig LP, Kluth DC, Walsh GM, Rees AJ (1998) Initial cytokine exposure determines function of macrophages and renders them unresponsive to other cytokines. *J Immunol* 161: 1983–1988

98  Nathan C, Sporn M (1991) Cytokines in context. *J Cell Biol* 113: 981–986

99  Sporn MB (1997) The importance of context in cytokine action. *Kidney Int* 51: 1352–1354

100  Noble PW, Henson PM, Lucas C, Mora-Worms M, Carre PC, Riches DW (1993) Transforming growth factor-beta primes macrophages to express inflammatory gene products in response to particulate stimuli by an autocrine/paracrine mechanism. *J Immunol* 151: 979–989

101  Vodovotz Y, Geiser AG, Chesler L, Letterio JJ, Campbell A, Lucia MS, Sporn MB, Roberts AB (1996) Spontaneously increased production of nitric oxide and aberrant expression of the inducible nitric oxide synthase *in vivo* in the transforming growth factor beta 1 null mouse. *J Exp Med* 183: 2337–2342

102  Vodovotz Y, Kopp JB, Takeguchi H, Shrivastav S, Coffin D, Lucia MS, Mitchell JB, Webber R, Letterio J, Wink D et al (1998) Increased mortality, blunted production of nitric oxide, and increased production of TNF-alpha in endotoxemic TGF-beta1 transgenic mice. *J Leukoc Biol* 63: 31–39

103  Turner M, Chantry D, Katsikis P, Berger A, Brennan FM, Feldmann M (1991) Induction of the interleukin 1 receptor antagonist protein by transforming growth factor-beta. *Eur J Immunol* 21: 1635–1639

104  Wahl SM, Costa GL, Corcoran M, Wahl LM, Berger AE (1993) Transforming growth factor-beta mediates IL-1-dependent induction of IL-1 receptor antagonist. *J Immunol* 150: 3553–3560

105  Hocevar BA, Howe PH (1998) Mechanisms of TGF-beta-induced cell cycle arrest. *Miner Electrolyte Metab* 24: 131–135

106  Christ M, McCartney-Francis NL, Kulkarni AB, Ward JM, Mizel DE, Mackall CL, Gress RE, Hines KL, Tian H, Karlsson S et al (1994) Immune dysregulation in TGF-beta 1-deficient mice. *J Immunol* 153: 1936–1946

107  Takeuchi M, Kosiewicz MM, Alard P, Streilein JW (1997) On the mechanisms by which transforming growth factor-beta 2 alters antigen-presenting abilities of macrophages on T cell activation. *Eur J Immunol* 27: 1648–1656

108  King C, Davies J, Mueller R, Lee MS, Krahl T, Yeung B, O'Connor E, Sarvetnick N

(1998) TGF-beta1 alters APC preference, polarizing islet antigen responses toward a Th2 phenotype. *Immunity* 8: 601–613

109  Takeuchi M, Alard P, Streilein JW (1998) TGF-beta promotes immune deviation by altering accessory signals of antigen-presenting cells. *J Immunol* 160: 1589–1597

110  van Ginkel FW, Wahl SM, Kearney JF, Kweon MN, Fujihashi K, Burrows PD, Kiyono H, McGhee JR (1999) Partial IgA-deficiency with increased Th2-type cytokines in TGF-beta1 knockout mice. *J Immunol* 163: 1951–1957

111  Mangan DF, Wahl SM (1991) Differential regulation of human monocyte programmed cell death (apoptosis) by chemotactic factors and pro-inflammatory cytokines. *J Immunol* 147: 3408–3412

112  Chin BY, Petrache I, Choi AM, Choi ME (1999) Transforming growth factor beta1 rescues serum deprivation-induced apoptosis *via* the mitogen-activated protein kinase (MAPK) pathway in macrophages. *J Biol Chem* 274: 11362–11368

113  Yanagisawa K, Osada H, Masuda A, Kondo M, Saito T, Yatabe Y, Takagi K, Takahashi T (1998) Induction of apoptosis by Smad3 and down-regulation of Smad3 expression in response to TGF-beta in human normal lung epithelial cells. *Oncogene* 17: 1743–1747

114  Cox G, Crossley J, Xing Z (1995) Macrophage engulfment of apoptotic neutrophils contributes to the resolution of acute pulmonary inflammation *in vivo*. *Am J Respir Cell Mol Biol* 12: 232–237

115  Fadok VA, Henson PM (1998) Apoptosis: getting rid of the bodies. *Curr Biol* 8: R693–695

116  Fadok VA, Bratton DL, Konowal A, Freed PW, Westcott JY, Henson PM (1998) Macrophages that have ingested apoptotic cells *in vitro* inhibit proinflammatory cytokine production through autocrine/paracrine mechanisms involving TGF-beta, PGE2, and PAF. *J Clin Invest* 101: 890–898

117  McCallion R, Ferguson M (1996) Fetal wound healing and the development of antiscarring therapies for adult wound healing. In: R Clark (ed): *The molecular and cellular biology of wound repair*. Plenum Press, New York, 561–600

118  Whitby DJ, Ferguson MW (1991) The extracellular matrix of lip wounds in fetal, neonatal and adult mice. *Development* 112: 651–668

119  Whitby DJ, Ferguson MW (1991) Immunohistochemical localization of growth factors in fetal wound healing. *Dev Biol* 147: 207–215

120  Shah M, Foreman DM, Ferguson MW (1995) Neutralisation of TGF-beta 1 and TGF-beta 2 or exogenous addition of TGF-beta 3 to cutaneous rat wounds reduces scarring. *J Cell Sci* 108: 985–1002

121  Shah M, Revis D, Herrick S, Baillie R, Thorgeirson S, Ferguson M, Roberts A (1999) Role of elevated plasma transforming growth factor-beta1 levels in wound healing. *Am J Pathol* 154: 1115–1124

122  Song XY, Zeng L, Pilo C, Zagorski J, Wahl SM (1999) Inhibition of rat leukocyte recruitment and hepatic granuloma formation by TGF-β gene transfer. *J Immunol* 163: 4020–4026

123  Song XY, Gu M, Jin WW, Klinman DM, Wahl SM (1998) Plasmid DNA encoding trans-

forming growth factor-beta1 suppresses chronic disease in a streptococcal cell wall-induced arthritis model. *J Clin Invest* 101: 2615–2621

124 Brown RL, Ormsby I, Doetschman TC, Greenhalgh DG (1995) Wound healing in the transforming growth factor-β1-deficient mouse. *Wound Rep Reg* 3: 25–36

125 O'Kane S, Ferguson MWJ (1996) Transforming growth factor βs and wound healing. *Int J Biochem Cell Biol* 29: 63–78

126 Letterio JJ, Roberts AB (1996) Transforming growth factor-beta1-deficient mice: identification of isoform-specific activities *in vivo*. *J Leukoc Biol* 59: 769–774

127 Borkowski TA, Letterio JJ, Farr AG, Udey MC (1996) A role for endogenous transforming growth factor beta 1 in Langerhans cell biology: the skin of transforming growth factor beta 1 null mice is devoid of epidermal Langerhans cells. *J Exp Med* 184: 2417–2422

128 Borkowski TA, Letterio JJ, Mackall CL, Saitoh A, Wang XJ, Roop DR, Gress RE, Udey MC (1997) A role for TGFbeta1 in langerhans cell biology. Further characterization of the epidermal Langerhans cell defect in TGFbeta1 null mice. *J Clin Invest* 100: 575–581

129 Strobl H, Knapp W (1999) TGF-β1 regulation of dendritic cells. *Microbes Infect* 1: 1283–1290

130 Wang XJ, Liefer KM, Tsai S, O'Malley BW, Roop DR (1999) Development of gene-switch transgenic mice that inducibly express transforming growth factor beta1 in the epidermis [In Process Citation]. *Proc Natl Acad Sci USA* 96: 8483–8488

131 Silva JS, Twardzik DR, Reed SG (1991) Regulation of Trypanosoma cruzi infections *in vitro* and *in vivo* by transforming growth factor beta (TGF-beta). *J Exp Med* 174: 539–545

132 Reed S (1999) TGF-β in infections and infectious diseases. *Microbes Infect* 1: 1313–1325

133 Gazzinelli RT, Oswald IP, Hieny S, James SL, Sher A (1992) The microbicidal activity of interferon-gamma-treated macrophages against Trypanosoma cruzi involves an L-arginine-dependent, nitrogen oxide-mediated mechanism inhibitable by interleukin-10 and transforming growth factor-beta. *Eur J Immunol* 22: 2501–2506

134 Silva JS, Aliberti JC, Martins GA, Souza MA, Souto JT, Padua MA (1998) The role of IL-12 in experimental Trypanosoma cruzi infection. *Braz J Med Biol Res* 31: 111–115

135 Green SJ, Scheller LF, Marletta MA, Seguin MC, Klotz FW, Slayter M, Nelson BJ, Nacy CA (1994) Nitric oxide: cytokine-regulation of nitric oxide in host resistance to intracellular pathogens. *Immunol Lett* 43: 87–94

136 Li J, Hunter CA, Farrell JP (1999) Anti-TGF-beta treatment promotes rapid healing of Leishmania major infection in mice by enhancing *in vivo* nitric oxide production. *J Immunol* 162: 974–979

137 Diefenbach A, Schindler H, Donhauser N, Lorenz E, Laskay T, MacMicking J, Rollinghoff M, Gresser I, Bogdan C (1998) Type 1 interferon (IFNalpha/beta) and type 2 nitric oxide synthase regulate the innate immune response to a protozoan parasite. *Immunity* 8: 77–87

138 Barral-Netto M, Barral A (1994) Transforming growth factor-beta in tegumentary leishmaniasis. *Braz J Med Biol Res* 27: 1–9

139 Locksley RM, Scott P (1991) Helper T-cell subsets in mouse leishmaniasis: induction, expansion and effector function. *Immunol Today* 12: A58–61

140 Barral-Netto M, Barral A, Brownell CE, Skeiky YA, Ellingsworth LR, Twardzik DR, Reed SG (1992) Transforming growth factor-beta in leishmanial infection: a parasite escape mechanism. *Science* 257: 545–548

141 Barral A, Teixeira M, Reis P, Vinhas V, Costa J, Lessa H, Bittencourt AL, Reed S, Carvalho EM, Barral-Netto M (1995) Transforming growth factor-beta in human cutaneous leishmaniasis. *Am J Pathol* 147: 947–954

142 Bermudez LE, Covaro G, Remington J (1993) Infection of murine macrophages with Toxoplasma gondii is associated with release of transforming growth factor beta and downregulation of expression of tumor necrosis factor receptors. *Infect Immun* 61: 4126–4130

143 Hirsch CS, Yoneda T, Averill L, Ellner JJ, Toossi Z (1994) Enhancement of intracellular growth of Mycobacterium tuberculosis in human monocytes by transforming growth factor-beta 1. *J Infect Dis* 170: 1229–1237

144 Hirsch CS, Ellner JJ, Blinkhorn R, Toossi Z (1997) *In vitro* restoration of T cell responses in tuberculosis and augmentation of monocyte effector function against Mycobacterium tuberculosis by natural inhibitors of transforming growth factor beta. *Proc Natl Acad Sci USA* 94: 3926–3931

145 Omer FM, Riley EM (1998) Transforming growth factor beta production is inversely correlated with severity of murine malaria infection. *J Exp Med* 188: 39–48

146 Brandes ME, Allen JB, Ogawa Y, Wahl SM (1991) Transforming growth factor beta 1 suppresses acute and chronic arthritis in experimental animals. *J Clin Invest* 87: 1108–1113

147 Kuruvilla AP, Shah R, Hochwald GM, Liggitt HD, Palladino MA, Thorbecke GJ (1991) Protective effect of transforming growth factor beta 1 on experimental autoimmune diseases in mice. *Proc Natl Acad Sci USA* 88: 2918–2921

148 Racke MK, Dhib-Jalbut S, Cannella B, Albert PS, Raine CS, McFarlin DE (1991) Prevention and treatment of chronic relapsing experimental allergic encephalomyelitis by transforming growth factor-beta 1. *J Immunol* 146: 3012–3017

149 Johns LD, Flanders KC, Ranges GE, Sriram S (1991) Successful treatment of experimental allergic encephalomyelitis with transforming growth factor-beta 1. *J Immunol* 147: 1792–1796

150 Wahl SM, Allen JB, Costa GL, Wong HL, Dasch JR (1993) Reversal of acute and chronic synovial inflammation by anti-transforming growth factor beta. *J Exp Med* 177: 225–230

151 Piccirillo CA, Chang Y, Prud'homme GJ (1998) TGF-beta1 somatic gene therapy prevents autoimmune disease in nonobese diabetic mice. *J Immunol* 161: 3950–3956

152 Raz E, Dudler J, Lotz M, Baird SM, Berry CC, Eisenberg RA, Carson DA (1995) Mod-

ulation of disease activity in murine systemic lupus erythematosus by cytokine gene delivery. *Lupus* 4: 286–292

153 Giladi E, Raz E, Karmeli F, Okon E, Rachmilewitz D (1995) Transforming growth factor-beta gene therapy ameliorates experimental colitis in rats. *Eur J Gastroenterol Hepatol* 7: 341–347

154 Isaka Y, Brees DK, Ikegaya K, Kaneda Y, Imai E, Noble NA, Border WA (1996) Gene therapy by skeletal muscle expression of decorin prevents fibrotic disease in rat kidney. *Nat Med* 2: 418–423

155 Isaka Y, Akagi Y, Ando Y, Tsujie M, Sudo T, Ohno N, Border WA, Noble NA, Kaneda Y, Hori M et al (1999) Gene therapy by transforming growth factor-beta receptor-IgG Fc chimera suppressed extracellular matrix accumulation in experimental glomerulonephritis. *Kidney Int* 55: 465–475

156 Suto TS, Fine LG, Shimizu F, Kitamura M (1997) *In vivo* transfer of engineered macrophages into the glomerulus: endogenous TGF-beta-mediated defense against macrophage-induced glomerular cell activation. *J Immunol* 159: 2476–2483

# TGF-β and the cardiovascular system

*David J. Grainger and David E. Mosedale*

Dept of Medicine, Box 157, Addenbrooke's Hospital, Cambridge, CB2 2QQ, UK

## Overview of the TGF-β superfamily

The TGF-β superfamily consists of a large number of structurally related cytokines, including activin/inhibin, the bone morphogenetic proteins (BMPs), the growth and differentiation factors (GDFs), the TGF-βs and a number of proteins involved in developmental patterning. Much of the research into the biology of the TGF-β superfamily has focused on TGF-$\beta_1$ (the first to be discovered), and it is this isoform about which most is known.

Three different isoforms of TGF-β have been identified in mammals and they are the products of different genes (*tgfb1*, *tgfb2* and *tgfb3*). These three isoforms have very high sequence homology within the C-terminal region which encodes the mature 25 kDa cytokine (see below), both across isoforms (64–82%) and across species (> 97%) [1]. Possibly as a result of this homology, their activities *in vitro* are usually similar.

A large number of processes are involved in the production and secretion of TGF-β including transcription, translation, intracellular processing and activation of the pro-protein (Fig. 1). Each of these processes can contribute to the regulation of TGF-β activity.

## Production of TGF-β

The promoter regions of the three mammalian TGF-β isoforms show little sequence similarity, suggesting that the transcription of each is differentially regulated. Consistent with this, the transcription factor AP-1 has been shown to regulate the transcription of the *tgfb1* gene [2], while Sp1 can regulate the transcription of both the *tgfb2* and *tgfb3* genes [3], and an activating transcription factor (ATF) binding site has been identified only in the promoter of the *tgfb2* gene [4]. However, under most

TGF-β and Related Cytokines in Inflammation, edited by Samuel N. Breit and Sharon M. Wahl
© 2001 Birkhäuser Verlag Basel/Switzerland

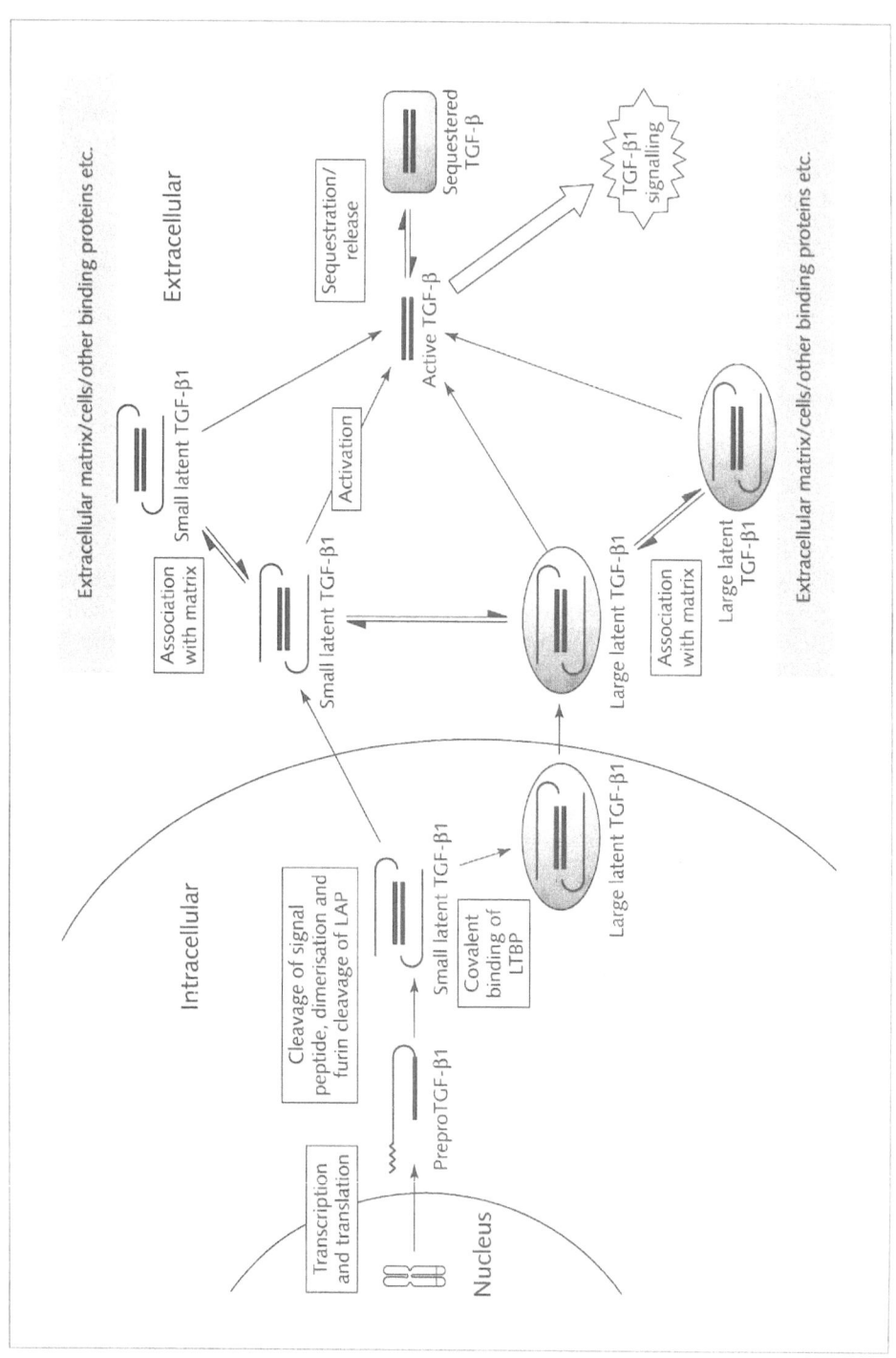

conditions, the combination of transcription factors which regulate the transcription of the TGF-β genes has not been well characterised. Furthermore, many different signalling molecules have been shown to regulate the transcription of TGF-β *in vitro*, but it is not clear which of these pathways have a physiological role. Notably, van Obberghen-Schilling and colleagues [5] showed that TGF-β$_1$ positively regulates its own expression in a number of cultured cell types, leading to a positive feedback loop. This mechanism has subsequently been shown to occur in cultures of cardiac myocytes and cardiac fibroblasts for both TGF-β$_1$ and TGF-β$_3$, and to a lesser extent TGF-β$_2$ [6]. Clearly, however, some restraining mechanism must be present in the intact organism, since the levels of TGF-β do not increase exponentially *in vivo*.

TGF-β$_2$ mRNA may be alternatively spliced, at least in cultured cells, to generate a 28 amino acid insertion in the pro-region [7, 8]. Furthermore, the stability of TGF-β mRNA may be altered by various treatments, including pre-incubation with TGF-β$_1$ itself [9]. During heart formation, an antisense RNA complementary to the mRNA encoding TGF-β$_3$ is present [10] which may negatively regulate TGF-β$_3$ production. Furthermore, both the 5' and 3' untranslated regions of TGF-β mRNAs have marked effects on the translation efficiency of the TGF-β mRNAs [11-13], which may provide another level of regulation.

The TGF-β mRNAs are translated to yield prepro-TGF-β consisting of a 29 amino acid signal sequence, a propeptide region (termed the latency associated peptide or LAP) and the mature protein at the C-terminus. The signal sequence is then cleaved [14] to generate pro-TGF-β (amino acids 30 to 390). The pro-TGF-β protein forms a dimer, with one intermolecular disulphide bond forming between the LAP regions and a second between the mature regions. Folding and dimerisation of both TGF-β$_1$ and activin (and presumably other members of the TGF-β family) is dependent upon the presence of the LAP. When the mature 112 aa TGF-β$_1$ molecule is expressed independently of the LAP, TGF-β$_1$ does not dimerise, and is therefore not exported [15]. The pro-TGF-β dimer is then proteolytically cleaved at a dibasic site between the LAP and mature TGF-β, by the proprotein convertase furin [16]. Other members of the TGF-β superfamily have also been shown to be processed by proprotein convertases: furin proteolytically cleaves the LAP from the mature protein of BMP-4 and nodal [17, 18], and Mullerian inhibiting substance may be cleaved by PC5 or furin during gonadal development [19]. Recently, TGF-β$_1$ has

*Figure 1*
*TGF-β activity is regulated on many levels. The C-terminal mature TGF-β peptide is shown as a thick bar, with the LAP region shown as a thin bar. The large shaded oval represents members of the LTBP family, while the shaded square represents lipoproteins. Arrows indicate possible interconversion processes between the TGF-β complexes shown. Boxes indicate processes for which direct evidence has been accumulated (see text).*

been shown to positively regulate the gene expression of furin [20], which may result in the generation of more cleaved TGF-$\beta_1$. N-linked glycosylation of the LAP region also takes place at some stage prior to secretion [21], mainly at two asparagine residues (Asn-82, Asn-136), and to a lesser degree at a third (Asn-177), although any physiological role for this glycosylation remains unclear. At least *in vitro*, the TGF-$\beta$ may then be secreted from cells as a complex consisting of disulphide-linked mature TGF-$\beta$ dimer non-covalently linked to glycosylated LAP dimer [22], termed the small latent complex.

## Bioavailability of TGF-$\beta$

In many cases the small latent complex becomes associated with additional component(s) prior to secretion. The best characterised of these components are the latent TGF-$\beta$ binding proteins (LTBPs) [23]. Four isoforms of LTBP have now been identified, each of which has been shown to bind to TGF-$\beta$ [24–28]. Furthermore, LTBP-1, -3 and -4 have been shown to undergo alternative splicing [27, 29, 30], leading to the production of an array of large latent TGF-$\beta$ complexes. The binding of LTBP to TGF-$\beta_1$ is mediated through a disulphide bond between an 8-cysteine repeat motif in LTBP and the LAP of small latent TGF-$\beta$ [31, 32]. The functions of the LTBPs *in vivo* have not been fully elucidated, but they have been shown to localise TGF-$\beta$ to elastic fibrils in the extracellular matrix [33, 34], and to form part of the extracellular matrix itself [35]. TGF-$\beta$ upregulates the transcription of LTBP-2 [36], which suggests that TGF-$\beta$ and the LTBPs may be co-ordinately regulated to generate large latent TGF-$\beta$ complexes.

In addition to the LTBP family, many other proteins have been shown to form complexes with TGF-$\beta$. As well as the high-affinity signalling receptors, there are many other cell surface components which have been shown to bind TGF-$\beta$, as well as various extracellular matrix proteins and components of blood plasma (see Tab. 1).

## TGF-$\beta$ activation

Neither the small or large latent TGF-$\beta$ complexes bind to the high-affinity signalling receptors. However, *in vitro* many different treatments of the latent forms of TGF-$\beta$ have been shown to activate TGF-$\beta$, yielding the mature 25 kDa dimer which is capable of binding to the signalling receptors. These include treatment with extremes of pH, denaturing agents, and various proteins such as proteases or thrombospondin (for review see [37]). *In vitro*, the serine protease plasmin cleaves the LAP, releasing active, mature TGF-$\beta$ from the small latent complex [38]. However, the cleavage of the LAP may also be mediated by other proteases, such as calpain [39], raising the possibility that this mechanism of activation may be an artefact due to the relative resistance to proteases of the active TGF-β dimer compared with the LAP. Activation of latent TGF-β by extremes of pH or denaturing agents is unlikely to have a broad physiological role. Similarly, thrombospondin, a large trimeric glycoprotein released from platelet α-granules, may bind to, and activate TGF-β *in vivo* [40] as well as *in vitro* [41], although the specificity of this effect is also doubtful [42].

Both before and after activation, TGF-β may be sequestered into pools which differ in their bioavailability. For example, TGF-β can be associated with a number of extracellular matrix components and to lipoproteins [43, 44]. Thus, a further mechanism regulating TGF-β activity may be by release from extracellular stores [45, 46].

## TGF-β signalling

Once activated, TGF-βs transduce signals to their target cells using a complex array of cell surface receptors (see Tab. 1). Much of the work has focused on the type I, II and III families of receptors (for review see [47, 48]). The type I and type II receptor families are serine/threonine kinases. Following ligand binding to an oligomeric receptor complex, the type II receptor phosphorylates the type I receptor, which in turn phosphorylates intracellular components of the TGF-β signal transduction pathway [49]. In general, the ligand specificity of the receptor complex is determined by the type II receptor present, while the type I receptor in the complex determines the signal produced [50]. The type III receptors (betaglycan and endoglin) do not appear to transduce a signal, but instead may localise TGF-β to the cell surface where betaglycan presents ligand to the signalling receptors [51, 52], and endoglin inhibits the transfer of TGF-β to the signalling receptors [52]. The putative type V receptor is a very large (400 kDa) protein which is internalised upon ligand binding, and contains an intracellular kinase [53].

Intracellular transduction of the TGF-β signal is mediated, at least in part, by a family of proteins known as Smads. At least nine different Smads have now been identified, and they have very different roles. One class of Smads (including Smad 1, 2 and 3) are phosphorylated by various type I receptors (for example, BMP-4 stimulates Smad 1 phosphorylation [54] while TGF-β/activin stimulates phosphorylation of Smad 2 and 3 [55]). Once activated, these Smads interact with Smad 4 and migrate into the nucleus [56] where they interact with the DNA binding proteins FAST-1 or tinman [57]. The third class of Smad proteins, which includes Smad 6 and 7, are termed inhibitory Smads: they bind to either the type I receptors [58] or to Smad 1, 2 or 3 [59], preventing signal transduction.

Over the past decade it has become increasingly clear that the members of the TGF-β superfamily play an important role in both the physiology and pathology of the cardiovascular system. There is a large amount of circumstantial evidence that

Table 1

TGF-β binding proteins. For each binding protein, the molecular weight given has been calculated from the protein sequence (where known). The list of "TGF-β family members bound"

| Binding protein | Synonyms | Binding protein size (kDa) | TGF-β family member(s) bound |
|---|---|---|---|
| **Receptors** | | | |
| TGF-β type I receptor | Alk5 | 54 | TGF-$\beta_1$, TGF-$\beta_2$, TGF-$\beta_3$ |
| TGF-β type I receptor | Alk2/Tsk7L | 55 | TGF-$\beta_1$, TGF-$\beta_2$, TGF-$\beta_3$ |
| TGF-β type II receptor | | 62 | TGF-$\beta_1$, TGF-$\beta_2$, TGF-$\beta_3$ |
| TGF-β type III receptor | Betaglycan | 92 | TGF-$\beta_1$, TGF-$\beta_2$, TGF-$\beta_3$ |
| TGF-β type III receptor | Endoglin | 68 | TGF-$\beta_1$, TGF-$\beta_3$ |
| TGF-β receptor type V | Insulin-like growth factor binding protein 3 receptor | 400 | TGF-$\beta_1$, TGF-$\beta_2$ |
| **Other cell surface proteins** | | | |
| GH3 pituitary cells surface component | | 70–74 (complexed with TGF-β) | TGF-$\beta_1$, activin, inhibin A and inhibin B |
| Porcine uterus membrane proteins | | 40, 60, 80, 160 | TGF-$\beta_1$ |
| FGF receptor | E-selectin ligand, MG-160, LTCP-1, FGF-receptor | 140 | TGF-$\beta_1$ |
| Cell surface glycoproteins | | 80, 150 & 180 | TGF-$\beta_1$, not TGF-$\beta_2$ |
| Cell surface glycoproteins | | 110 (homodimer of 60) & 140 | TGF-$\beta_2$, not TGF-$\beta_1$ |
| Cell surface glycoproteins | | 90–100 and 180 | TGF-$\beta_1$, not TGF-$\beta_2$ |
| **Extracellular matrix proteins** | | | |
| $\alpha_v\beta_1$ integrin | CD51/29 | 199 | TGF-$\beta_1$-LAP |
| $\alpha_v\beta_6$ integrin | | 197 | TGF-$\beta_1$-LAP |
| Decorin | | 38 | TGF-$\beta_1$ |
| Fibronectin | | 259 | TGF-$\beta_1$ |
| Ficolin | Hucolin | 40 | TGF-$\beta_1$ |
| LTBP-1 | | 125 (platelets) 170–190 (fibroblasts) | TGF-$\beta_1$, TGF-$\beta_2$, TGF-$\beta_3$ |
| LTBP-2 | | 260–310 | TGF-$\beta_1$ |
| LTBP-3 | | 180 | TGF-$\beta_1$ |
| LTBP-4 | | 215 | TGF-$\beta_1$? |
| Type IV collagen | | 175–185 | TGF-$\beta_1$, TGF-$\beta_2$ |
| **Blood components** | | | |
| $\alpha_2$-macroglobulin | | Multimeric | TGF-$\beta_1$ |
| Heparin | | varies | TGF-$\beta_1$ |
| Thrombospondin | | 420 | TGF-$\beta_1$ |
| Pregnancy zone protein | | Multimeric | TGF-$\beta_1$, TGF-$\beta_2$ |
| **Miscellaneous** | | | |
| β-amyloid precursor protein (soluble derivatives of) | | 110 | TGF-$\beta_2$ |
| Glomeruli | | 90–320 | TGF-$\beta_1$ and -$\beta_2$ |
| Glioblastoma cell line protein | | 210 (complexed with TGF-β | TGF-$\beta_1$, -$\beta_2$ and -$\beta_3$ |

*indicates the family members which have been investigated – those omitted from the list are not necessarily unable to bind. The affinity constant is for binding of labelled TGF-β to an excess of the binding protein. n/d, not determined*

| Affinity constant | Notes | Refs. |
|---|---|---|
| 5–50 pM | Forms oligomeric signalling complex. | [50] |
| 5–50 pM | Forms oligomeric signalling complex. | [50] |
| 5–50 pM | Forms oligomeric signalling complex. | [50] |
| 50–200 pM | No direct signalling function. | [273] |
| 50 pM | No direct signalling function. | [112] |
| ≤ 1 nM | | [274, 275] |
| 90 pM | Identified from rat pituitary tumour cell line. | [276] |
| n/d | 40 kDa component later identified as ficolin (see below). | [277] |
| n/d | Identified from Chinese hamster ovary cells. Previously observed, but not identified in chicken, rat and mouse systems. | [278] |
| 4.4 pM | Identified from cultured human umbilical vein endothelial cells, A549, MvLu, MG-63 and MS-C-1 cells. | [279, 280] |
| 0.5-1 nM | Identified from foetal bovine heart endothelial cells and MG-63 human osteosarcoma cells. | [281, 282] |
| 0.1–0.2 nM | Identified from foetal bovine heart endothelial cells and MG-63 human osteosarcoma cells. | [282] |
| n/d | | [283] |
| n/d | | [284] |
| 0.3 nM and 5 nM | Two binding sites are present. | [285] |
| 1 nM | | [286] |
| n/d | Identified from porcine uterus membranes. | [287] |
| n/d | Major component of TGF-β complex in platelets. Alternatively spliced. | [24] |
| n/d | | [33] |
| n/d | | [26] |
| n/d | | [27] |
| 19 pM | Binding not interfered with by laminin or fibronectin, which bind type IV collagen. | [43] |
| 10–100 nM | A major TGF-β complex in plasma. Binds with higher affinity to "activated" α₂-macroglobulin. | [288] |
| Varies | Dissociates TGF-β from α₂-macroglobulin complexes. | [289] |
| n/d | Bind to both the dimeric and tetrameric forms of PZP. Affinity for TGF-β₂ > TGF-β₁. Related to α₂-macroglobulin. | [291] |
| n/d | | [292] |
| | Four bands under non-reducing conditions yield many others upon reduction. | [293] |
| n/d | Identified from U-1240 MG cells. | [294] |

97

TGF-$\beta_1$ activity is important throughout the cardiovascular system in maintenance of normal tissue architecture: in the heart, the vascular smooth muscle and the endothelium.

## TGF-$\beta$ related cytokines in the normal heart

### Cardiac development

Members of the TGF-$\beta$ superfamily participate in cardiac development from the earliest specification of the left-right axis shortly after fertilisation, through to regulation of cardiac myocyte differentiation in the first few weeks after birth. The heart, like most mammalian organ systems, is positioned asymmetrically with respect to the organism's midline. The specification of this left-right asymmetry depends on asymmetric expression of a number of TGF-$\beta$ superfamily members, including activin, nodal and lefty [60–63]. There are complex interactions between vgr-1, activin, lefty and nodal during left-right axis specification. The order in which these proteins act is currently unclear, although a recent report demonstrated that lefty-1 acted upstream of both lefty-2 and nodal [64]. Interestingly, a recent report suggested that fluid shear stress (generated by leftward flow from the extra-embryonic cilia) might be the extrinsic signal responsible for the asymmetric expression of TGF-$\beta$ superfamily members at the earliest stage of development [65], mirroring one of the regulation mechanisms of TGF-$\beta$ in endothelial cells from the adult [66].

The heart develops from the middle of the three embryonic cell layers, the mesoderm. Induction of mesoderm occurs at the late blastula stage, and may be induced by activin [67], although a variety of other signalling molecules including $\beta$-catenin and members of the fibroblast growth factor (FGF) superfamily may also be required [68]. From *Xenopus* to mammals, activin (or its homologues) are thought to be responsible for mesoderm patterning that will give rise to both skeletal and cardiac muscle.

TGF-$\beta$ superfamily members also play a role in the next stage of cardiac development, when a tube forms which subsequently turns and loops in a complex morphogenetic sequence to generate the four chambered mammalian heart. Constitutive mutation of Alk5 (a type I TGF-$\beta$ signalling receptor) disrupts cardiac looping and morphogenesis in mice, while homozygous deletion of the immunophilin FKBP12, a component of the signal transduction pathway initiated by type I TGF-$\beta$ receptor activation, leads to developmentally-induced dilated cardiomyopathy [69].

During cardiac development, the TGF-$\beta$ isoforms participate in the fine morphological changes as well as the earlier specification of left-right axis and induction of mesoderm. TGF-$\beta$, and in particular the TGF-$\beta_3$ isoform have been implicated in the formation of the endocardial cushions and in the formation of the complex valve structures which regulate blood flow out of the heart [70–72]. The regulation of

TGF-$\beta_3$ expression during valve formation is particularly intriguing, with a recent study demonstrating that the *tgfb3* gene is expressed in both sense and antisense directions during cardiac development, suggesting that the expression of TGF-$\beta_3$ protein (essential for normal valve morphogenesis) depends on the relative amounts of the sense and antisense transcripts [10].

The lack of developmental abnormalities in the heart of either TGF-$\beta_1$ or TGF-$\beta_3$ null embryos [73] suggests that the TGF-β isoforms can substitute for one another during development of the heart, since any maternal transfer of TGF-β during development is unlikely to participate in exquisite spatial patterning events.

Retinoids (like other nuclear hormone receptor ligands) have significant effects on TGF-β transcription. Consequently, the profound effects of retinoid depletion or excess on cardiac development [74, 75] may relate to the complex roles played by members of the TGF-β superfamily. Disturbance of the highly regulated expression of TGF-$\beta_1$ in the heart [76, 77] could plausibly contribute to the development abnormalities resulting from inappropriate levels of retinoids [78].

## Post-natal development

Cardiac development continues after birth, with dramatic changes in the levels of a number of contractile proteins occurring in the first few weeks post-partum [79]. TGF-β isoforms have been implicated in this process [80], since TGF-$\beta_1$ regulates the expression of muscle isoforms of actin and myosin in a wide range of cell types, at least *in vitro* [81, 82]. We have recently shown that TGF-$\beta_1$ levels increase by three to four fold in the mouse myocardium over the first ten days after birth, with the most dramatic changes occurring in the first 72 hours [83]. Accumulation of cardiac α-actin by the myocytes is correlated with this increase in TGF-$\beta_1$ (Fig. 2), consistent with the *in vitro* data suggesting that TGF-β regulates cardiac α-actin expression.

Recent data from experiments examining the response of the adult myocardium to increased loading, for example during pressure-induced hypertrophy, have suggested that TGF-$\beta_1$ production is elevated in response to increased loading on the myocardial cells (see below). Following birth, the peripheral resistance that the heart must work against is markedly increased, as a result of the closure of the ductus arteriosus and foramen ovalis (which ensures that the lungs are fully perfused for the first time in the life of the organism [84]). It is therefore plausible, but presently unproven, that TGF-$\beta_1$ rapidly accumulates in the myocardium in the hours and days following birth in response to this increase in peripheral resistance. According to this model, members of the TGF-β superfamily act to couple elevated expression of contractile proteins to the sudden increase in imposed load.

The mechanisms by which levels of various TGF-β isoforms may be elevated in response to imposed load, as well as the mechanisms by which TGF-β increases levels of contractile proteins, are largely unknown although some circumstantial evi-

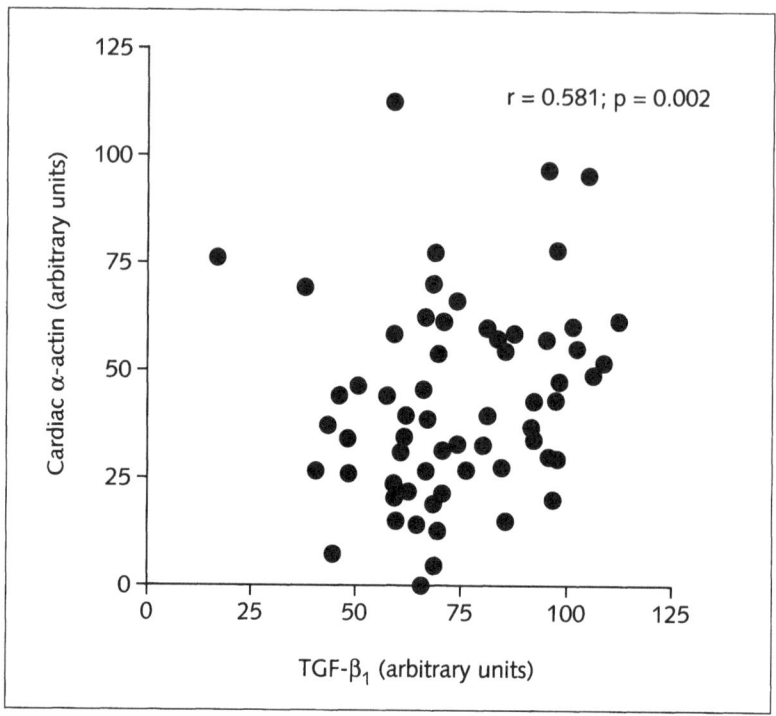

**Figure 2**
*Levels of TGF-$\beta_1$ in the myocardium correlate with levels of cardiac $\alpha$-actin. The levels of TGF-$\beta_1$ and cardiac-$\alpha$-actin were measured in the myocardium from mice 1, 3, 5, 7 and 10 days after birth (n = 10 at each time point) by quantitative immunofluoresence [272]. Higher levels of TGF-$\beta_1$ were significantly associated with higher levels of cardiac $\alpha$-actin (r = 0.581; p = 0.002; Pearson's r test). Data from D.J. Grainger and A.A. Grace, unpublished observations.*

dence permits speculation. We recently demonstrated that mice heterozygous for a deletion of the gene encoding the retinoid receptor RXR$\alpha$ have altered kinetics of cardiac growth in the perinatal period. In particular, the RXR$\alpha$ +/– pups accumulated TGF-$\beta_1$ more slowly during the first few days after birth, with accumulation of cardiac $\alpha$-actin delayed to a similar extent [83]. These observations provide further circumstantial evidence for the hypothesis that TGF-$\beta_1$ causes the increases in levels of contractile proteins seen in the early post-natal period. RXR$\alpha$, along with its heterodimer transcription factor partners, may therefore play a role in translating the increase in imposed load into an increase in TGF-$\beta_1$ accumulation.

The mechanism(s) by which TGF-$\beta$ increases contractile protein expression has not been extensively studied for the cardiac specific genes, such as cardiac $\alpha$-actin, although progress has been made in studying the analogous process in cultured smooth muscle cells. Hautmann and colleagues [85] have identified key TGF-β regulatory motifs in the upstream sequences of the smooth muscle α-actin promoter and it is likely that similar transcriptional controls regulate cardiac gene expression. Recent data on the mechanism of TGF-β signalling suggest that an additional mechanism may also be operating, in which TGF-β stimulates general protein synthesis. TGF-β receptors interact with the immunophilin FKBP12 which may participate in TGF-β signalling [86]. Immunophilins (FKBP12 and cyclophilin) interact with the calcineurin pathway which in turn regulates activation of the S6 kinase $p70^{s6k}$ (see Fig. 3). Such a pathway would provide a mechanism by which TGF-β signalling could directly stimulate general protein synthesis, although at present no data is available which directly supports this hypothesis. Matrix proteins (such as collagen type I) and contractile proteins (such as cardiac α-actin), which are two major classes of proteins whose synthesis is known to be stimulated by TGF-β, represent the major gene products of a muscle cell *in vivo*, and therefore a stimulation of general protein synthesis would lead to a marked increase in accumulation of these gene products. Hence, both non-specific (stimulated protein synthesis) and specific mechanisms (stimulated transcription of particular target genes, such as α-actin) may contribute to the accumulation of contractile proteins in response to TGF-β, but the relative contribution of each process under any given circumstances has yet to be determined.

## The adult heart

The regulation of cardiac contractile protein levels by TGF-β does not end with post-natal development. Similar mechanisms to those we have proposed to occur when the heart is first exposed to full loading immediately after birth may operate to match expression of cardiac gene expression to the imposed load throughout adult life. It has been known for more than a century that cardiac muscle, like skeletal muscle, undergoes adaptive hypertrophy in response to the demands placed upon it ([84] and references therein). This results in the increase in cardiac force-generating capacity induced by continuous aerobic exercise, but can also participate in several cardiac pathologies where inappropriate hypertrophy eventually leads to loss of function and ultimately to heart failure [87].

We have recently extended the hypothesis originally put forward by Schneider [71], and proposed a model whereby TGF-β is produced in response to increased load, which in turn leads to increased expression of contractile proteins (such as cardiac-α-actin) as well as matrix components ([88] and Fig. 4). In this way, TGF-β expression would couple cardiac hypertrophy to the extent of the workload imposed upon the heart on a time scale of days or longer (as opposed to the shorter time scale coupling which is controlled by neurendocrine signals). To investigate

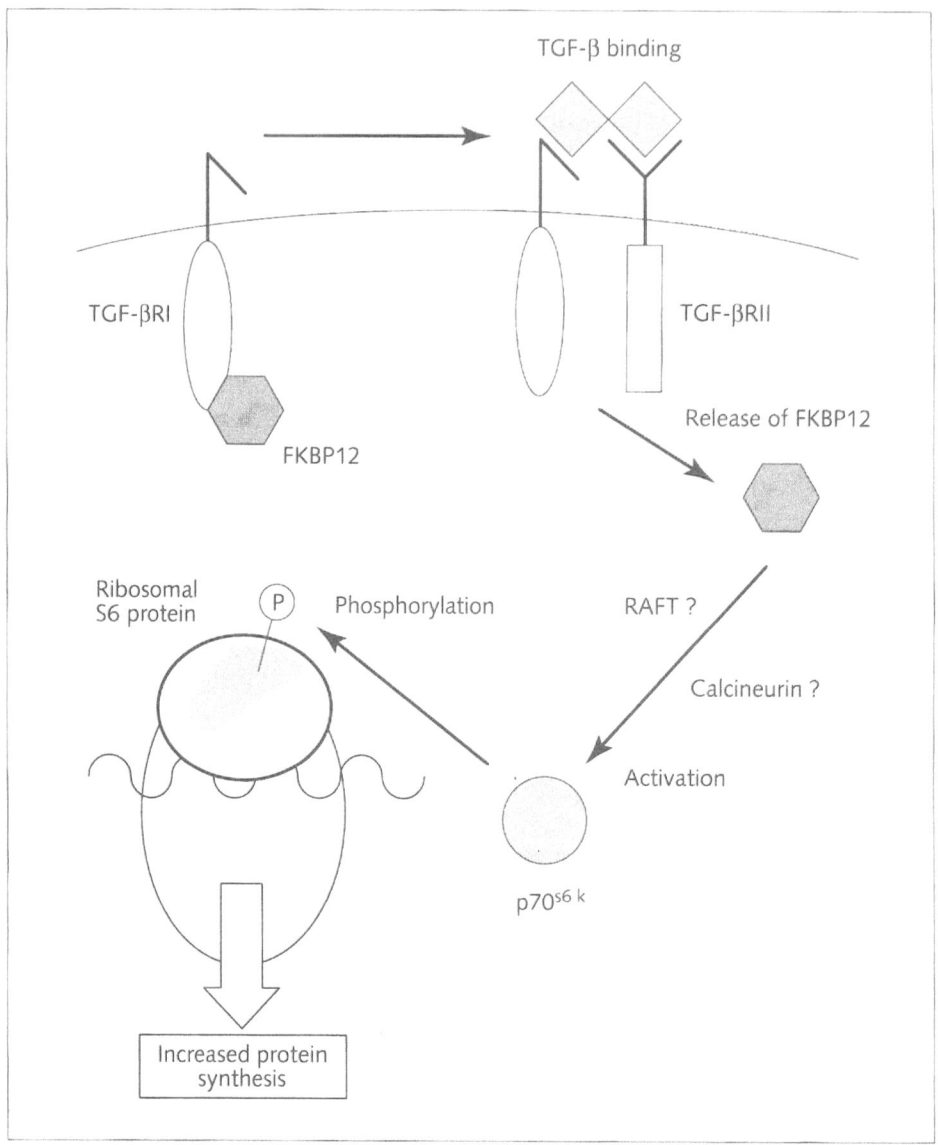

*Figure 3*
*Pathway mediating increased general protein synthesis in response to TGF-β. TGF-β (shaded diamonds) binds to the cell surface, inducing oligomerisation of the receptors (type I: open oval; type II: open rectangle). Activation of the type I receptor leads to dissociation of FKBP12 (shaded hexagon). FKBP may mediate activation of $p70^{s6k}$, possibly through interactions with calcineurin and/or RAFT. Once activated $p70^{s6k}$ phosphorylates the ribosomal S6 protein (stippled area) leading to general stimulation of protein synthesis.*

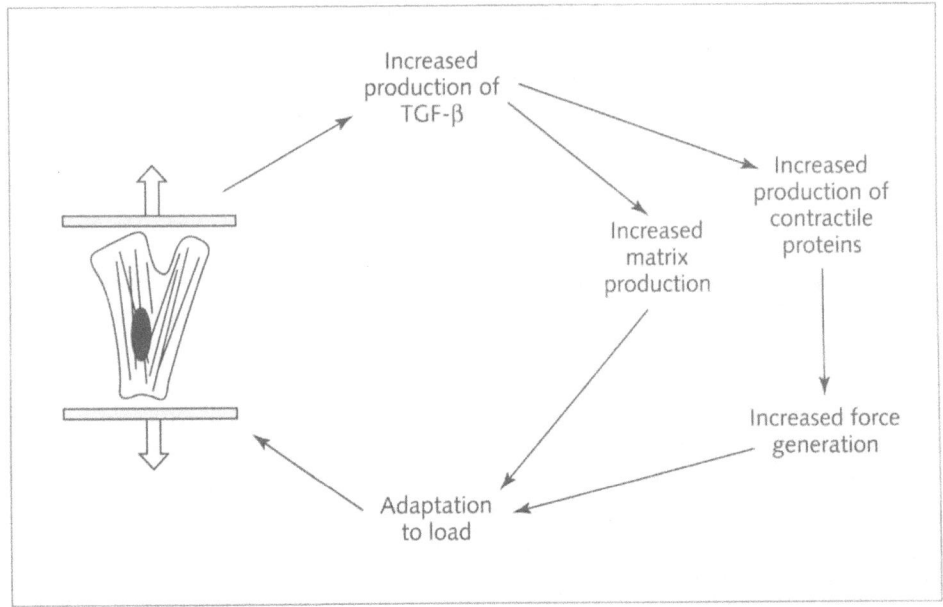

*Figure 4*

*The "load-coupling" hypothesis applied to the myocardium. When the myocytes are subjected to an increase in loading (such as due to increased blood volume, or increased peripheral resistance), TGF-β₁ activity is increased. This leads to an increase in both matrix production and accumulation of proteins composing the contractile apparatus, which together adapt the myocardium to the changed loading.*

this proposal further, we examined a model of pressure overload hypertrophy in the mouse. A ligature was applied round the aortic arch between the carotid and innominate arteries to restrict blood flow. After seven days, the left ventricle had undergone marked hypertrophy as a result of the increased peripheral resistance and cardiac workload [89]. Consistent with previous reports of other models of overload induced hypertrophy [90–92], we found that TGF-$\beta_1$ levels in the left ventricle were elevated by two-fold. The extent to which levels of TGF-$\beta_1$ were elevated was directly correlated with the extent of aortic constriction (assessed by measuring the pressure gradient between the proximal and distal carotid arteries). Furthermore, the increase in cardiac $\alpha$-actin and type I collagen accumulation which occurred in response to pressure overload also correlated with the increase in TGF-$\beta$ and the imposed load.

The mechanisms which regulate TGF-$\beta$ production by the myocytes and fibroblasts in the healthy adult heart are largely unknown. However, studies of pathological hypertrophy, both in animal models and in man, have suggested that angiotensin II may play an important role in stimulating TGF-β expression which in turn leads to myocyte hypertrophy and excessive extracellular matrix deposition. Angiotensin converting enzyme inhibitors, and more recently antagonists selective for the AT-1 angiotensin receptor, have been shown to both reduce TGF-β production and to ameliorate the response to hypertrophic stimuli [89, 93]. Whether angiotensin II, possibly acting through AT-1 receptors, has any role in regulating TGF-$β_1$ expression in the normal myocardium is not known but has been the subject of recent speculation [94].

A recent paper by Li and colleagues provided direct evidence that stretch stimulates TGF-β activity in an organ culture system [95]. In the Langendorff perfused heart system, an intraventricular balloon was inflated to an end diastolic load of 35 mmHg. This increased load resulted in a six-fold increase in expression of vascular endothelial growth factor (VEGF), and this stretch-induced VEGF expression could be abolished by neutralising antibodies to TGF-β, but not by inhibitors of endothelin or of angiotensin II. These observations provide direct evidence that increased stretch regulates TGF-β production (probably independently of angiotensin II), consistent with the load coupling hypothesis. Furthermore, Li et al. [95] noted that the protein kinase C inhibitor staurosporine blocked the stretch-induced VEGF expression but that this inhibition could be relieved by addition of TGF-$β_1$ to the perfusate. This experiment provides indirect evidence that protein kinase C activity may be involved in the transduction mechanism which increases TGF-β activity in response to stretch, although concerns over the specificity of agents such as staurosporine prevent firm conclusions being drawn.

VEGF is a potent stimulator of angiogenesis, and may play an important role in ensuring adequate oxygenation of the entire myocardium. Since hypoxia is known to stimulate TGF-β production, at least in some cell types [96, 97], and TGF-β activity regulates VEGF expression in the heart, it is possible that TGF-β production in regions of low oxygen tension leads to VEGF expression. This could result in the development and maintenance of a network of capillaries which allows homogenous oxygenation of the whole cardiac muscle.

Studies of TGF-$β_1$ null mice have recently revealed a further role for TGF-$β_1$ which may have implications for cardiac physiology. Loss of TGF-$β_1$ activity results in a marked increase in the activity of the inducible nitric oxide synthase, NOS2, in the cardiac myocytes [98]. This suggests that TGF-$β_1$ is an endogenous inhibitor of inducible nitric oxide synthase activity [99]. Since cyclical strain inhibits NOS2 expression in an amplitude-dependent pattern [100], it is plausible that strain-induced TGF-β mediates this effect, although Yamamoto and colleagues found no evidence for this mechanism [100]. It should be noted that the effects of TGF-β (and in particular TGF-$β_3$) on endothelial NOS synthase activity (mediated by NOS3) are opposite to the effects on NOS2 in cardiac myocytes. Endothelial NOS3 activity is stimulated by TGF-β, at least during glomerular pressure-induced fibrosis [101]. As a result, the overall impact of increased myocyte loading on cardiac nitric oxide production will depend on the balance between NOS2 activity in myocytes and NOS3 activity on the endothelium. It is possible that increased strain will inhibit production of nitric oxide in the myocardium during increased loading, reducing its relaxing effects on the muscle and allowing greater strength of contraction [99]. In contrast, increasing nitric oxide production in the vasculature may lead to local vasodilatation and an increased blood supply to support the increased work rate of the myocytes.

## TGF-β in the normal vasculature

### Vascular development

One of the earliest stages in vascular development is the differentiation of mesoderm tissue to give rise to endothelial cells (for review see [102]). These early endothelial cells aggregate around the haematopoietic progenitor cells, to give structures termed blood islands. Further development of the vascular system consists of two distinct processes, vasculogenesis and angiogenesis, which act in parallel on the blood islands to form the blood vessels of the early embryo [103]. Vasculogensis is the process whereby a new vessel is generated *de novo* by the organisation of endothelial cells into tubes, whereas angiogenesis is the process of elongation of existing blood vessels. Locally-derived smooth muscle cells, possibly recruited by the endothelium, then form the medial layer of the developing vessel [104].

*In vitro*, TGF-β markedly inhibits both endothelial cell proliferation and migration (reviewed in [105]). Furthermore, TGF-β also has effects on the expression of many different endothelial gene products, including matrix components, integrins, proteases and protease inhibitors. Based on this *in vitro* evidence, TGF-β is likely to modulate the process of angiogenesis *in vivo*.

There are two widely used experimental models for angiogenesis *in vivo*, the chick embryo chorioallantoic membrane and the rabbit corneal micropocket. Unexpectedly, in both of these models [106, 107], and in other models of angiogenesis [107], TGF-$\beta_1$ has been shown to be angiogenic. Furthermore, application of anti-TGF-$\beta_1$ antibodies reduces spontaneous vascular growth into implanted sponges to below the level of controls [108].

TGF-$\beta_1$ is expressed in the haemangioblasts [76], a cellular component of the blood islands and in the early endothelial cell during tube formation [109]. However, the most important evidence for the role of TGF-$\beta_1$ in vasculogenesis comes from studies of mice with a deletion of one or both alleles of the gene encoding TGF-$\beta_1$ [110]. Approximately 50% of mice with both alleles of the *tgfb1* gene deleted (*tgfb1 –/–* mice) die *in utero* as a result of a specific defect in yolk sac vasculogenesis. This defect ranges in severity from a delay in vasculogenesis to a phenotype where regions of the yolk sac are completely lacking in vessels. As many as 20% of mice with only a single allele of the *tgfb1* gene deleted show similar defects in vasculogenesis.

Mice lacking the TGF-β type II receptor (TGF-β RII) have a similar, although more severe, phenotype to mice lacking TGF-$\beta_1$ ligand – loss of TGF-β RII is lethal *in utero*, and death is due to defects in yolk sac haematopoiesis and vasculogenesis [111]. In addition, in man, mutations in either of the genes encoding endoglin (a TGF-β type III receptor related to betaglycan [112]) or Alk-1 (a TGF-$\beta_1$ type I receptor; [113]) result in hereditary haemorrhagic telangectasia (HHT; [114, 115]). HHT is characterised by vascular lesions, in which the post-capillary venules of the skin dilate, although the endothelial cells appear normal (for review see [116]).

Angiogenesis, though not vasculogenesis, can occur in the adult. It contributes to revascularisation during wound healing, and is essential for tumour growth. The TGF-βs are highly expressed in a large number of different tumour types [117], possibly because many tumours accumulate mutations in TGF-β receptors [118], making them unresponsive to the growth inhibitory action of TGF-β. In these tumours, TGF-β may now promote angiogenesis and lead to an increase in vascularity of the tumour and hence tumour size [119, 120]. However, data on whether TGF-β levels correlate with tumour vascularity *in vivo* are conflicting [121].

## Post-natal development

Major changes in the vasculature continue after birth. Firstly, there must be growth of the vascular system to support the increasing mass of the organism and secondly the vessels must adapt to the large increase in peripheral resistance that occurs when the lungs are first perfused.

Vascular smooth muscle differentiation increases markedly throughout post-natal development [122]. The smooth muscle cells increase their volume fraction of myofilaments, which results in an increase in their force-generating capacity [123, 124]. We have shown that during this period of post-natal development there is also an increase in the levels of TGF-$\beta_1$ in the artery wall (in mouse arteries there is an eight-fold increase in TGF-$\beta_1$ levels between 2 and 8 weeks of age [125]). The increase in smooth muscle differentiation during post-natal development is very likely to be due to the increase in TGF-$\beta_1$ [88]. One possible mechanism for the increase in levels of TGF-$\beta_1$ is increased shear stress. *In vitro*, sheer stress upregulates TGF-$\beta_1$ production by endothelial cells [126] and smooth muscle cells [127]. Following birth, the increased peripheral resistance leads to increased mechanical forces acting on the vessel wall which may lead to upregulation of TGF-$\beta_1$ levels. This in turn promotes the differentiation of the smooth muscle, contributing to the adaptation in response to increased load.

## The adult vessel wall

As chronic changes in blood pressure occur throughout life, the structure of the vessel wall adapts to them. Thus, although the structure of the vessel wall cannot change rapidly, it is constantly being matched to chronic changes in local haemodynamics.

The same TGF-β-dependent mechanisms (discussed earlier) which may participate in the increased smooth muscle differentiation in the post-natal period would be sufficient to match vessel wall structure to local haemodynamics. Moreover, based on its properties *in vitro*, TGF-β would also be expected to act in other ways to maintain the normal structure of the vessel wall. In addition to its effects on smooth muscle differentiation, TGF-β is a potent inhibitor of smooth muscle migration [128] and proliferation [129, 130], at least under most conditions *in vitro*. Furthermore, TGF-β maintains the endothelium in a differentiated state (both *in vitro* [131] and *in vivo*[132]) which not only inhibits platelet adhesion and inappropriate thrombus formation but also reduces leukocyte trafficking and inflammation.

The cardiovascular system provides a major conduit for cellular traffic, with many leukocyte subsets residing for significant periods in the bloodstream. As a result, the blood vessel wall plays a central role not only regulating blood pressure but also regulating the passage of leukocytes both into and out of the bloodstream. Present knowledge would suggest that much of this "gatekeeper" function is played by the vascular endothelium.

Under normal circumstances, the vascular endothelium does not express high levels of the adhesion molecules involved in leukocyte trafficking, but instead expresses proteins characteristic of a differentiated endothelium (such as factor VIII and von Willebrand factor). However, at sites where leukocyte extravasation is occurring, the endothelium is de-differentiated, expressing both adhesion molecules (such as intercellular adhesion molecule (ICAM), vascular cell adhesion molecule (VCAM) and the selectins) and leukocyte chemoattractants (chemokines and tumour necrosis factor (TNF)-α). The factors which regulate endothelial differentiation *in vivo* are not well understood (reviewed in [133]), but a variety of studies *in vitro* suggest that TGF-β family members may have an important role [134]. For example, TGF-$\beta_1$ inhibits expression of a wide variety of adhesion molecules that are upregulated in response to pro-inflammatory signals. Moreover, we have shown that the effects of TGF-$\beta_1$ on cultured endothelial cells have functional consequences, inhibiting adhesion of platelets and neutrophils to endothelial cells [135].

Based on these *in vitro* observations it is tempting to speculate that TGF-β may play a central role in maintaining a differentiated endothelium *in vivo* and that it acts to prevent systemic extravasation of leukocytes primarily at the level of the vascular endothelium. For example, loss of the endothelium-specific TGF-β type III receptor endoglin leads to disruption of the capillary endothelium and hereditary haemorrhagic telangectasia [115]. Additionally, mice with a homozygous deletion of the *tgfb1* gene die shortly after birth from multi-organ inflammation with leukocyte-rich cuffs around the smaller blood vessels [136], suggesting that the excessive inflammation was caused by disregulated leukocyte extravasation. However, two more recent observations refute this simplest interpretation. Firstly, Diebold and colleagues demonstrated that endothelial activation and leukocyte extravasation were lymphocyte-dependent, since neither occur in SCID mice (which completely lack lymphocytes) when the *tgfb1* gene is deleted [73]. More recently, we have examined endothelial cell activation (marked by expression of ICAM-1, VCAM-1 and monocyte chemoattractant protein-1 (MCP-1)) in mice with a single allele of the *tgfb1* gene deleted, which lack the inflammatory response seen in the *tgfb1* –/– mice. As in Diebold's experiment, we found no evidence for endothelial activation induced by lowered levels of TGF-$\beta_1$ [73]. In contrast, where an inflammatory response is ongoing, for example following feeding with a lipid-enriched diet, endothelial cell activation and vascular macrophage accumulation both occur to a much greater extent in *tgfb1* +/– mice than in animals with normal levels of TGF-$\beta_1$ [125].

These experiments suggest that leukocyte extravasation is controlled by a complex interaction between pro-inflammatory stimuli and loss of TGF-$\beta_1$ activity. Reduced TGF-$\beta_1$ activity alone does not cause endothelial cell activation, but it is plausible that it decreases the resistance to activation in response to pro-inflammatory stimuli.

TGF-$\beta$ may also play a role in the regulation of leukocyte numbers in the blood. In addition to the well-studied endothelial transmigration of leukocytes that occurs at sites of inflammation, each leukocyte must cross the endothelium to reach the blood stream in the first place. Systemic levels of TGF-$\beta_1$ may therefore regulate the entry of leukocytes into the blood, as well as their subsequent exit, and hence participate in the homeostasis of leukocyte numbers in the blood. Since leukocytes are a major source of TGF-$\beta$ protein [137], it is possible that leukocyte-derived TGF-$\beta$ acts to increase endothelial differentiation, thereby reducing the flux of further leukocytes from bone marrow to blood in a negative feedback loop (Fig. 5). Under circumstances where tissue inflammation is occurring and many leukocytes undergo extravasation and are lost from the circulation, a drop in the level of leukocyte-derived TGF-$\beta$ would allow a degree of endothelial activation and hence increased efflux of leukocytes from the bone marrow to replenish the leukocyte pool in the blood. Such a model could account for the large increase in total (that is, blood plus tissue) leukocyte numbers which occurs in mice *tgfb1* –/– mice [136]. Presumably, leukocyte flux from the bone marrow through the blood and into the periphery is accelerated in the absence of TGF-$\beta_1$.

Regulation of leukocyte trafficking across the vascular endothelium may also play a role in physiological processes other than inflammation. For example, regulation of bone mineral density depends on the balance between mineral deposition by osteoblastic cells and its subsequent resorption by osteoclasts [138]. The osteoclast population is derived from precursor cells which co-purify with, and may be

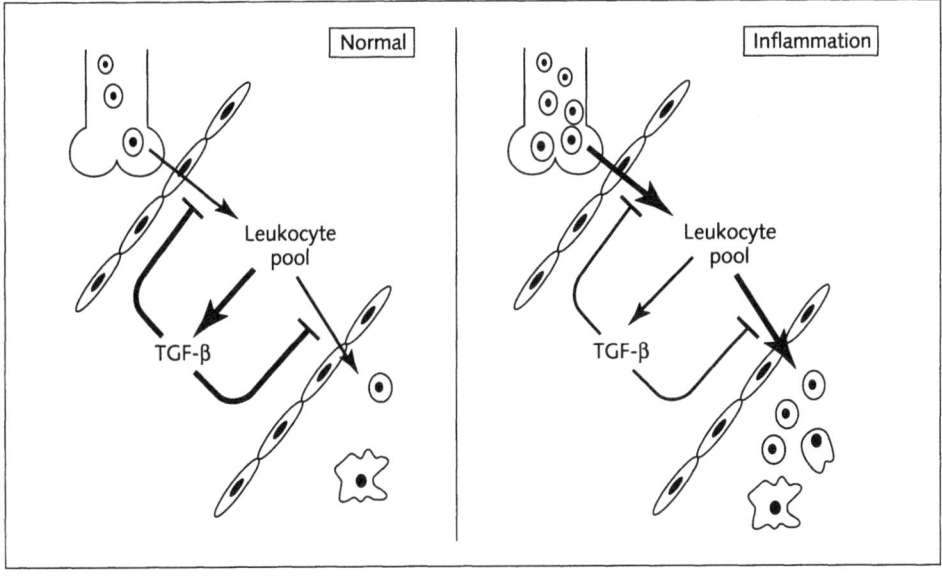

*Figure 5*
*A model of leukocyte flux from bone marrow to the periphery. According to this model, leukocyte flux from the blood into peripheral tissues occurs only slowly (thin arrow), under normal circumstances (left panel), as a result of TGF-β activity contributed in part by the leukocytes in the blood (thick arrow). This leukocyte-derived TGF-β also maintains a low flux of leukocytes from the bone marrow into the blood (thin arrow). When inflammation occurs (right panel), the flux of leukocytes into peripheral tissue is greatly increased (thick arrow), temporarily reducing the circulating leukocyte pool, and hence the supply of leuko-cyte-derived TGF-β (thin arrow). This will promote flux of leukocytes from the bone marrow into the blood (thick arrow) normalising the circulating leukocyte numbers.*

identical to, monocytes. Osteoclast recruitment may therefore resemble other mono-cyte extravasation processes (such as Kupffer cell formation in the liver or vascular macrophage accumulation during atherogenesis). In the same way that TGF-$\beta_1$ may regulate vascular macrophage accumulation, it may also reduce osteoclast recruit-ment and so reduce bone turnover. There is circumstantial evidence to support this proposition. Oestrogen and the triphenylethylene raloxifene decrease bone resorp-tion *via* a mechanism that is likely to depend on TGF-β [139, 140], and oestrogen regulates osteoclast number *in vivo* in a TGF-β-dependent fashion [141]. However, as with the regulation of trans-endothelial migration during local inflammation, the impact of TGF-β on endothelial cell differentiation is likely to be only one of a num-ber of mechanisms contributing to the regulation of bone mineral density *in vivo*.

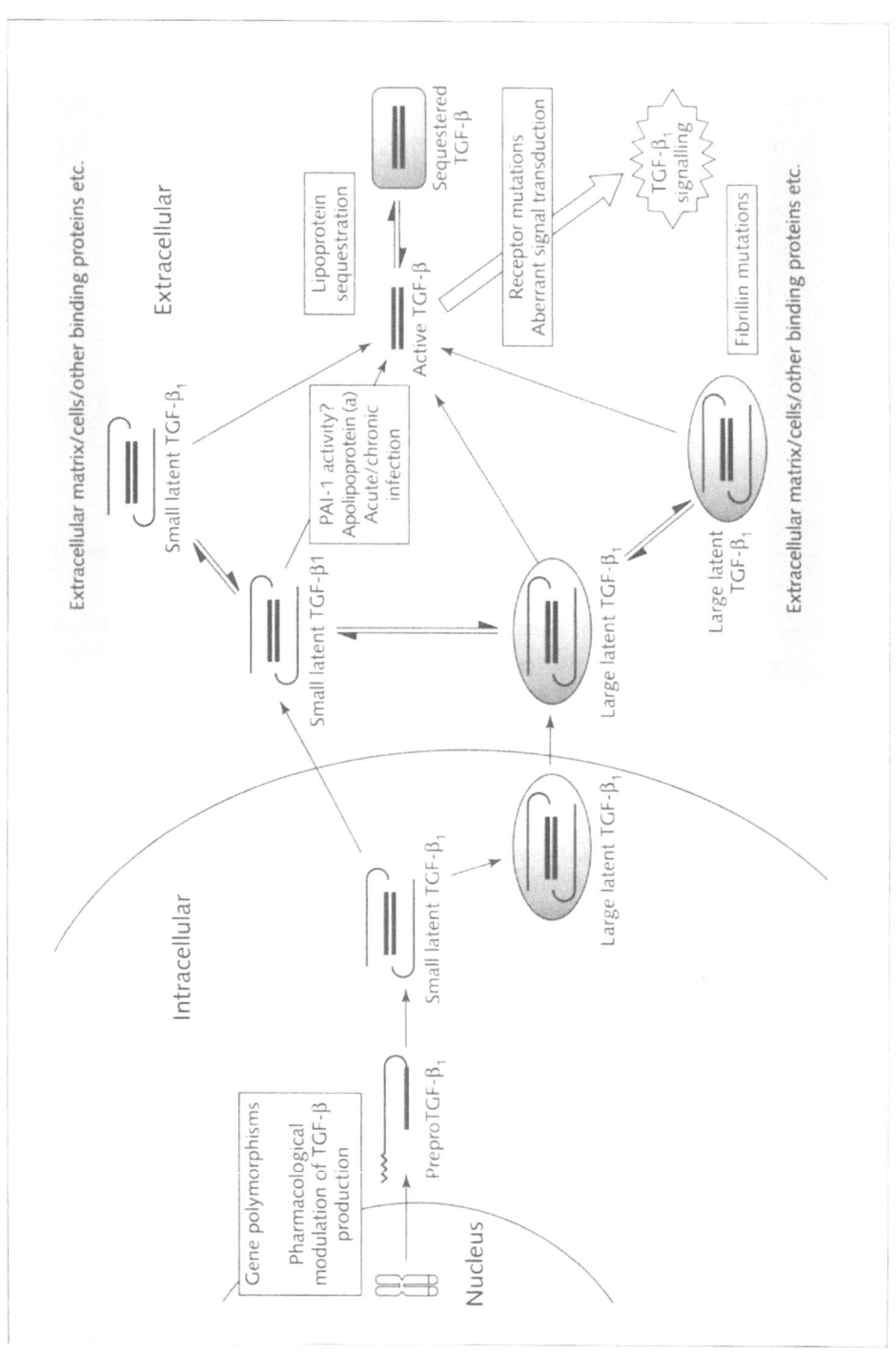

## Aberrant regulation of the TGF-β system

Since TGF-β activity is regulated on such a wide variety of levels, a range of molecular pathways impinge on TGF-β activity in both physiological (Fig. 1) and pathological situations (Fig. 6). These pathways may therefore contribute to the changes in tissue architecture which characterise cardiovascular diseases such as atherosclerosis, hypertrophic cardiomyopathies or Marfan syndrome.

## Production of TGF-β

Although much work has been done on the regulation of TGF-$\beta_1$ transcription *in vitro*, relatively little is known about factors regulating transcription of this gene in human tissues *in vivo*. The most informative studies have come from molecular genetic analysis of cohorts for whom circulating levels of TGF-$\beta_1$ have been measured. Recently, three independent studies have indicated that polymorphisms in the promoter region of the *tgfb1* gene are associated with either cellular production of TGF-$\beta_1$ or circulating levels of TGF-$\beta_1$ [142–144]. Taken together, these studies strongly suggest that cellular production of TGF-$\beta_1$ depends on the *tgfb1* gene haplotype and that circulating levels of TGF-$\beta_1$ protein are likely to be influenced by cellular production of TGF-$\beta_1$.

Several studies have extended these observations to examine any association between *tgfb1* gene haplotypes and disease phenotypes which might be expected to result from misregulation of TGF-$\beta_1$ activity. Cambien et al. reported a weak association between *tgfb1* gene haplotype and both myocardial infarction and hypertension [145]. While a subsequent study confirmed the association between *tgfb1* genotype and blood pressure [144], other more recent studies provided conflicting evidence as to whether there is any association between *tgfb1* haplotype and myocardial infarction [146, 147]. Although association studies do not exclude a role for a particular locus in determining the risk of the disease under investigation, nevertheless the molecular genetic data obtained to date provide little support for the hypothesis that cellular production of TGF-$\beta_1$ is a major determinant of atherosclerosis risk, at least in Europeans, although it may be more important in other pathologies associated with alterations in vascular architecture or function [148, 149], including hypertension [144, 145].

---

*Figure 6*
*Aberrant regulation of TGF-β signalling. Since TGF-β activity is regulated on many levels (Fig. 1), there are many potential mechanisms which can interfere with normal signalling. Boxed text indicates those processes which are known to be modulated during cardiovascular disease development or progression.*

Environment, as well as genes, is likely to affect TGF-β production. In particular a range of pharmacological agents which are associated with reduced incidence of cardiovascular disease have been shown to stimulate TGF-β production both *in vitro* and *in vivo*. These include aspirin [88, 150], vitamin E [151, 152] and triphenylethylenes (such as Tamoxifen [153–155] or raloxifene [141]). Each of these agents stimulates TGF-β production by cultured cells or increases levels of TGF-β in the blood vessel wall in animals. However, the extent to which TGF-β elevation contributes to any beneficial effects of these agents on the cardiovascular system remains unclear.

## Bioavailability of TGF-β

A number of lines of evidence suggest that retention in the extracellular matrix may be an important determinant of tissue levels of TGF-β. The best characterised TGF-β binding proteins are members of the LTBP/fibrillin superfamily and both LTBP and fibrillin are assembled into fibrillar extracellular matrix structures *in vitro* and *in vivo* [156–158]. Such structures have been shown to act as a repository for TGF-β in the extracellular matrix [35, 159]. Mutations in the fibrillin gene cause Marfan syndrome, a disease with characteristic cardiovascular complications [160]. It is plausible, but unproven, that reduced TGF-β in the extracellular matrix of the vascular wall contributes to the disease phenotype (see below).

In mice, mutations in the fibrillin gene have also been implicated in a disease with a phenotype opposite to Marfan syndrome – excessive matrix deposition. The *tightskin (tsk)* phenotype in mice [161] has been attributed to a partial duplication of the fibrillin gene, which results in the region of fibrillin homologous to the TGF-β-binding region of LTBP being repeated [162, 163]. In contrast to the deletions and point mutations in the fibrillin gene associated with Marfan syndrome, such a partial duplication could lead to increased TGF-β deposition in the matrix and ultimately to excessive matrix deposition and fibrogenesis.

In addition to association with insoluble matrix proteins, TGF-β family members have also been shown to bind to a number of soluble proteins, particularly in the bloodstream (see Tab. 1). In most cases, the consequences of these interactions (physiological or pathological) are unclear. However, the association between TGF-β and lipoprotein particles [44] could plausibly participate in cardiovascular disease pathology. A proportion (10–20%) of plasma TGF-$\beta_1$ is associated with the lipoprotein fraction in blood from normal individuals [44]. Interestingly, the proportion of plasma TGF-$\beta_1$ associated with lipoprotein was markedly higher in individuals with diabetes (who have an increased incidence of cardiovascular diseases). It is likely that this interaction between TGF-$\beta_1$ and lipoproteins explains the inverse correlation between plasma TGF-$\beta_1$ levels and LDL-cholesterol concentrations which we reported [150]. However, any functional consequence of TGF-$\beta_1$ binding to lipoproteins in plasma is more speculative. *In vitro*, lipoproteins inhibit the activity of recombinant TGF-$\beta_1$ [44] and it is possible that even mild dyslipidemia could promote atherogenic changes in the blood vessel wall architecture at least in part through reduced levels of TGF-$\beta_1$.

## TGF-β activation

In addition to its effects on bioavailability of TGF-β, lipoproteins may affect TGF-β activity in other ways. We recently reported the suppression of TGF-β activity for at least 8 h following a standardised lipid-rich meal [164]. However, this suppression is unlikely to be due to binding of TGF-β to lipoprotein particles, since the proportion of plasma TGF-β in the lipoprotein fraction did not change over the 8 h period studied [164]. Instead, it is more likely that a lipoprotein-induced increase in plasminogen activator inhibitor-1 (PAI-1), a well characterised inhibitor of TGF-β activation [165–168], was responsible. We observed marked effects of the PAI-1 promoter genotype (at the 4G/5G polymorphic site [169]) on both the increase in PAI-1 activity and the decrease in TGF-β activity in response to the lipid-rich meal [164]. Irrespective of the molecular mechanism(s) behind the diet-induced reduction in TGF-β activity, this suppression could promote pro-atherogenic changes in vessel wall architecture.

A wide variety of other factors may regulate PAI-1 levels, and hence impinge on TGF-β activation. The adipose cell has recently been identified as a major source of PAI-1 [170-172] and this may contribute to the higher prevalence of cardiovascular disease among individuals with a high body mass index [170, 171]. PAI-1 (which is a positive acute phase reactant) is also upregulated by acute and possibly chronic infections [173]. Individuals with chronic infections (such as herpes simplex virus (HSV), cytomegalovirus (CMV), *Chlamydia* or *Helicobacter pylori*) may therefore have a small chronic elevation of PAI-1 activity, resulting in a mild reduction in TGF-β activity [166, 173]. This might promote pro-atherogenic changes in vessel wall structure, providing a molecular mechanism to explain the weak epidemiological associations between chronic infection and atherosclerosis [174].

Proteins other than PAI-1 may modulate TGF-β activation and thus contribute to pathological changes in vessel wall structure. One of the best characterised of these is apolipoprotein(a), apo(a), the protein component of the atherogenic lipoprotein Lp(a) that distinguishes it from LDL. Initially reported by Rifkin and colleagues [175], a large number of reports have now confirmed that apo(a), and indeed Lp(a), markedly inhibit TGF-β activation *in vitro* [176–178]. Apo(a) also inhibits TGF-β activation in the vessel wall *in vivo*, at least in transgenic mice which express the human gene that encodes apo(a) [179, 180]. Like PAI-1, apo(a) can inhibit the generation of plasmin activity, and *in vitro* there is strong circumstantial evidence that this inhibition of plasmin is responsible for the reduced TGF-β activation [176]. The situation *in vivo*, however, is clearly much more complex, since plasmin is probably not a major activator of TGF-β (based on the phenotype of plasminogen knock-out mice [181]). Thus, the molecular pathways responsible for reduced TGF-β activity in the presence of apo(a), or indeed PAI-1, *in vivo* remained to be defined.

## TGF-β signalling

Even if the levels of active TGF-β ligand in the tissues of the cardiovascular system are normal, this may not be sufficient for the homeostatsis of vessel wall structure. Some evidence is now accumulating for alterations in the TGF-β receptors and signalling pathway which may lead to pathological loss of the homeostatic signal. One such change is somatic mutation of the gene encoding the type II TGF-β signalling receptor. Such loss-of-function mutations have been well characterised in a wide range of tumours [182, 183], since they were first reported by Markowitz in replication error-prone colon cancers [184]. Recently, McCaffrey et al. [185] reported that the same somatic mutations can be found at higher levels in atherosclerotic vessel wall tissue than in normal vessel wall segments. Although there are a number of technical caveats which preclude a conclusive statement that somatic mutation of TGF-β RII is occurring during atherogenesis, nevertheless it is tempting to speculate that loss of this TGF-β signalling receptor contributes to the loss of normal vessel wall structure in atherosclerosis.

In addition to somatic mutations in the gene encoding TGF-β RII, other mechanisms may result in altered expression of TGF-β receptors in cardiovascular diseases. A number of studies have demonstrated that the levels of both the type II and type I signalling receptors are modulated in diseased tissue, including atherosclerotic vessel wall segments [186] and hypertrophic myocardium [187]. In the atherosclerotic plaque there is an increased ratio of levels of the type I receptor to the type II receptor: a change which leads to a switch from an anti-proliferative to a profibrotic response to TGF-β in cultured smooth muscle cells [186]. In addition, levels of both receptor types are increased during cardiac hypertrophy which could exacerbate any effects of excess ligand. The importance of the TGF-β signal transduction pathway in the maintenance of normal cardiac architecture was highlighted recently by the cardiac defects seen in mice lacking the protein FKBP12 [69], which interacts with the TGF-β RI [188] and may play an important role in transducing at least some signals in response to TGF-β [86].

In addition to FKBP12, the Smad family of transcription factors have also been identified as components of the TGF-β signal transduction pathway (see above). Although activation of the Smads seems to occur predominantly in response to interaction between TGF-β superfamily members and their receptors [50], the factors which regulate levels of the inhibitory Smads (Smad 6 and 7) are less well defined. The original description of Smad 6 and 7 suggested they were regulated by shear stress [189], which may be especially important in the cardiovascular system, and in particular for the vascular endothelium. For many decades, it has been known that changes in vessel wall architecture associated with atherosclerosis occur preferentially at particular sites throughout the vascular tree, and these sites are commonly in regions of turbulent flow (such as vessel branch points) where shear stress is low [190, 191]. Even in the absence of atherosclerotic changes in vessel architecture, vessel branch points have low levels of the smooth muscle differentiation marker smooth muscle α-actin, indicative of reduced TGF-β signalling locally [88]. This may be due either to lower levels of tissue TGF-β ligand [88] or to increased levels of inhibitory Smads [189]. Whichever (or possibly both) of these mechanisms is responsible for the reduced TGF-β activity at these sites, it is possible that loss of the homeostatic TGF-β signal contributes to the increased risk of atheroma formation at low shear stress sites in the vasculature.

## Consequences for the heart

### Hypertrophic cardiomyopathy

Hypertrophic cardiomyopathy is the term used to describe diseases characterised by left and/or right ventricular hypertrophy [192]. The hypertrophy is usually asymmetric, with the interventricular septum commonly affected. Disease progression leads to an increase in the amount of extracellular matrix in the affected heart, which eventually results in breakdown of the normal tissue architecture potentially leading to arrhythmias and premature death [192].

The most common cause of hypertrophic cardiomyopathy is genetic, with an autosomal dominant pattern of inheritance. Mutations in at least seven genes are associated with familial hypertrophic cardiomyopathy (FHC), all of which encode components of the sarcomere [193]. Many different mutations have been identified in each of these genes, contributing to the phenotypic heterogeneity of FHC [194]. The mutated genes are translated and incorporated into the sarcomere, explaining the observed genetic dominance. In most cases, the mutations result in a reduction in the force-generating capacity of the sarcomere [194], although several lead to a hypercontractile state [194].

The "hypomorphic alleles" will result in a lower force generation capacity for the whole myocardium, such that in response to a normal workload the muscle will be overstretched. The normal physiological response to work overload will then occur: we have proposed that this involves upregulation of TGF-β. In response to the increase in TGF-β signalling there will be myocyte hypertrophy and increased expression of contractile proteins which will increase the work capacity of the myocardium, but there will also be extracellular matrix deposition. Thus, the level of TGF-β needed to maintain a normal workload will be higher, and the more sub-functional the allele, the higher the level of TGF-β in the tissue. Over a long period of time, this slightly higher level of TGF-β activity will lead to excessive matrix deposition and what might be considered benign hypertrophy.

However, if the loss of function is sufficiently severe there may become a point when extracellular matrix deposition is so great that it disrupts the myocyte organisation and prevents the co-ordinated contraction of all of the myocytes [192]. At this point, a rubicon is crossed and the hypertrophy could no longer be considered benign. A positive feedback loop is established in which disruption of the myocardial architecture leads to reduced force generation that in turn leads to increased TGF-β production, increased matrix deposition and further disruption to the myocyte organisation (Fig. 7). After years of benign hypertrophy, progression to heart failure would occur rapidly and irreversibly.

Such a model describes accurately the natural history of cardiac hypertrophies, whether familial or idiopathic [192]. There is substantial evidence consistent with this role for TGF-β in the pathogenesis of hypertrophic cardiomyopathy. Firstly, in cell culture experiments, TGF-$\beta_1$ is involved in the hypertrophic responses to both β-adrenoceptor stimulation [195] and angiotensin II [196]. Secondly, levels of TGF-$\beta_1$ mRNA and protein have been shown to be up-regulated in several animal models of cardiac hypertrophy [91, 92, 197, 198]. Furthermore, the myocardium of patients with idiopathic hypertrophic cardiomyopathy contains elevated levels of TGF-$\beta_1$ mRNA and protein compared to controls [95].

As well as TGF-$\beta_1$, levels of its receptors are also elevated in the myocardium of patients with myocardial hypertrophy [187] as are levels of the enzyme type II transglutaminase [199] (an enzyme which has been suggested to have a role in the processing of TGF-β [200]). In contrast, levels of TGF-$\beta_2$ are unchanged in a rat model of left ventricular hypertrophy, while levels of TGF-$\beta_3$ protein are decreased transiently in the same model [198].

There is, therefore, considerable evidence that in hypertrophic cardiomyopathy the normal physiological pathway coupling myocyte hypertrophy to imposed load is driven to destroy the tissue architecture through overproduction of TGF-$\beta_1$. Such a hypothesis also provides a molecular explanation for the predisposition of the left ventricle (which is subject to the largest workload) to malignant hypertrophy in patients with FHC even though the whole muscle is equally affected by the primary genetic lesion.

## Other cardiac pathologies

Following myocardial infarction, the injured area of the muscle is unable to generate the necessary force to meet the imposed workload and is overstretched. The cells surrounding the infarct will therefore respond by upregulating TGF-$\beta_1$ that in turn

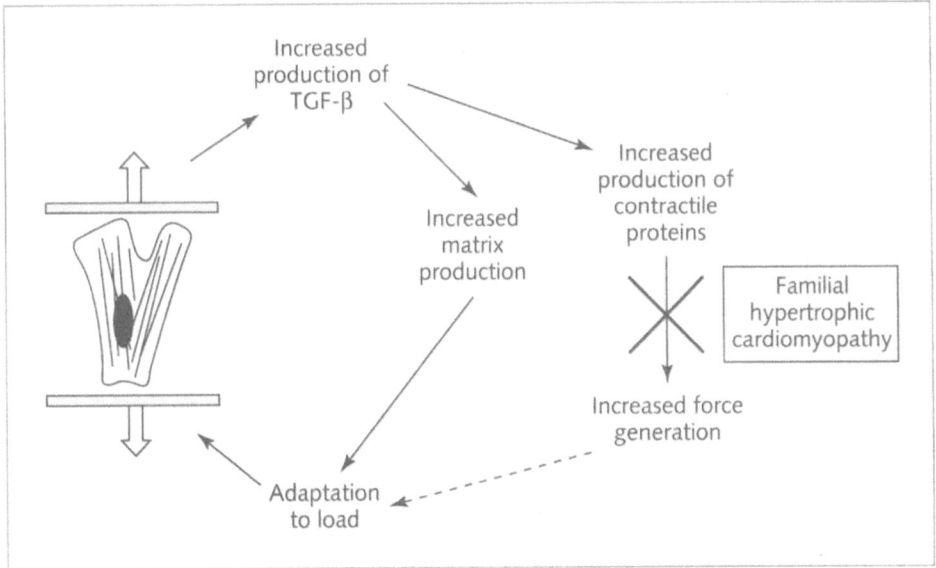

*Figure 7*

*The pathogenesis of familial hypertrophic cardiomyopathy: impact of the "load-coupling" hypothesis. In familial hypertrophic cardiomyopathy, associated with the presence of hypomorphic alleles in genes encoding components of the contractile proteins, any increase in load results in stimulation of contractile protein accumulation, but insufficient force generation. The increase in matrix proteins in response to TGF-β, however, still occurs normally. Over an extended period of time this may lead to disruption of muscle architecture and malignant hypertrophy (see text).*

increases extracellular matrix formation, which contributes to the formation of the fibrotic scar tissue [201, 202]. While this may be beneficial in the infarct zone (by preventing the damaged tissue from ballooning out with each heartbeat), it is likely to progressively impair the performance of the surrounding functioning myocardium and may contribute substantially, at least in the most severe cases, to left ventricular hypertrophy and ultimately heart failure in the post-myocardial infarction patient [201, 203].

Furthermore, TGF-β production by invading leukocytes [137] may contribute to myocardial scarring seen following severe local infections (such as pericarditis [204, 205]) or severe systemic infection (such as following abdominal sepsis or pancreatitis [206]). In each case, leukocyte-derived TGF-β would be expected to drive inappropriate cardiac fibrosis. If this is severe enough to disrupt myocyte organisation this could induce the malignant hypertrophic pathway shown in Figure 7.

Although TGF-$\beta_1$ may participate in the pathogenesis of these cardiac disorders, it is through the inappropriate application of the normal physiological mechanism for matching muscle function to imposed workload that normal cardiac structure is lost. Direct misregulation of TGF-$\beta$ activity (such as in response to elevated PAI-1 or apo(a) or sequestration by lipoproteins, for example) does not seem to be a principal cause of cardiac pathology.

## Consequences for the vasculature

### Atherosclerosis

Many different processes are thought to contribute to the development of atherosclerosis including endothelial dysfunction or injury, smooth muscle cell de-differentiation and migration, monocyte recruitment and differentiation into tissue macrophages, recruitment and activation of other inflammatory cells, lipid accumulation and thrombogenesis [207]. Members of the TGF-$\beta$ superfamily may participate in a number of these processes.

There are numerous studies in the literature that describe the *in vitro* effects of TGF-$\beta$ on the cell types which compose the atherosclerotic plaque. However, it is difficult to draw general conclusions from these studies about the role of TGF-$\beta$ in the pathogenesis of the disease *in vivo* because of the large amount of conflicting evidence. For example, several reports clearly demonstrate that TGF-$\beta_1$ promotes the proliferation of smooth muscle cells [208-211], while others show the opposite [128–130, 212, 213]. Such variability is likely to be attributable to small differences in the culture conditions used (see for example [208, 214]).

Unfortunately, even with the publication of a range of *in vivo* studies, a consensus opinion on the role of TGF-$\beta$ in atherogenesis is yet to form. For example, transfection of a gene encoding constitutively active TGF-$\beta$ into the vessel wall leads to the formation of a neointima [215, 216], whereas mice with one allele of the TGF-$\beta_1$ gene deleted are more prone to lipid lesion formation when fed a high fat diet [125].

This apparent conflict may arise in part because the animal models used for the study of vascular disease fall broadly into two types. One class is characterised by smooth muscle cell proliferation and neointima formation. For example, vascular injury (either caused by a balloon catheter or by air drying of the endothelium) in a variety of different species leads to the formation of a smooth muscle cell-rich neointima over a period of several weeks [217]. The other class of animal models is characterised by inappropriate vascular lipid deposition and local inflammation in the vessel wall. For example, over a period of months, mice with a broad range of defects in lipoprotein metabolism develop fatty streak lesions that resemble early human atherosclerosis [218]. The available *in vivo* data strongly suggests that TGF-β exacerbates neointima formation in the injury-type models [219, 220], but ameliorates lipid lesion formation and inflammation in the models more closely resembling atherosclerosis (reviewed in [155]).

In all the animal models examined to date (C57Bl/6 in-bred mice [221], apo(a) transgenic mice [180] and apoE knockout mice [222]), as well as in aortic tissue from humans with atherosclerosis (H.L. Kirschenlohr, J.C. Metcalfe, D.E. Mosedale and D.J. Grainger, unpublished observations), levels of active TGF-β are reduced in the vessel wall. Furthermore, McCaffrey and colleagues have shown that expression of the TGF-β type II receptor is selectively lost in smooth muscle cells cultured from atherosclerotic lesions compared to smooth muscle cells from the normal vessel wall, whereas levels of the TGF-β type I receptor are similar in smooth muscle cells from both sources [186]. Taken together, it is likely that the TGF-β signal involved in vessel wall homeostasis is reduced or lost during atherogenesis.

Partly as a result of this reduced TGF-β signal, the endothelium becomes locally activated and expresses adhesion molecules such as ICAM-1, VCAM-1 and E-selectin [125, 132]. Leukocyte extravasation is presumably, therefore, increased at these sites, contributing to the local inflammatory response characteristic of atherosclerosis [207]. Furthermore, the recruited leukocytes are themselves a source of pro-inflammatory cytokines [223], contributing to local increases in PAI-1 [224, 225] and possibly, therefore, greater suppression of TGF-β signalling. Such a positive feedback mechanism (depicted in Fig. 8) could contribute to the highly focal nature of atherosclerotic changes in vessel architecture.

It is important, however, to keep the role of TGF-β in this process in context. Reduced levels of TGF-β signalling alone are not sufficient for endothelial activation or monocyte recruitment. Endothelial activation does not result from deficiency of TGF-$\beta_1$ in the absence of lymphocytes [73], nor from reduction of TGF-$\beta_1$ levels in the absence of inflammation (either in *tgfb1* +/– mice [125] or apo(a) transgenic mice [180]). In all cases studied to date, a pro-inflammatory stimulus is also required for endothelial activation. At least in mice, it is likely that a significant part of this pro-inflammatory stimulus comes from expression of the chemokine MCP-1, since deletion of MCP-1 [226] or its receptor [227] leads to a reduction in vascular macrophage accumulation and reduced lipid lesion formation.

TGF-β may regulate other processes involved in atherogenesis, including smooth muscle cell differentiation, migration and extracellular matrix deposition. Smooth muscle differentiation is well known to be reduced in both human plaques [207] and fatty streak lesions in animals [180, 221, 222], and this reduction in differentiation is probably a direct consequence of reduced TGF-β signalling [88]. In the atherosclerotic plaque, as in the normal vessel wall, TGF-β is likely to be important in regulating the amount and composition of the extracellular matrix, although this role may be more prominent in the plaque due to the changes in TGF-β receptor expression that have occurred [186]. Failure to maintain a sufficiently strong extracellular matrix is likely to contribute to the risk of plaque rupture [228, 229], leading to

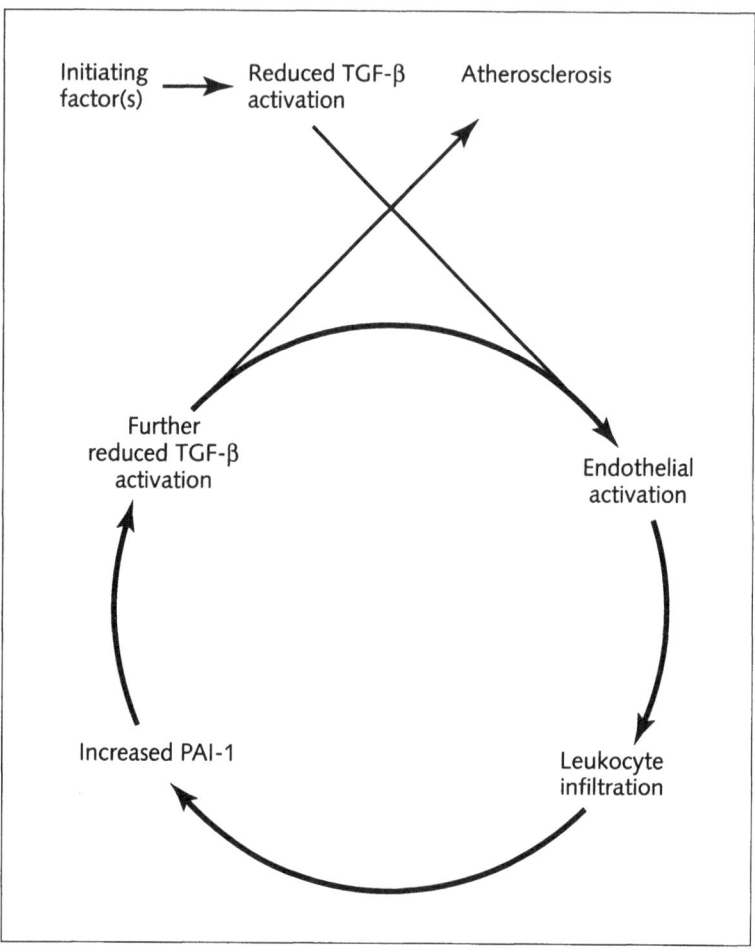

*Figure 8*

*A feedback loop in atherogenesis. One example of a feedback loop that may operate during atherogenesis is shown. Once TGF-β activity is locally depressed, even to a small extent, by initiating factors (such as low shear stress, apo(a) etc.), the endothelium is locally more prone to activation, promoting leukocyte infiltration. The presence of leukocytes leads to increased PAI-1 production which further reduces TGF-β activation, leading to a positive feedback loop. This, and similar positive feedback loops [180], may contribute to the highly focal nature of atherosclerotic plaques.*

thrombus formation, vessel occlusion and myocardial infarction. As a result, any residual TGF-β activity in the advanced atherosclerotic plaque may still be an important determinant of the clinical consequences of atherosclerosis.

## Restenosis

Restenosis is an iatrogenic disease, due to the narrowing of the vessel wall which may occur following angioplasty (a surgical intervention used to widen the vessel lumen in a region affected by atherosclerosis using a balloon catheter). In approximately 30% of cases, restenosis occurs, usually within six months, which may necessitate a further angioplasty [230]. Although superficially similar to atherosclerosis, in that it results in lumen narrowing, the pathogenesis (and time scale) of restenosis differs markedly.

Various processes are involved in the development of a restenotic lesion (for review see [231]). These include platelet adhesion and aggregation, growth factor production and release by smooth muscle cells, macrophages and platelets, smooth muscle cell migration and proliferation and production of extracellular matrix. All of these processes may perpetuate the lumen narrowing caused by any vessel spasm that occurs in the first few days after the intervention.

In animal models of neointima formation (which are not necessarily good models of restenosis), TGF-β is thought to have a major role. In the widely used balloon-injury model, a balloon catheter is dragged through the healthy common carotid artery, causing significant injury to the endothelium and vessel media. TGF-β mRNA and protein may be upregulated in arteries injured in this way, both in rats [232] and rabbits [233], although different results have been obtained using different analytical methods [88]. Despite any upregulation in the level of TGF-$\beta_1$ protein, the level of active TGF-β is reduced by balloon-injury, at least at 14 days after injury of the rat carotid artery [88]. Interventional experiments suggest that the role of this TGF-β is to promote neointima formation. Neutralising antibodies against TGF-$\beta_1$ suppress neointima formation in the rat balloon-injury model [219]. Furthermore, direct transfer of a gene encoding constitutively active TGF-$\beta_1$ into normal arteries results in intimal and medial hyperplasia together with increased matrix production [215, 216] and administration of TGF-$\beta_1$ protein intravenously potentiates the increase in intimal area caused by balloon-injury of rabbit arteries [220]. In addition, Tranilast, a drug used to reduce the frequency of restenosis after angioplasty in humans [234], reduces the levels of the mRNA encoding TGF-$\beta_1$ and -$\beta_3$, as well as the type I and type II TGF-β receptors in rats [235].

In humans, the level of mRNA encoding for TGF-$\beta_1$ is elevated in restenotic tissues compared with control tissues [236, 237], and the levels of a TGF-β-inducible protein, βig-h3, have been shown to be upregulated in restenotic tissue [238]. Taken together, it is probable that TGF-β plays a similar role in human restenosis as in neointima formation in animal models.

The mechanism by which TGF-β promotes neointima formation, either in animal models or in man, is less well understood, although there are a number of possibilities. Enhanced expression of TGF-$\beta_1$ leads to elevated extracellular matrix production and deposition, but may not increase cell number in the neointima [220]. TGF-$\beta$ may also promote neointima formation indirectly through its inhibitory action on endothelial cell proliferation [239]. If the rate of endothelial regrowth over the injury site is reduced, smooth muscle migration and/or proliferation may be exacerbated. Consistent with this hypothesis, Lehmann-Bruinsma et al. found that treatment with TGF-$\beta_2$ (which inhibits proliferation of smooth muscle cells but not endothelial cells) inhibited neointima formation [240]. The balance of the TGF-$\beta$ activity on smooth muscle cells versus endothelial cells may therefore be an important determinant of the extent of neointima formation *in vivo*.

## Hypertension

The majority (> 90%) of patients with hypertension (diastolic pressures greater than 90 mm Hg) have "primary" hypertension, which is defined by the lack of an identified cause, with the remainder having "secondary" hypertension, whose cause is known. Hypertension causes arterial damage, especially to the eyes, brain, kidney and heart and may eventually cause death of the patient [241].

Many factors may be involved in the development of primary hypertension, such as mild changes in kidney function leading to increased blood volume, and increased peripheral vascular resistance, both of which then lead to increased blood pressure. Accompanying the increase in blood pressure is an increase in the media/lumen ratio of the arteries [242]. This increase in media/lumen ratio may be a consequence of the increase in blood pressure (for example, if changes in kidney function were the initiating factor) or may itself be the primary defect leading to the hypertension. One component of the increase in media/lumen ratio is an increase in medial mass, which, in the small arteries, is due to smooth muscle cell hyperplasia, which, in animal models of hypertension, occurs very early in the development of the disease [243]. However, in the large arteries the increase in media/lumen ratio is predominantly caused by smooth muscle cell hypertrophy, which may be accompanied by hyperploidy [244].

It has been suggested that TGF-$\beta$ contributes to the development of smooth muscle cell hypertrophy in hypertension [245, 246]. TGF-$\beta$ gene expression is upregulated in the vessels wall in many different animal models of hypertension [247, 248] and levels of TGF-$\beta$ receptors are modulated in hypertensive rats compared to control rats [249].

Two recent reports described an association between polymorphisms of the *tgfb1* gene and blood pressure [144, 145], although no association was detected in a third study [146]. In the report by Li and colleagues [144] levels of TGF-$\beta_1$ in the blood, in addition to polymorphisms in the *tgfb1* gene, correlated with blood pressure, although the population they studied was not randomly selected. In addition, levels of TGF-$\beta_1$ protein [246] are modulated in arteries from hypertensive individuals. Furthermore, TGF-β production by monocytes of hypertensive patients is greater than that by monocytes from normotensive controls [250], suggesting that a widespread tendency to overproduce TGF-β may be associated with hypertension.

The mechanism(s) underlying the increase in TGF-β seen in hypertension may be genetic or, by extrapolation from the load-coupling hypothesis presented earlier (Figs. 4 and 7), may result from the increased load placed on the smooth muscle cells. Irrespective of the mechanism, the paradox highlighted by Cambien's report remains unresolved: hypertension is associated with elevated TGF-β production, while atherosclerosis is associated with reduced TGF-β signalling, yet hypertension is a major risk factor for atherosclerosis.

## Marfan syndrome

Marfan syndrome is a systemic connective tissue disorder with autosomal dominant inheritance. It is characterised by a collection of physical manifestations in the skeletal, cardiovascular, pulmonary and ocular systems, including arachnodactyly, ectopia lentis and dilation of the aortic root [251]. Premature death often results from aortic dissection. Marfan syndrome is caused by mutations in the extracellular matrix protein, fibrillin [160], which forms microfibrils around which elastin associates during elastic fibre formation [252].

Two fibrillin genes have now been identified [253, 254], which have strong homology with each other and with the LTBPs. Both protein families consist of many repeats of three different types: EGF-like repeats, 8-cysteine repeats and hybrid repeats. The 8-cysteine and hybrid repeats have not been identified in any other proteins. It has recently been shown that LTBP-1 binds to the pro-region of TGF-β through one of these 8-cysteine repeats ([31, 32]; see earlier). However, it is not known whether either fibrillin-1 or 2 bind TGF-β directly. However, it has been shown that LTBP-1, like fibrillin, is a component of elastic microfibrils [255]. It is possible, therefore, that heteropolymers may exist consisting of both LTBP and fibrillin, and that fibrillin may have a role in the localisation of the large latent TGF-β complex to the extracellular matrix.

As a consequence, there are at least two potential mechanisms by which mutations in fibrillin may lead to aortic dilation and eventually to dissection. Firstly, the mutation may cause defects in the formation and/or function of the fibrillin fibres, which may in turn affect elastin deposition and hence vessel strength. Secondly (or in addition), mutations in either of the genes encoding fibrillin may reduce the capacity of the elastic fibre to act as a store for TGF-β, either through a reduction in the capacity of fibrillin to bind to TGF-β directly or a reduction in the levels of

LTBP copolymerised with the fibrillin. Reduced capacity of the extracellular matrix to store TGF-β may lead to a lower level of TGF-β activity in the vessel wall. This in turn would result in a decline in the levels of smooth muscle-specific contractile proteins [88] and to a reduction in the levels of extracellular matrix proteins in the vessel wall [256]. Both of these effects would contribute to a weakening of the structure of the vessel wall, predisposing it to dilation and dissection.

At present, however, there is little direct evidence to support a role for TGF-β in the pathogenesis of Marfan syndrome. Fibrillin has not been shown to bind TGF-β, nor have LTBP and fibrillin been shown to copolymerise. Furthermore, it may be difficult to distinguish between a TGF-β independent mechanism (reduced vessel strength due to altered structure and/or function of the fibrillin fibres) and a TGF-β dependent mechanism (reduced TGF-β binding to fibrillin fibres). If the load-coupling hypothesis applies to the vessel wall, then altered structure and/or function of the fibrillin fibre would lead to altered TGF-β signalling, even if TGF-β binding to fibrillin fibres remained unaltered.

If Marfan syndrome results from reduced TGF-β signalling in the vessel wall, one might ask: why do the vessel wall changes in Marfan syndrome not resemble atherosclerosis? One possibility is that development of an atherosclerotic plaque depends on the action of a positive feedback loop leading to severe focal deficiency in TGF-β signalling (see Fig. 8). In contrast, in Marfan syndrome the primary defect (altered fibrillin) is present throughout the vessel wall and may lead to a mild, homogeneous reduction in TGF-β levels.

## Moyamoya disease

Moyamoya disease is a progressive cerebrovascular disease, characterised by occlusion of certain cerebral arteries, particularly the circle of Willis, beginning in childhood [257]. Moyamoya disease is quite rare, with a total of about 3000 cases described in Japan where it is most prevalent, but less than 300 described in the United States.

The occlusive vascular lesion is composed of a multilayered intimal thickening [258], a histological feature usually attributed to repeated mural thrombus formation [259]. Smooth muscle cells cultured from patients with Moyamoya disease have several characteristic features: they have a longer doubling time [260] than smooth muscle cells from control patients, and respond differently to cytokines [261]. Furthermore, in smooth muscle cell cultures from patients with Moyamoya disease, elastin mRNA and protein levels are elevated, and the smooth muscle cells secrete significantly more TGF-$\beta_1$ into the culture medium than control smooth muscle cells [262]. Furthermore, the levels of TGF-$\beta_1$ are elevated in serum from patients with Moyamoya disease compared with controls [263], although the levels of TGF-$\beta_1$ in cerebrospinal fluid is similar in patients and controls [264].

## Concluding remarks

In smooth muscle, and probably cardiac muscle, TGF-β signalling regulates expression of proteins which compose the contractile apparatus [88, 265]. This has led us to propose the load-coupling hypothesis, suggesting that in both muscle types (and possibly in skeletal muscle as well [266]) the imposed workload regulates myocyte hypertrophy *via* increases in TGF-$\beta_1$ activity. Although there is currently only circumstantial evidence to support this hypothesis, it has implications for a number of cardiovascular pathologies and provides an attractive molecular description of the natural history of cardiac hypertrophy. This parallel between cardiac and smooth muscle suggests that the molecular pathogenesis of hypertension may resemble that of cardiac hypertrophy more closely than had previously been realised. Such analogy may prove a useful guide in the continuing search to identify genes which predispose to hypertension in the human population [267] since the class of genes which predispose to cardiac hypertrophy are already well characterised [193, 194].

If normal levels of TGF-$\beta_1$ are required to maintain normal vessel wall function, it is possible that aberrant regulation of TGF-$\beta_1$ may lead to the changes in tissue architecture which occur in the pathogenesis of diseases such as atherosclerosis. Rifkin and colleagues first proposed that factors which reduced TGF-β activity, such as apolipoprotein(a), might predispose to atherogenesis [175], and we later extended this concept in the protective cytokine hypothesis [155, 268], suggesting that TGF-β was essential for the maintenance of normal vessel wall structure and that loss of this protective signal (by whatever mechanism) would promote atherogenic changes in vessel wall structure.

There seems little doubt now that altered TGF-$\beta_1$ signalling contributes to pathogenic changes in the cardiovascular system in animal models [125, 198, 216]. However, an important question for the future is to determine what contribution TGF-$\beta_1$-dependent processes make to cardiovascular disease processes in man. This review has focused on the role of TGF-$\beta_1$ family members in the cardiovascular system to the exclusion of many other important contributing mechanisms. For example, pathways such as lipoprotein metabolism and thrombosis are undoubtedly important in the pathogenesis of atherosclerosis independently of TGF-β [207]. The challenge is to begin to define the relative contributions of these individual mechanisms to the whole complex disease process.

Finally, if misregulation of TGF-β signalling contributes to the pathogenesis of cardiovascular diseases, modulating TGF-β activity would be a potential target for therapeutic intervention. Some progress has been made using gene therapy techniques to transfect cells in the cardiovascular system with either the *tgfb1* gene to elevate levels of TGF-$\beta_1$ or its antisense sequence to reduce levels of TGF-β. This approach has advanced furthest in the field of trauma-induced neointima formation in animals [215, 269], but it seems unlikely that this approach will proceed into the clinic until gene therapy is well established for more serious diseases which may be decades rather than years into the future. As a pharmacological approach, a number of agents already in use to combat cardiovascular disease have been shown to modulate TGF-β activity, either *in vitro* or *in vivo*, including red wine, aspirin, fish oils and vitamin E [88, 150, 151]. One class of compounds, however, which may hold particular promise (the triphenylethylenes such as Tamoxifen) have not yet found utility in the cardiovascular clinic. Molecules of this class stimulate TGF-β activity in the vessel wall of animals to a greater extent than do agents such as aspirin [180, 221, 222]. The extent to which TGF-β elevation contributes to the reduction in cardiovascular disease seen among women taking Tamoxifen for breast cancer [270, 271], however, remains uncertain. Whatever the mechanism, it is possible that triphenylethylenes will find use in the treatment and prevention of cardiovascular disease [155]. More specific modulation of TGF-β activity in the human cardiovascular system, however, remains a distant possibility.

# References

1    Massagué J (1990) The transforming growth factor-beta family. *Annu Rev Cell Biol* 6: 597–641
2    Birchenall-Roberts MC, Ruscetti FW, Kasper J, Lee HD, Friedman R, Geiser A, Sporn MB, Roberts AB, Kim SJ (1990) Transcriptional regulation of the transforming growth factor beta 1 promoter by v-src gene products is mediated through the AP-1 complex. *Mol Cell Biol* 10: 4978–4983
3    Geiser AG, Busam KJ, Kim SJ, Lafyatis R, O'Reilly MA, Webbink R, Roberts AB, Sporn MB (1993) Regulation of the transforming growth factor-beta 1 and -beta 3 promoters by transcription factor Sp1. *Gene* 129: 223–228
4    O'Reilly MA, Geiser AG, Kim SJ, Bruggeman LA, Luu AX, Roberts AB, Sporn MB (1992) Identification of an activating transcription factor (ATF) binding site in the human transforming growth factor-beta 2 promoter. *J Biol Chem* 267: 19938–19943
5    Van Obberghen-Schilling E, Roche NS, Flanders KC, Sporn MB, Roberts AB (1988) Transforming growth factor-beta-1 positively regulates its own expression in normal and transformed cells. *J Biol Chem* 263: 7741–7746
6    Flanders KC, Holder MG, Winokur TS (1995) Autoinduction of mRNA and protein expression for transforming growth factor-beta in cultured cardiac cells. *J Mol Cell Cardiol* 27: 805–812
7    Madisen L, Lioubin MN, Finerty PJ Jr, Sutter K, Blake J, Frederick J, Purchio AF (1991) Expression of recombinant TGF-beta 2(442) precursor and detection in BSC-40 cells. *Growth Factors* 5: 317–325
8    Webb NR, Madisen L, Rose TM, Purchio AF (1988) Structural and sequence analysis of TGF-beta 2 cDNA clones predicts two different precursor proteins produced by alternative mRNA splicing. *DNA* 7: 493–497

9    Liu C, Wallace K, Shi C, Heyner S, Komm B, Haddad JG (1996) Post-transcriptional stimulation of transforming growth factor beta 1 mRNA by TGF-beta 1 treatment of transformed human osteoblasts. *J Bone Miner Res* 11: 211–217

10   Potts JD, Vincent EB, Runyan RB, Weeks DL (1992) Sense and antisense TGF beta 3 mRNA levels correlate with cardiac valve induction. *Dev Dyn* 193: 340–345

11   Scotto L, Assoian RK (1993) A GC-rich domain with bifunctional effects on mRNA and protein levels: implications for control of transforming growth factor beta 1 expression. *Mol Cell Biol* 13: 3588–3597

12   Arrick BA, Lee AL, Grendell RL, Derynck R (1991) Inhibition of translation of transforming growth factor-beta 3 mRNA by its 5' untranslated region. *Mol Cell Biol* 11: 4306–4313

13   Kim SJ, Park K, Koeller D, Kim KY, Wakefield LM, Sporn MB, Roberts AB (1992) Post-transcriptional regulation of the human transforming growth factor-beta 1 gene. *J Biol Chem* 267: 13702–13707

14   Gentry LE, Lioubin MN, Purchio AF, Marquardt H (1988) Molecular events in the processing of recombinant type 1 pre-pro-transforming growth factor beta to the mature polypeptide. *Mol Cell Biol* 8: 4162–4168

15   Gray AM, Mason AJ (1990) Requirement for activin A and transforming growth factor-beta 1 pro-regions in homodimer assembly. *Science* 247: 1328–1330

16   Dubois CM, Laprise MH, Blanchette F, Gentry LE, Leduc R (1995) Processing of transforming growth factor beta 1 precursor by human furin convertase. *J Biol Chem* 270: 10618–10624

17   Cui Y, Jean F, Thomas G, Christian JL (1998) BMP-4 is proteolytically activated by furin and/or PC6 during vertebrate embryonic development. *EMBO J* 17: 4735–4743

18   Constam DB, Robertson EJ (1999) Regulation of bone morphogenetic protein activity by pro domains and proprotein convertases. *J Cell Biol* 144: 139–149

19   Nachtigal MW, Ingraham HA (1996) Bioactivation of Mullerian inhibiting substance during gonadal development by a kex2/subtilisin-like endoprotease. *Proc Natl Acad Sci USA* 93: 7711–7716

20   Blanchette F, Day R, Dong W, Laprise MH, Dubois CM (1997) TGFbeta1 regulates gene expression of its own converting enzyme furin. *J Clin Invest* 99: 1974–1983

21   Purchio AF, Cooper JA, Brunner AM, Lioubin MN, Gentry LE, Kovacina KS, Roth RA, Marquardt H (1988) Identification of mannose 6-phosphate in two asparagine-linked sugar chains of recombinant transforming growth factor-beta 1 precursor. *J Biol Chem* 263: 14211–14215

22   Bonewald LF, Wakefield L, Oreffo RO, Escobedo A, Twardzik DR, Mundy GR (1991) Latent forms of transforming growth factor-beta (TGF beta) derived from bone cultures: identification of a naturally occurring 100-kDa complex with similarity to recombinant latent TGF beta. *Mol Endocrinol* 5: 741–751

23   Miyazono K, Olofsson A, Colosetti P, Heldin CH (1991) A role of the latent TGF-beta-1-binding protein in the assembly and secretion of TGF-beta-1. *EMBO J* 10: 1091–1101

24   Kanzaki T, Olofsson A, Moren A, Wernstedt C, Hellman U, Miyazono K, Claesson-

welsh L, Heldin CH (1990) TGF-beta-1 binding-protein: a component of the large latent complex of TGF-beta-1 with multiple repeat sequences. *Cell* 61: 1051–1061

25  Moren A, Olofsson A, Stenman G, Sahlin P, Kanzaki T, Claesson-Welsh L, ten Dijke P, Miyazono K, Heldin CH (1994) Identification and characterization of LTBP-2, a novel latent transforming growth factor-beta-binding protein. *J Biol Chem* 269: 32469–32478

26  Yin W, Smiley E, Germiller J, Mecham RP, Florer JB, Wenstrup RJ, Bonadio J (1995) Isolation of a novel latent transforming growth factor-beta binding protein gene (LTBP-3). *J Biol Chem* 270: 10147–10160

27  Saharinen J, Taipale J, Monni O, Keski-Oja J (1998) Identification and characterization of a new latent transforming growth factor-beta-binding protein, LTBP-4. *J Biol Chem* 273: 18459–18469

28  Yin W, Fang J, Smiley E, Bonadio J (1998) 8-Cysteine TGF-BP structural motifs are the site of covalent binding between mouse LTBP-3, LTBP-2, and latent TGF-beta 1. *Biochim Biophys Acta* 1383: 340–350

29  Yin W, Smiley E, Bonadio J (1998) Alternative splicing of LTBP-3. *Biochem Biophys Res Commun* 245: 454–458

30  Oklu R, Hesketh TR, Metcalfe JC, Kemp PR (1998) Expression of alternatively spliced human latent transforming growth factor beta binding protein-1. *FEBS Lett* 435: 143–148

31  Saharinen J, Taipale J, Keski-Oja J (1996) Association of the small latent transforming growth factor-beta with an eight cysteine repeat of its binding protein LTBP-1. *EMBO J* 15: 245–253

32  Gleizes PE, Beavis RC, Mazzieri R, Shen B, Rifkin DB (1996) Identification and characterization of an eight-cysteine repeat of the latent transforming growth factor-beta binding protein-1 that mediates bonding to the latent transforming growth factor-beta1. *J Biol Chem* 271: 29891–29896

33  Gibson MA, Hatzinikolas G, Davis EC, Baker E, Sutherland GR, Mecham RP (1995) Bovine latent transforming growth factor beta 1-binding protein 2: molecular cloning, identification of tissue isoforms, and immunolocalization to elastin-associated microfibrils. *Mol Cell Biol* 15: 6932–6942

34  Taipale J, Miyazono K, Heldin CH, Keski-Oja J (1994) Latent transforming growth-factor-beta-1 associates to fibroblast extracellular-matrix *via* latent TGF-beta binding-protein. *J Cell Biol* 124: 171–181

35  Dallas SL, Miyazono K, Skerry TM, Mundy GR, Bonewald LF (1995) Dual role for the latent transforming growth-factor-beta binding-protein in storage of latent TGF-beta in the extracellular matrix and as a structural matrix protein. *J Cell Biol* 131: 539–549

36  Ahmed W, Kucich U, Abrams W, Bashir M, Rosenbloom J, Segade F, Mecham R (1998) Signaling pathway by which TGF-beta1 increases expression of latent TGF-beta binding protein-2 at the transcriptional level. *Connect Tissue Res* 37: 263–276

37  Munger JS, Harpel JG, Gleizes PE, Mazzieri R, Nunes I, Rifkin DB (1997) Latent transforming growth factor-beta: Structural features and mechanisms of activation. *Kidney Int* 51: 1376–1382

38  Lyons RM, Gentry LE, Purchio AF, Moses HL (1990) Mechanism of activation of latent recombinant transforming growth factor-beta-1 by plasmin. *J Cell Biol* 110: 1361–1367

39  Abe M, Oda N, Sato Y (1998) Cell-associated activation of latent transforming growth factor-beta by calpain. *J Cell Physiol* 174: 186–193

40  Crawford SE, Stellmach V, Murphy-Ullrich JE, Ribeiro SM, Lawler J, Hynes RO, Boivin GP, Bouck N (1998) Thrombospondin-1 is a major activator of TGF-beta1 *in vivo*. *Cell* 93: 1159–1170

41  Schultz-Cherry S, Murphy-Ullrich JE (1993) Thrombospondin causes activation of latent transforming growth factor-beta secreted by endothelial cells by a novel mechanism. *J Cell Biol* 122: 923–932

42  Grainger DJ, Frow EK (2000) Thrombospondin-1 does not activate transforming growth factor-β1 in a chemically defined system or in smooth muscle cell cultures. *Biochem J* 350: 291–298

43  Paralkar VM, Vukicevic S, Reddi AH (1991) Transforming growth factor beta type 1 binds to collagen IV of basement membrane matrix: implications for development. *Dev Biol* 143: 303–308

44  Grainger DJ, Byrne CD, Witchell CM, Metcalfe JC (1997) Transforming growth factor beta is sequestered into an inactive pool by lipoproteins. *J Lipid Res* 38: 2344–2352

45  Taipale J, Lohi J, Saarinen J, Kovanen PT, Keski-Oja J (1995) Human mast cell chymase and leukocyte elastase release latent transforming growth factor-beta 1 from the extracellular matrix of cultured human epithelial and endothelial cells. *J Biol Chem* 270: 4689–4696

46  Imai K, Hiramatsu A, Fukushima D, Pierschbacher MD, Okada Y (1997) Degradation of decorin by matrix metalloproteinases: identification of the cleavage sites, kinetic analyses and transforming growth factor-beta1 release. *Biochem J* 322: 809–814

47  Kolodziejczyk SM, Hall BK (1996) Signal transduction and TGF-beta superfamily receptors. *Biochem Cell Biol* 74: 299–314

48  Derynck R, Feng XH (1997) TGF-beta receptor signaling. *Biochim Biophys Acta* 1333: F105–150

49  Wrana JL, Attisano L, Carcamo J, Zentella A, Doody J, Laiho M, Wang XF, Massagué J (1992) TGF beta signals through a heteromeric protein kinase receptor complex. *Cell* 71: 1003–1014

50  Massagué J (1998) TGF-beta signal transduction. *Annu Rev Biochem* 67: 753–791

51  López-Casillas F, Wrana JL, Massagué J (1993) Betaglycan presents ligand to the TGF-beta signaling receptor. *Cell* 73: 1435–1444

52  Letamendia A, Lastres P, Botella LM, Raab U, Langa C, Velasco B, Attisano L, Bernabeu C (1998) Role of endoglin in cellular responses to transforming growth factor-beta. A comparative study with betaglycan. *J Biol Chem* 273: 33011–33019

53  O'Grady P, Liu Q, Huang SS, Huang JS (1992) Transforming growth factor beta (TGF-beta) type V receptor has a TGF-beta-stimulated serine/threonine-specific autophosphorylation activity. *J Biol Chem* 267: 21033–21037

54  Hoodless PA, Haerry T, Abdollah S, Stapleton M, O'Connor MB, Attisano L, Wrana JL

(1996) MADR1, a MAD-related protein that functions in BMP2 signaling pathways. *Cell* 85: 489–500

55  Baker JC, Harland RM (1996) A novel mesoderm inducer, Madr2, functions in the activin signal transduction pathway. *Genes Dev* 10: 1880–1889

56  Liu F, Pouponnot C, Massagué J (1997) Dual role of the Smad4/DPC4 tumor suppressor in TGFbeta-inducible transcriptional complexes. *Genes Dev* 11: 3157–3167

57  Chen X, Weisberg E, Fridmacher V, Watanabe M, Naco G, Whitman M (1997) Smad4 and FAST-1 in the assembly of activin-responsive factor. *Nature* 389: 85–89

58  Hayashi H, Abdollah S, Qiu Y, Cai J, Xu YY, Grinnell BW, Richardson MA, Topper JN, Gimbrone MA Jr., Wrana JL et al (1997) The MAD-related protein Smad7 associates with the TGFbeta receptor and functions as an antagonist of TGFbeta signaling. *Cell* 89: 1165–1173

59  Hata A, Lagna G, Massagué J, Hemmati-Brivanlou A (1998) Smad6 inhibits BMP/Smad1 signaling by specifically competing with the Smad4 tumor suppressor. *Genes Dev* 12: 186–197

60  Lohr JL, Danos MC, Groth TW, Yost HJ (1998) Maintenance of asymmetric nodal expression in *Xenopus laevis*. *Dev Genet* 23: 194–202

61  Oh SP, Li E (1997) The signaling pathway mediated by the type IIB activin receptor controls axial patterning and lateral asymmetry in the mouse. *Genes Dev* 11: 1812–1826

62  Collignon J, Varlet I, Robertson EJ (1996) Relationship between asymmetric nodal expression and the direction of embryonic turning. *Nature* 381: 155–158

63  Meno C, Saijoh Y, Fujii H, Ikeda M, Yokoyama T, Yokoyama M, Toyoda Y, Hamada H (1996) Left-right asymmetric expression of the TGF beta-family member lefty in mouse embryos. *Nature* 381: 151–155

64  Meno C, Shimono A, Saijoh Y, Yashiro K, Mochida K, Ohishi S, Noji S, Kondoh H, Hamada H (1998) lefty-1 is required for left-right determination as a regulator of lefty-2 and nodal. *Cell* 94: 287–297

65  Nonaka S, Tanaka Y, Okada Y, Takeda S, Harada A, Kanai Y, Kido M, Hirokawa N (1998) Randomization of left-right asymmetry due to loss of nodal cilia generating leftward flow of extraembryonic fluid in mice lacking KIF3B motor protein. *Cell* 95: 829–837

66  Ohno I, Nitta Y, Yamauchi K, Hoshi H, Honma M, Woolley K, O'Byrne P, Tamura G, Jordana M, Shirato K (1996) Transforming growth factor beta 1 (TGF beta 1) gene expression by eosinophils in asthmatic airway inflammation. *Am J Respir Cell Mol Biol* 15: 404–409

67  Gurdon JB, Harger P, Mitchell A, Lemaire P (1994) Activin signalling and response to a morphogen gradient. *Nature* 371: 487–492

68  Lough J, Barron M, Brogley M, Sugi Y, Bolender DL, Zhu X (1996) Combined BMP-2 and FGF-4, but neither factor alone, induces cardiogenesis in non-precardiac embryonic mesoderm. *Dev Biol* 178: 198–202

69  Shou W, Aghdasi B, Armstrong DL, Guo Q, Bao S, Charng MJ, Mathews LM, Schnei-

der MD, Hamilton SL, Matzuk MM (1998) Cardiac defects and altered ryanodine receptor function in mice lacking FKBP12. *Nature* 391: 489–492

70  Nakajima Y, Yamagishi T, Nakamura H, Markwald RR, Krug EL (1998) An autocrine function for transforming growth factor (TGF)-beta3 in the transformation of atrioventricular canal endocardium into mesenchyme during chick heart development. *Dev Biol* 194: 99–113

71  MacLellan WR, Brand T, Schneider MD (1993) Transforming growth factor-beta in cardiac ontogeny and adaptation. *Circ Res* 73: 783–791

72  Engelmann GL, Grutkoski PS (1994) Coordinate TGF-beta receptor gene expression during rat heart development. *Cell Mol Biol Res* 40: 93–104

73  Diebold RJ, Eis MJ, Yin M, Ormsby I, Boivin GP, Darrow BJ, Saffitz JE, Doetschman T (1995) Early-onset multifocal inflammation in the transforming growth factor beta 1-null mouse is lymphocyte mediated. *Proc Natl Acad Sci USA* 92: 12215–12219

74  Davis LA, Sadler TW (1981) Effects of vitamin A on endocardial cushion development in the mouse heart. *Teratology* 24: 139–148

75  Kastner P, Messaddeq N, Mark M, Wendling O, Grondona JM, Ward S, Ghyselinck N, Chambon P (1997) Vitamin A deficiency and mutations of RXRalpha, RXRbeta and RARalpha lead to early differentiation of embryonic ventricular cardiomyocytes. *Development* 124: 4749–4758

76  Akhurst RJ, Lehnert SA, Faissner A, Duffie E (1990) TGF beta in murine morphogenetic processes: the early embryo and cardiogenesis. *Development* 108: 645–656

77  Millan FA, Denhez F, Kondaiah P, Akhurst RJ (1991) Embryonic gene expression patterns of TGF beta 1, beta 2 and beta 3 suggest different developmental functions *in vivo*. *Development* 111: 131–143

78  Mahmood R, Flanders KC, Morriss-Kay GM (1992) Interactions between retinoids and TGF betas in mouse morphogenesis. *Development* 115: 67–74

79  Anderson PA (1989) Maturation and cardiac contractility. *Cardiol Clin* 7: 209–225

80  Engelmann GL, Boehm KD, Birchenall-Roberts MC, Ruscetti FW (1992) Transforming growth factor-beta 1 in heart development. *Mech Dev* 38: 85–97

81  Kocher O, Madri JA (1989) Modulation of actin mRNAs in cultured vascular cells by matrix components and TGF-beta 1. *In Vitro Cell Dev Biol* 25: 424–434

82  Hales AM, Schulz MW, Chamberlain CG, McAvoy JW (1994) TGF-beta 1 induces lens cells to accumulate alpha-smooth muscle actin, a marker for subcapsular cataracts. *Curr Eye Res* 13: 885–890

83  Grace AA, Grainger DJ, Mao L, Ross J, Chien KR (1996) RXR-alpha dependent signalling pathways are required for the activation of TGF-beta during cardiac growth and hypertrophy. *Circulation* 94: 3229

84  Guyton AC (1991) *Textbook of medical physiology*. W.B. Saunders, London

85  Hautmann MB, Madsen CS, Owens GK (1997) A transforming growth factor beta (TGFbeta) control element drives TGFbeta-induced stimulation of smooth muscle alpha-actin gene expression in concert with two CArG elements. *J Biol Chem* 272: 10948–10956

86  Wang T, Li BY, Danielson PD, Shah PC, Rockwell S, Lechleider RJ, Martin J, Manganaro T, Donahoe PK (1996) The immunophilin FKBP12 functions as a common inhibitor of the TGF beta family type I receptors. *Cell* 86: 435–444

87  Geisterfer-Lowrance AA, Kass S, Tanigawa G, Vosberg HP, McKenna W, Seidman CE, Seidman JG (1990) A molecular basis for familial hypertrophic cardiomyopathy: a beta cardiac myosin heavy chain gene missense mutation. *Cell* 62: 999–1006

88  Grainger DJ, Metcalfe JC, Grace AA, Mosedale DE (1998) Transforming growth factor-beta dynamically regulates vascular smooth muscle differentiation *in vivo. J Cell Sci* 111: 2977–2988

89  Rockman HA, Wachhorst SP, Mao L, Ross J Jr (1994) ANG II receptor blockade prevents ventricular hypertrophy and ANF gene expression with pressure overload in mice. *Am J Physiol* 266: H2468–2475

90  Takahashi N, Calderone A, Izzo NJ, Jr., Maki TM, Marsh JD, Colucci WS (1994) Hypertrophic stimuli induce transforming growth factor-beta 1 expression in rat ventricular myocytes. *J Clin Invest* 94: 1470–1476

91  Villarreal FJ, Dillmann WH (1992) Cardiac hypertrophy-induced changes in mRNA levels for TGF-beta 1, fibronectin, and collagen. *Am J Physiol* 262: H1861–1866

92  Wunsch M, Sharma HS, Markert T, Bernotat-Danielowski S, Schott RJ, Kremer P, Bleese N, Schaper W (1991) In situ localization of transforming growth factor beta 1 in porcine heart: enhanced expression after chronic coronary artery constriction. *J Mol Cell Cardiol* 23: 1051–1062

93  Nishikawa K (1998) Angiotensin AT1 receptor antagonism and protection against cardiovascular end-organ damage. *J Hum Hypertens* 12: 301–309

94  Hudlicka O, Brown MD (1996) Postnatal growth of the heart and its blood vessels. *J Vasc Res* 33: 266–287

95  Li RK, Li G, Mickle DA, Weisel RD, Merante F, Luss H, Rao V, Christakis GT, Williams WG (1997) Overexpression of transforming growth factor-beta1 and insulin-like growth factor-I in patients with idiopathic hypertrophic cardiomyopathy. *Circulation* 96: 874–881

96  Patel B, Khaliq A, Jarvis-Evans J, McLeod D, Mackness M, Boulton M (1994) Oxygen regulation of TGF-beta 1 mRNA in human hepatoma (Hep G2) cells. *Biochem Mol Biol Int* 34: 639–644

97  Behzadian MA, Wang XL, Shabrawey M, Caldwell RB (1998) Effects of hypoxia on glial cell expression of angiogenesis-regulating factors VEGF and TGF-beta. *Glia* 24: 216–225

98  Vodovotz Y, Geiser AG, Chesler L, Letterio JJ, Campbell A, Lucia MS, Sporn MB, Roberts AB (1996) Spontaneously increased production of nitric oxide and aberrant expression of the inducible nitric oxide synthase *in vivo* in the transforming growth factor beta 1 null mouse. *J Exp Med* 183: 2337–2342

99  Vodovotz Y (1997) Control of nitric oxide production by transforming growth factor-beta1: mechanistic insights and potential relevance to human disease. *Nitric Oxide* 1: 3–17

100 Yamamoto K, Dang QN, Kelly RA, Lee RT (1998) Mechanical strain suppresses inducible nitric-oxide synthase in cardiac myocytes. *J Biol Chem* 273: 11862–11866

101 Ying WZ, Sanders PW (1998) Dietary salt enhances glomerular endothelial nitric oxide synthase through TGF-beta1. *Am J Physiol* 275: F18–24

102 Noden DM (1989) Embryonic origins and assembly of blood vessels. *Am Rev Respir Dis* 140: 1097–1103

103 Poole TJ, Coffin JD (1989) Vasculogenesis and angiogenesis: two distinct morphogenetic mechanisms establish embryonic vascular pattern. *J Exp Zool* 251: 224–231

104 Topouzis S, Majesky MW (1996) Smooth muscle lineage diversity in the chick embryo. Two types of aortic smooth muscle cell differ in growth and receptor-mediated transcriptional responses to transforming growth factor-beta. *Dev Biol* 178: 430–445

105 Pepper MS (1997) Transforming growth factor-beta: vasculogenesis, angiogenesis, and vessel wall integrity. *Cytokine Growth Factor Rev* 8: 21–43

106 Yang EY, Moses HL (1990) Transforming growth factor beta 1-induced changes in cell migration, proliferation, and angiogenesis in the chicken chorioallantoic membrane. *J Cell Biol* 111: 731–741

107 Ribatti D, Vacca A, Roncali L, Dammacco F (1991) Angiogenesis under normal and pathological conditions. *Haematologica* 76: 311–320

108 Fajardo LF, Prionas SD, Kwan HH, Kowalski J, Allison AC (1996) Transforming growth factor beta1 induces angiogenesis *in vivo* with a threshold pattern. *Lab Invest* 74: 600–608

109 Lehnert SA, Akhurst RJ (1988) Embryonic expression pattern of TGF beta type-1 RNA suggests both paracrine and autocrine mechanisms of action. *Development* 104: 263–273

110 Dickson MC, Martin JS, Cousins FM, Kulkarni AB, Karlsson S, Akhurst RJ (1995) Defective haematopoiesis and vasculogenesis in transforming growth factor-beta 1 knock out mice. *Development* 121: 1845–1854

111 Oshima M, Oshima H, Taketo MM (1996) TGF-beta receptor type II deficiency results in defects of yolk sac hematopoiesis and vasculogenesis. *Dev Biol* 179: 297–302

112 Cheifetz S, Bellon T, Cales C, Vera S, Bernabeu C, Massagué J, Letarte M (1992) Endoglin is a component of the transforming growth factor-beta receptor system in human endothelial cells. *J Biol Chem* 267: 19027–19030

113 ten Dijke P, Ichijo H, Franzen P, Schulz P, Saras J, Toyoshima H, Heldin CH, Miyazono K (1993) Activin receptor-like kinases: a novel subclass of cell-surface receptors with predicted serine/threonine kinase activity. *Oncogene* 8: 2879–2887

114 Johnson DW, Berg JN, Baldwin MA, Gallione CJ, Marondel I, Yoon SJ, Stenzel TT, Speer M, Pericak-Vance MA, Diamond A et al (1996) Mutations in the activin receptor-like kinase 1 gene in hereditary haemorrhagic telangiectasia type 2. *Nat Genet* 13: 189–195

115 McAllister KA, Grogg KM, Johnson DW, Gallione CJ, Baldwin MA, Jackson CE, Helmbold EA, Markel DS, McKinnon WC, Murrell J et al (1994) Endoglin, a TGF-beta bind-

ing protein of endothelial cells, is the gene for hereditary haemorrhagic telangiectasia type 1. *Nat Genet* 8: 345–351

116 Shovlin CL (1997) Molecular defects in rare bleeding disorders: hereditary haemorrhagic telangiectasia. *Thromb Haemost* 78: 145–150

117 Norgaard P, Hougaard S, Poulsen HS, Spang-Thomsen M (1995) Transforming growth factor beta and cancer. *Cancer Treat Rev* 21: 367–403

118 Markowitz SD, Roberts AB (1996) Tumor suppressor activity of the TGF-beta pathway in human cancers. *Cytokine Growth Factor Rev* 7: 93–102

119 Choi YH, Choi KC, Park YE (1997) Relationship of transforming growth factor beta 1 to angiogenesis in gastric carcinoma. *J Korean Med Sci* 12: 427–432

120 Wikstrom P, Stattin P, Franck-Lissbrant I, Damber JE, Bergh A (1998) Transforming growth factor beta1 is associated with angiogenesis, metastasis, and poor clinical outcome in prostate cancer. *Prostate* 37: 19–29

121 de Jong JS, van Diest PJ, van der Valk P, Baak JP (1998) Expression of growth factors, growth-inhibiting factors, and their receptors in invasive breast cancer. II: Correlations with proliferation and angiogenesis. *J Pathol* 184: 53–57

122 Kocher O, Skalli O, Cerutti D, Gabbiani F, Gabbiani G (1985) Cytoskeletal features of rat aortic cells during development. An electron microscopic, immunohistochemical, and biochemical study. *Circ Res* 56: 829–838

123 Owens GK, Thompson MM (1986) Developmental changes in isoactin expression in rat aortic smooth muscle cells *in vivo*. Relationship between growth and cytodifferentiation. *J Biol Chem* 261: 13373–13380

124 Seidel CL, Allen JC (1979) Pharmacologic characteristics and actomyosin content of aorta from neonatal rats. *Am J Physiol* 237: C81–86

125 Grainger DJ, Mosedale DE, Metcalfe JC, Bottinger EP (2000) Dietary fat and reduced levels of TGF-beta1 act synergistically to promote activation of the vascular endothelium and formation of vascular lipid lesions. *J Cell Sci* 113: 2355–2361

126 Ohno M, Cooke JP, Dzau VJ, Gibbons GH (1995) Fluid shear-stress induces endothelial transforming growth-factor-beta-1 transcription and production – modulation by potassium channel blockade. *J Clin Invest* 95: 1363–1369

127 Ueba H, Kawakami M, Yaginuma T (1997) Shear stress as an inhibitor of vascular smooth muscle cell proliferation. Role of transforming growth factor-beta 1 and tissue-type plasminogen activator. *Arterioscler Thromb Vasc Biol* 17: 1512–1516

128 Mii S, Ware JA, Kent KC (1993) Transforming growth factor-beta inhibits human vascular smooth muscle cell growth and migration. *Surgery* 114: 464–470

129 Morisaki N, Kawano M, Koyama N, Koshikawa T, Umemiya K, Saito Y, Yoshida S (1991) Effects of transforming growth factor-beta 1 on growth of aortic smooth muscle cells. Influences of interaction with growth factors, cell state, cell phenotype, and cell cycle. *Atherosclerosis* 88: 227–234

130 Grainger DJ, Kemp PR, Witchell CM, Weissberg PL, Metcalfe JC (1994) Transforming growth factor beta decreases the rate of proliferation of rat vascular smooth muscle cells

by extending the G2 phase of the cell cycle and delays the rise in cyclic AMP before entry into M phase. *Biochem J* 299: 227–235

131 RayChaudhury A, D'Amore PA (1991) Endothelial cell regulation by transforming growth factor-beta. *J Cell Biochem* 47: 224–229

132 Lefer AM, Tsao P, Aoki N, Palladino MA Jr (1990) Mediation of cardioprotection by transforming growth factor-beta. *Science* 249: 61–64

133 Risau W (1995) Differentiation of endothelium. *FASEB J* 9: 926–933

134 Pintavorn P, Ballermann BJ (1997) TGF-beta and the endothelium during immune injury. *Kidney Int* 51: 1401–1412

135 Grainger DJ, Metcalfe JC (1997) Transforming growth factor-beta and cardiovascular protection. In: GM Rubanyi, VJ Dzau (eds): *The endothelium in clinical practice. Source and target of novel therapies.* Marcel Dekker, Inc., New York, 203–243

136 Shull MM, Ormsby I, Kier AB, Pawlowski S, Diebold RJ, Yin MY, Allen R, Sidman C, Proetzel G, Calvin D et al (1992) Targeted disruption of the mouse transforming growth factor-beta-1 gene results in multifocal inflammatory disease. *Nature* 359: 693–699

137 Grotendorst GR, Smale G, Pencev D (1989) Production of transforming growth factor beta by human peripheral blood monocytes and neutrophils. *J Cell Physiol* 140: 396–402

138 Rodan GA (1998) Control of bone formation and resorption: biological and clinical perspective. *J Cell Biochem* 31: 55–61

139 Wronski TJ, Cintron M, Doherty AL, Dann LM (1988) Estrogen treatment prevents osteopenia and depresses bone turnover in ovariectomized rats. *Endocrinology* 123: 681–686

140 Black LJ, Sato M, Rowley ER, Magee DE, Bekele A, Williams DC, Cullinan GJ, Bendele R, Kauffman RF, Bensch WR et al (1994) Raloxifene (LY139481 HCI) prevents bone loss and reduces serum cholesterol without causing uterine hypertrophy in ovariectomized rats. *J Clin Invest* 93: 63–69

141 Yang NN, Bryant HU, Hardikar S, Sato M, Galvin RJ, Glasebrook AL, Termine JD (1996) Estrogen and raloxifene stimulate transforming growth factor-beta 3 gene expression in rat bone: a potential mechanism for estrogen- or raloxifene-mediated bone maintenance. *Endocrinology* 137: 2075–2084

142 Awad MR, El-Gamel A, Hasleton P, Turner DM, Sinnott PJ, Hutchinson IV (1998) Genotypic variation in the transforming growth factor-beta1 gene: association with transforming growth factor-beta1 production, fibrotic lung disease, and graft fibrosis after lung transplantation. *Transplantation* 66: 1014–1020

143 Grainger DJ, Heathcote K, Chiano M, Snieder H, Kemp PR, Metcalfe JC, Carter ND and Spector TD (1999) Genetic control of the circulating concentration of transforming growth factor type beta1. *Hum Mol Genet* 8: 93–97

144 Li B, Khanna A, Sharma V, Singh T, Suthanthiran M, August P (1999) TGF-beta1 DNA polymorphisms, protein levels, and blood pressure. *Hypertension* 33: 271–275

145 Cambien F, Ricard S, Troesch A, Mallet C, Généréaz L, Evans A, Arveiler D, Luc G, Ruidavets JB, Poirier O (1996) Polymorphisms of the transforming growth factor-beta

1 gene in relation to myocardial infarction and blood pressure. The Etude Cas-Témoin de l'Infarctus du Myocarde (ECTIM) Study. *Hypertension* 28: 881–887

146 Syrris P, Carter ND, Metcalfe JC, Kemp PR, Grainger DJ, Kaski JC, Crossman DC, Francis SE, Gunn J, Jeffery S et al (1998) Transforming growth factor-beta1 gene polymorphisms and coronary artery disease. *Clin Sci (Colch)* 95: 659–667

147 Yokota M, Ichihara S, Lin TL, Nakashima N, Yamada Y (2000) Association of a T29→C polymorphism of the transforming growth factor-β1 gene with genetic susceptibility to myocardial infarction in Japanese. *Circulation* 101: 2783–2787

148 Langdahl BL, Knudsen JY, Jensen HK, Gregersen N, Eriksen EF (1997) A sequence variation: 713-8delC in the transforming growth factor-beta 1 gene has higher prevalence in osteoporotic women than in normal women and is associated with very low bone mass in osteoporotic women and increased bone turnover in both osteoporotic and normal women. *Bone* 20: 289–294

149 Hobbs K, Negri J, Klinnert M, Rosenwasser LJ, Borish L (1998) Interleukin-10 and transforming growth factor-beta promoter polymorphisms in allergies and asthma. *Am J Respir Crit Care Med* 158: 1958–1962

150 Grainger DJ, Kemp PR, Metcalfe JC, Liu AC, Lawn RM, Williams NR, Grace AA, Schofield PM, Chauhan A (1995) The serum concentration of active transforming growth factor-beta is severely depressed in advanced atherosclerosis. *Nat Med* 1: 74–79

151 Charpentier A, Groves S, Simmons-Menchaca M, Turley J, Zhao B, Sanders BG, Kline K (1993) RRR-alpha-tocopheryl succinate inhibits proliferation and enhances secretion of transforming growth factor-beta (TGF-beta) by human breast cancer cells. *Nutr Cancer* 19: 225–239

152 Turley JM, Funakoshi S, Ruscetti FW, Kasper J, Murphy WJ, Longo DL, Birchenall-Roberts MC (1995) Growth inhibition and apoptosis of RL human B lymphoma cells by vitamin E succinate and retinoic acid: role for transforming growth factor beta. *Cell Growth Differ* 6: 655–663

153 Colletta AA, Wakefield LM, Howell FV, van Roozendaal KE, Danielpour D, Ebbs SR, Sporn MB, Baum M (1990) Anti-oestrogens induce the secretion of active transforming growth factor beta from human fetal fibroblasts. *Br J Cancer* 62: 405–409

154 Grainger DJ, Weissberg PL, Metcalfe JC (1993) Tamoxifen decreases the rate of proliferation of rat vascular smooth-muscle cells in culture by inducing production of transforming growth factor beta. *Biochem J* 294: 109–112

155 Grainger DJ, Metcalfe JC (1996) Tamoxifen: teaching an old drug new tricks? *Nat Med* 2: 381–385

156 Nakajima Y, Miyazono K, Kato M, Takase M, Yamagishi T, Nakamura H (1997) Extracellular fibrillar structure of latent TGF beta binding protein-1: role in TGF beta-dependent endothelial-mesenchymal transformation during endocardial cushion tissue formation in mouse embryonic heart. *J Cell Biol* 136: 193–204

157 Sinha S, Nevett C, Shuttleworth CA, Kielty CM (1998) Cellular and extracellular biology of the latent transforming growth factor-beta binding proteins. *Matrix Biol* 17: 529–545

158 Nakajima Y, Miyazono K, Nakamura H (1999) Immunolocalization of latent transforming growth factor-beta binding protein-1 (LTBP1) during mouse development: possible roles in epithelial and mesenchymal cytodifferentiation. *Cell Tissue Res* 295: 257–267

159 Pedrozo HA, Schwartz Z, Gomez R, Ornoy A, Xin-Sheng W, Dallas SL, Bonewald LF, Dean DD, Boyan BD (1998) Growth plate chondrocytes store latent transforming growth factor (TGF)-beta 1 in their matrix through latent TGF-beta 1 binding protein-1. *J Cell Physiol* 177: 343–354

160 Dietz HC, Cutting GR, Pyeritz RE, Maslen CL, Sakai LY, Corson GM, Puffenberger EG, Hamosh A, Nanthakumar EJ, Curristin SM et al (1991) Marfan syndrome caused by a recurrent de novo missense mutation in the fibrillin gene. *Nature* 352: 337–339

161 Green MC, Sweet HO, Bunker LE (1976) Tight-skin, a new mutation of the mouse causing excessive growth of connective tissue and skeleton. *Am J Pathol* 82: 493–512

162 Siracusa LD, McGrath R, Ma Q, Moskow JJ, Manne J, Christner PJ, Buchberg AM, Jimenez SA (1996) A tandem duplication within the fibrillin 1 gene is associated with the mouse tight skin mutation. *Genome Res* 6: 300–313

163 Kielty CM, Raghunath M, Siracusa LD, Sherratt MJ, Peters R, Shuttleworth CA, Jimenez SA (1998) The Tight skin mouse: demonstration of mutant fibrillin-1 production and assembly into abnormal microfibrils. *J Cell Biol* 140: 1159–1166

164 Byrne CD, Wareham NJ, Martensz ND, Humphries SE, Metcalfe JC, Grainger DJ (1998) Increased PAI activity and PAI-1 antigen occurring with an oral fat load: associations with PAI-1 genotype and plasma active TGF-beta levels. *Atherosclerosis* 140: 45–53

165 Sato Y, Tsuboi R, Lyons R, Moses H, Rifkin DB (1990) Characterization of the activation of latent TGF-beta by co-cultures of endothelial cells and pericytes or smooth muscle cells: a self-regulating system. *J Cell Biol* 111: 757–763

166 Kojima S, Vernooy R, Moscatelli D, Amanuma H, Rifkin DB (1995) Lipopolysaccharide inhibits activation of latent transforming growth factor-beta in bovine endothelial cells. *J Cell Physiol* 163: 210–219

167 Nackman GB, Bech FR, Fillinger MF, Wagner RJ, Cronenwett JL (1996) Endothelial cells modulate smooth muscle cell morphology by inhibition of transforming growth factor-beta 1 activation. *Surgery* 120: 418–425; discussion 425–426

168 Rifkin DB, Mazzieri R, Munger JS, Noguera I, Sung J (1999) Proteolytic control of growth factor availability. *Apmis* 107: 80–85

169 Dawson S, Hamsten A, Wiman B, Henney A, Humphries S (1991) Genetic variation at the plasminogen activator inhibitor-1 locus is associated with altered levels of plasma plasminogen activator inhibitor-1 activity. *Arterioscler Thromb* 11: 183–190

170 Lundgren CH, Brown SL, Nordt TK, Sobel BE, Fujii S (1996) Elaboration of type-1 plasminogen activator inhibitor from adipocytes. A potential pathogenetic link between obesity and cardiovascular disease. *Circulation* 93: 106–110

171 Shimomura I, Funahashi T, Takahashi M, Maeda K, Kotani K, Nakamura T, Yamashita

S, Miura M, Fukuda Y, Takemura K et al (1996) Enhanced expression of PAI-1 in visceral fat: possible contributor to vascular disease in obesity. *Nat Med* 2: 800–803

172  Alessi MC, Peiretti F, Morange P, Henry M, Nalbone G, Juhan-Vague I (1997) Production of plasminogen activator inhibitor 1 by human adipose tissue: possible link between visceral fat accumulation and vascular disease. *Diabetes* 46: 860–867

173  Woodhouse PR, Meade TW, Khaw KT (1997) Plasminogen activator inhibitor-1, the acute phase response and vitamin C. Atherosclerosis 133: 71–76

174  Mehta JL, Saldeen TG, Rand K (1998) Interactive role of infection, inflammation and traditional risk factors in atherosclerosis and coronary artery disease. *J Am Coll Cardiol* 31: 1217–1225

175  Kojima S, Harpel PC, Rifkin DB (1991) Lipoprotein (a) inhibits the generation of transforming growth factor beta: an endogenous inhibitor of smooth muscle cell migration. *J Cell Biol* 113: 1439–1445

176  Grainger DJ, Kirschenlohr HL, Metcalfe JC, Weissberg PL, Wade DP, Lawn RM (1993) Proliferation of human smooth muscle cells promoted by lipoprotein(a). *Science* 260: 1655–1658

177  Miyata M, Biro S, Kaieda H, Tanaka H (1995) Lipoprotein(a) stimulates the proliferation of cultured human arterial smooth muscle cells through two pathways. *FEBS Lett* 377: 493–496

178  Sato Y, Kobori S, Sakai M, Yano T, Higashi T, Matsumura T, Morikawa W, Terano T, Miyazaki A, Horiuchi S et al (1996) Lipoprotein(a) induces cell growth in rat peritoneal macrophages through inhibition of transforming growth factor-beta activation. *Atherosclerosis* 125: 15–26

179  Grainger DJ, Kemp PR, Liu AC, Lawn RM, Metcalfe JC (1994) Activation of transforming growth factor-beta is inhibited in transgenic apolipoprotein(a) mice. *Nature* 370: 460–462

180  Lawn RM, Pearle AD, Kunz LL, Rubin EM, Reckless J, Metcalfe JC, Grainger DJ (1996) Feedback mechanism of focal vascular lesion formation in transgenic apolipoprotein(a) mice. *J Biol Chem* 271: 31367–31371

181  Carmeliet P, Collen D (1998) Development and disease in proteinase-deficient mice: role of the plasminogen, matrix metalloproteinase and coagulation system. *Thromb Res* 91: 255–285

182  Izumoto S, Arita N, Ohnishi T, Hiraga S, Taki T, Tomita N, Ohue M, Hayakawa T (1997) Microsatellite instability and mutated type II transforming growth factor-beta receptor gene in gliomas. *Cancer Lett* 112: 251–256

183  Goggins M, Shekher M, Turnacioglu K, Yeo CJ, Hruban RH, Kern SE (1998) Genetic alterations of the transforming growth factor beta receptor genes in pancreatic and biliary adenocarcinomas. *Cancer Res* 58: 5329–5332

184  Markowitz S, Wang J, Myeroff L, Parsons R, Sun L, Lutterbaugh J, Fan RS, Zborowska E, Kinzler KW, Vogelstein B et al (1995) Inactivation of the type II TGF-beta receptor in colon cancer cells with microsatellite instability. *Science* 268: 1336–1338

185  McCaffrey TA, Du B, Consigli S, Szabo P, Bray PJ, Hartner L, Weksler BB, Sanborn TA,

Bergman G, Bush HL Jr (1997) Genomic instability in the type II TGF-beta1 receptor gene in atherosclerotic and restenotic vascular cells. *J Clin Invest* 100: 2182–2188

186  McCaffrey TA, Consigli S, Du B, Falcone DJ, Sanborn TA, Spokojny AM, Bush HL, Jr. (1995) Decreased type II/type I TGF-beta receptor ratio in cells derived from human atherosclerotic lesions. Conversion from an antiproliferative to profibrotic response to TGF-beta1. *J Clin Invest* 96: 2667–2675

187  Li G, Li RK, Mickle DA, Weisel RD, Merante F, Ball WT, Christakis GT, Cusimano RJ, Williams WG (1998) Elevated insulin-like growth factor-I and transforming growth factor-beta 1 and their receptors in patients with idiopathic hypertrophic obstructive cardiomyopathy. A possible mechanism. *Circulation* 98: II 144–149

188  Wang T, Donahoe PK, Zervos AS (1994) Specific interaction of type I receptors of the TGF-beta family with the immunophilin FKBP-12. *Science* 265: 674–676

189  Topper JN, Cai J, Qiu Y, Anderson KR, Xu YY, Deeds JD, Feeley R, Gimeno CJ, Woolf EA, Tayber O et al (1997) Vascular MADs: two novel MAD-related genes selectively inducible by flow in human vascular endothelium. *Proc Natl Acad Sci USA* 94: 9314–9319

190  Schwartz C, Mitchell J (1962) Observations on the localisation of arterial plaques. *Circ Res* 11: 63–73

191  Friedman MH, Brinkman AM, Qin JJ, Seed WA (1993) Relation between coronary artery geometry and the distribution of early sudanophilic lesions. *Atherosclerosis* 98: 193–199

192  Davies MJ, McKenna WJ (1995) Hypertrophic cardiomyopathy – pathology and pathogenesis. *Histopathology* 26: 493–500

193  Towbin JA (1998) The role of cytoskeletal proteins in cardiomyopathies. *Curr Opin Cell Biol* 10: 131–139

194  Bonne G, Carrier L, Richard P, Hainque B, Schwartz K (1998) Familial hypertrophic cardiomyopathy: from mutations to functional defects. *Circ Res* 83: 580–593

195  Schlüter KD, Zhou XJ, Piper HM (1995) Induction of hypertrophic responsiveness to isoproterenol by TGF-beta in adult rat cardiomyocytes. *Am J Physiol* 269: C1311–1316

196  Gray MO, Long CS, Kalinyak JE, Li HT, Karliner JS (1998) Angiotensin II stimulates cardiac myocyte hypertrophy *via* paracrine release of TGF-beta 1 and endothelin-1 from fibroblasts. *Cardiovasc Res* 40: 352–363

197  Everett AD, Tufro-McReddie A, Fisher A, Gomez RA (1994) Angiotensin receptor regulates cardiac hypertrophy and transforming growth factor-beta 1 expression. *Hypertension* 23: 587–592

198  Li JM, Brooks G (1997) Differential protein expression and subcellular distribution of TGFbeta1, beta2 and beta3 in cardiomyocytes during pressure overload-induced hypertrophy. *J Mol Cell Cardiol* 29: 2213–2224

199  Iwai N, Shimoike H, Kinoshita M (1995) Genes up-regulated in hypertrophied ventricle. *Biochem Biophys Res Commun* 209: 527–534

200  Nunes I, Gleizes PE, Metz CN, Rifkin DB (1997) Latent transforming growth factor-

beta binding protein domains involved in activation and transglutaminase-dependent cross-linking of latent transforming growth factor-beta. *J Cell Biol* 136: 1151–1163

201 Sun Y, Zhang JQ, Zhang J, Ramires FJ (1998) Angiotensin II, transforming growth factor-beta1 and repair in the infarcted heart. *J Mol Cell Cardiol* 30: 1559–1569

202 Hao J, Ju H, Zhao S, Junaid A, Fleur TS, Dixon IM (1999) Elevation of expression of Smads 2, 3, and 4, decorin and TGF-beta in the chronic phase of myocardial infarct scar healing. *J Mol Cell Cardiol* 31: 667–678

203 Yue P, Massie BM, Simpson PC, Long CS (1998) Cytokine expression increases in non-myocytes from rats with postinfarction heart failure. *Am J Physiol* 275: H250–258

204 Sekiguchi M, Yu ZX, Hasumi M, Hiroe M, Morimoto S, Nishikawa T (1985) Histopathologic and ultrastructural observations of acute and convalescent myocarditis: a serial endomyocardial biopsy study. *Heart Vessels* 1: 143–153

205 Okada R, Kawai S, Kasyuya H (1989) Nonspecific myocarditis: a statistical and clinicopathological study of autopsy cases. *Jpn Circ J* 53: 40–48

206 Clowes GH, Jr., Farrington GH, Zuschneid W, Cossette GR, Saravis C (1970) Circulating factors in the etiology of pulmonary insufficiency and right heart failure accompanying severe sepsis (peritonitis). *Ann Surg* 171: 663–678

207 Ross R (1993) The pathogenesis of atherosclerosis: a perspective for the 1990s. *Nature* 362: 801–809

208 Assoian RK, Sporn MB (1986) Type beta transforming growth factor in human platelets: release during platelet degranulation and action on vascular smooth muscle cells. *J Cell Biol* 102: 1217–1223

209 Battegay EJ, Raines EW, Seifert RA, Bowen-Pope DF, Ross R (1990) TGF-beta induces bimodal proliferation of connective tissue cells *via* complex control of an autocrine PDGF loop. *Cell* 63: 515–524

210 Stouffer GA, LaMarre J, Gonias SL, Owens GK (1993) Activated alpha 2-macroglobulin and transforming growth factor-beta 1 induce a synergistic smooth muscle cell proliferative response. *J Biol Chem* 268: 18340–18344

211 Grainger DJ, Witchell CM, Weissberg PL, Metcalfe JC (1994) Mitogens for adult rat aortic vascular smooth muscle cells in serum-free primary culture. *Cardiovasc Res* 28: 1238–1242

212 Owens GK, Geisterfer AA, Yang YW, Komoriya A (1988) Transforming growth factor-beta-induced growth inhibition and cellular hypertrophy in cultured vascular smooth muscle cells. *J Cell Biol* 107: 771–780

213 Björkerud S (1991) Effects of transforming growth factor-beta 1 on human arterial smooth muscle cells *in vitro*. *Arterioscler Thromb* 11: 892–902

214 Kirschenlohr HL, Metcalfe JC, Weissberg PL, Grainger DJ (1995) Proliferation of human aortic vascular smooth muscle cells in culture is modulated by active TGF beta. *Cardiovasc Res* 29: 848–855

215 Nabel EG, Shum L, Pompili VJ, Yang ZY, San H, Shu HB, Liptay S, Gold L, Gordon D, Derynck R et al (1993) Direct transfer of transforming growth factor beta 1 gene into arteries stimulates fibrocellular hyperplasia. *Proc Natl Acad Sci USA* 90: 10759–10763

216 Schulick AH, Taylor AJ, Zuo W, Qiu CB, Dong G, Woodward RN, Agah R, Roberts AB, Virmani R, Dichek DA (1998) Overexpression of transforming growth factor beta1 in arterial endothelium causes hyperplasia, apoptosis, and cartilaginous metaplasia. *Proc Natl Acad Sci USA* 95: 6983–6988

217 de Meyer GR, Bult H (1997) Mechanisms of neointima formation – lessons from experimental models. *Vasc Med* 2: 179–189

218 Breslow JL (1996) Mouse models of atherosclerosis. *Science* 272: 685–688

219 Wolf YG, Rasmussen LM, Ruoslahti E (1994) Antibodies against transforming growth factor-beta 1 suppress intimal hyperplasia in a rat model. *J Clin Invest* 93: 1172–1178

220 Kanzaki T, Tamura K, Takahashi K, Saito Y, Akikusa B, Oohashi H, Kasayuki N, Ueda M, Morisaki N (1995) *In vivo* effect of TGF-beta 1. Enhanced intimal thickening by administration of TGF-beta 1 in rabbit arteries injured with a balloon catheter. *Arterioscler Thromb Vasc Biol* 15: 1951–1957

221 Grainger DJ, Witchell CM, Metcalfe JC (1995) Tamoxifen elevates transforming growth factor-beta and suppresses diet-induced formation of lipid lesions in mouse aorta. *Nat Med* 1: 1067–1073

222 Reckless J, Metcalfe JC, Grainger DJ (1997) Tamoxifen decreases cholesterol sevenfold and abolishes lipid lesion development in apolipoprotein E knockout mice. *Circulation* 95: 1542–1548

223 Perez-Perez GI, Shepherd VL, Morrow JD, Blaser MJ (1995) Activation of human THP-1 cells and rat bone marrow-derived macrophages by Helicobacter pylori lipopolysaccharide. *Infect Immun* 63: 1183–1187

224 Schneiderman J, Sawdey MS, Keeton MR, Bordin GM, Bernstein EF, Dilley RB, Loskutoff DJ (1992) Increased type 1 plasminogen activator inhibitor gene expression in atherosclerotic human arteries. *Proc Natl Acad Sci USA* 89: 6998–7002

225 Soeda S, Tsunoda T, Kurokawa Y, Shimeno H (1998) Tumor necrosis factor-alpha-induced release of plasminogen activator inhibitor-1 from human umbilical vein endothelial cells: involvement of intracellular ceramide signaling event. *Biochim Biophys Acta* 1448: 37–45

226 Gu L, Okada Y, Clinton SK, Gerard C, Sukhova GK, Libby P, Rollins BJ (1998) Absence of monocyte chemoattractant protein-1 reduces atherosclerosis in low density lipoprotein receptor-deficient mice. *Mol Cell* 2: 275–281

227 Boring L, Gosling J, Cleary M, Charo IF (1998) Decreased lesion formation in CCR2–/– mice reveals a role for chemokines in the initiation of atherosclerosis. *Nature* 394: 894–897

228 Shah PK, Falk E, Badimon JJ, Fernandez-Ortiz A, Mailhac A, Villareal-Levy G, Fallon JT, Regnstrom J, Fuster V (1995) Human monocyte-derived macrophages induce collagen breakdown in fibrous caps of atherosclerotic plaques. Potential role of matrix-degrading metalloproteinases and implications for plaque rupture. *Circulation* 92: 1565–1569

229 Libby P, Geng YJ, Aikawa M, Schoenbeck U, Mach F, Clinton SK, Sukhova GK, Lee RT (1996) Macrophages and atherosclerotic plaque stability. *Curr Opin Lipidol* 7: 330–335

230 Wurdeman RL, Hilleman DE, Mooss AN (1998) Restenosis, the Achilles' heel of coronary angioplasty. *Pharmacotherapy* 18: 1024–1040

231 Schwartz RS (1998) Pathophysiology of restenosis: interaction of thrombosis, hyperplasia, and/or remodeling. *Am J Cardiol* 81: 14E–17E

232 Majesky MW, Lindner V, Twardzik DR, Schwartz SM, Reidy MA (1991) Production of transforming growth factor-beta-1 during repair of arterial injury. *J Clin Invest* 88: 904–910

233 Grant MB, Wargovich TJ, Bush DM, Player DW, Caballero S, Foegh M, Spoerri PE (1999) Expression of IGF-1, IGF-1 receptor and TGF-beta following balloon angioplasty in atherosclerotic and normal rabbit iliac arteries: an immunocytochemical study. *Regul Pept* 79: 47–53

234 Kosuga K, Tamai H, Ueda K, Hsu YS, Ono S, Tanaka S, Doi T, Myou UW, Motohara S, Uehata H (1997) Effectiveness of tranilast on restenosis after directional coronary atherectomy. *Am Heart J* 134: 712–718

235 Ward MR, Sasahara T, Agrotis A, Dilley RJ, Jennings GL, Bobik A (1998) Inhibitory effects of tranilast on expression of transforming growth factor-beta isoforms and receptors in injured arteries. *Atherosclerosis* 137: 267–275

236 Nikol S, Isner JM, Pickering JG, Kearney M, Leclerc G, Weir L (1992) Expression of transforming growth factor-beta 1 is increased in human vascular restenosis lesions. *J Clin Invest* 90: 1582–1592

237 Nikol S, Weir L, Sullivan A, Sharaf B, White CJ, Zemel G, Hartzler G, Stack R, Leclerc G, Isner JM (1994) Persistently increased expression of the transforming growth-factor-beta-1 gene in human vascular restenosis – analysis of 62 patients with one or more episode of restenosis. *Cardiovasc Pathol* 3: 57–64

238 O'Brien ER, Bennett KL, Garvin MR, Zderic TW, Hinohara T, Simpson JB, Kimura T, Nobuyoshi M, Mizgala H, Purchio A et al (1996) Beta ig-h3, a transforming growth factor-beta-inducible gene, is overexpressed in atherosclerotic and restenotic human vascular lesions. *Arterioscler Thromb Vasc Biol* 16: 576–584

239 Frater-Schroder M, Muller G, Birchmeier W, Bohlen P (1986) Transforming growth factor-beta inhibits endothelial cell proliferation. *Biochem Biophys Res Commun* 137: 295–302

240 Lehmann-Bruinsma K, Higley H, Powell JS (1994) Transforming growth factor-beta(2) (TGF-beta(2)) suppression of smooth-muscle cell (SMC) proliferation after balloon angioplasty of rat carotid arteries. *Clin Res* 42: A4

241 Swales J (1994) Textbook of hypertension. Blackwell Scientific, Oxford

242 Lee R, Forrest JB, Garfield RE, Daniel EE (1983) Ultrastructural-changes in mesenteric-arteries from spontaneously hypertensive rats – a morphometric study. *Blood Vessels* 20: 72–91

243 de Mey J, Daemen M, Boonen H, Bosman FT, Dijkstra EH, Fazzi GE, Janssen G, Schiffers P, Struykerboudier H, Vrijdag M (1991) *In vivo* DNA-synthesis is not uniformly increased in arterial smooth-muscle of young spontaneously hypertensive rats. *J Hypertens* 9: 695–701

244 Owens GK (1989) Control of hypertrophic versus hyperplastic growth of vascular smooth-muscle cells. *Am J Physiol* 257: H1755–H1765

245 Agrotis A, Saltis J, Dilley R, Bray P, Bobik A (1995) Transforming growth factor-beta 1 and the development of vascular hypertrophy in hypertension. *Blood Press* (Suppl) 2: 43–48

246 Botney MD, Bahadori L, Gold LI (1994) Vascular remodeling in primary pulmonary hypertension. Potential role for transforming growth factor-beta. *Am J Pathol* 144: 286–295

247 Kim S, Ohta K, Hamaguchi A, Omura T, Yukimura T, Miura K, Inada Y, Wada T, Ishimura Y, Chatani F et al (1994) Contribution of renal angiotensin II type I receptor to gene expressions in hypertension-induced renal injury. *Kidney Int* 46: 1346–1358

248 Tamaki K, Okuda S, Nakayama M, Yanagida T, Fujishima M (1996) Transforming growth factor-beta 1 in hypertensive renal injury in Dahl salt-sensitive rats. *J Am Soc Nephrol* 7: 2578–2589

249 Fukuda N, Kubo A, Izumi Y, Soma M, Kanmatsuse K (1995) Distinct expression of transforming growth factor-beta receptor subtypes on vascular smooth muscle cells from spontaneously hypertensive rats and Wistar-Kyoto rats. *Clin Exp Pharmacol Physiol* (Suppl) 1: S120–122

250 Porreca E, Di Febbo C, Mincione G, Reale M, Baccante G, Guglielmi MD, Cuccurullo F, Colletta G (1997) Increased transforming growth factor-beta production and gene expression by peripheral blood monocytes of hypertensive patients. *Hypertension* 30: 134–139

251 Maron BJ, Moller JH, Seidman CE, Vincent GM, Dietz HC, Moss AJ, Sondheimer HM, Pyeritz RE, McGee G, Epstein AE (1998) Impact of laboratory molecular diagnosis on contemporary diagnostic criteria for genetically transmitted cardiovascular diseases:hypertrophic cardiomyopathy, long-QT syndrome, and Marfan syndrome. *Circulation* 98: 1460–1471

252 Sakai LY, Keene DR (1994) Fibrillin – monomers and microfibrils. *Meth Enzymol* 245: 29–52

253 Zhou J, Mochizuki T, Smeets H, Antignac C, Laurila P, Depaepe A, Tryggvason K, Reeders ST (1993) Deletion of the paired alpha-5(IV) and alpha-6(IV) collagen genes in inherited smooth-muscle tumors. *Science* 261: 1167–1169

254 Sakai LY, Keene DR, Engvall E (1986) Fibrillin, a new 350-kD glycoprotein, is a component of extracellular microfibrils. *J Cell Biol* 103: 2499–2509

255 Karonen T, Jeskanen L, Keski-Oja J (1997) Transforming growth factor beta 1 and its latent form binding protein-1 associate with elastic fibres in human dermis: accumulation in actinic damage and absence in anetoderma. *Br J Dermatol* 137: 51–58

256 Roberts AB, McCune BK, Sporn MB (1992) TGF-beta: regulation of extracellular matrix. *Kidney Int* 41: 557–559

257 Ueki K, Meyer FB, Mellinger JF (1994) Moyamoya disease: the disorder and surgical treatment. *Mayo Clin Proc* 69: 749–757

258 Hosoda Y, Ikeda E, Hirose S (1997) Histopathological studies on spontaneous occlusion

of the circle of Willis (cerebrovascular moyamoya disease). *Clin Neurol Neurosurg* 99 Suppl 2: S203–208

259 von Rokitansky C (1852) Abnormal conditions of the arteries. In: *Manual of pathological anatomy*. Sydenham Society, London, 261–275

260 Fukai N, Aoyagi M, Yamamoto M, Sakamoto H, Ogami K, Matsushima Y, Yamamoto K (1994) Human arterial smooth muscle cell strains derived from patients with moyamoya disease: changes in biological characteristics and proliferative response during cellular aging *in vitro*. *Mech Ageing Dev* 75: 21–33

261 Yamamoto M, Aoyagi M, Fukai N, Matsushima Y, Yamamoto K (1998) Differences in cellular responses to mitogens in arterial smooth muscle cells derived from patients with moyamoya disease. *Stroke* 29: 1188–1193

262 Yamamoto M, Aoyagi M, Tajima S, Wachi H, Fukai N, Matsushima Y, Yamamoto K (1997) Increase in elastin gene expression and protein synthesis in arterial smooth muscle cells derived from patients with Moyamoya disease. *Stroke* 28: 1733–1738

263 Hojo M, Hoshimaru M, Miyamoto S, Taki W, Nagata I, Asahi M, Matsuura N, Ishizaki R, Kikuchi H, Hashimoto N (1998) Role of transforming growth factor-beta1 in the pathogenesis of moyamoya disease. *J Neurosurg* 89: 623–629

264 Yoshimoto T, Houkin K, Takahashi A, Abe H (1996) Angiogenic factors in moyamoya disease. *Stroke* 27: 2160–2165

265 Owens GK (1998) Molecular control of vascular smooth muscle cell differentiation. *Acta Physiol Scand* 164: 623–635

266 MacLellan WR, Lee TC, Schwartz RJ, Schneider MD (1994) Transforming growth factor-beta response elements of the skeletal alpha-actin gene. Combinatorial action of serum response factor, YY1, and the SV40 enhancer-binding protein, TEF-1. *J Biol Chem* 269: 16754–16760

267 Marian AJ (1997) Genetic markers: genes involved in human hypertension. *J Cardiovasc Risk* 4: 341–345

268 Grainger DJ, Metcalfe JC (1995) A pivotal role for TGF-beta in atherogenesis? *Biol Rev Camb Philos Soc* 70: 571–596

269 Merrilees MJ, Scott L (1994) Antisense S-oligonucleotide against transforming growth factor-beta 1 inhibits proteoglycan synthesis in arterial wall. *J Vasc Res* 31: 322–329

270 McDonald CC, Stewart HJ (1991) Fatal myocardial infarction in the Scottish adjuvant tamoxifen trial. The Scottish Breast Cancer Committee. *Br Med J* 303: 435–437

271 McDonald CC, Alexander FE, Whyte BW, Forrest AP, Stewart HJ (1995) Cardiac and vascular morbidity in women receiving adjuvant tamoxifen for breast cancer in a randomised trial. The Scottish Cancer Trials Breast Group. *Br Med J* 311: 977–980

272 Mosedale DE, Metcalfe JC, Grainger DJ (1996) Optimization of immunofluorescence methods by quantitative image analysis. *J Histochem Cytochem* 44: 1043–1050

273 López-Casillas F, Cheifetz S, Doody J, Andres JL, Lane WS, Massagué J (1991) Structure and expression of the membrane proteoglycan betaglycan, a component of the TGF-beta receptor system. *Cell* 67: 785–795

274 Leal SM, Liu Q, Huang SS, Huang JS (1997) The type V transforming growth factor

beta receptor is the putative insulin-like growth factor-binding protein 3 receptor. *J Biol Chem* 272: 20572–20576

275 O'Grady P, Kuo MD, Baldassare JJ, Huang SS, Huang JS (1991) Purification of a new type high-molecular-weight receptor (type-V receptor) of transforming growth-factor-beta (TGF-beta) from bovine liver – identification of the type-V TGF-beta receptor in cultured-cells. *J Biol Chem* 266: 8583–8589

276 Cheifetz S, Ling N, Guillemin R, Massagué J (1988) A surface component on GH3 pituitary cells that recognizes transforming growth factor-beta, activin, and inhibin. *J Biol Chem* 263: 17225–17228

277 Ichijo H, Ronnstrand L, Miyagawa K, Ohashi H, Heldin CH, Miyazono K (1991) Purification of transforming growth factor-beta 1 binding proteins from porcine uterus membranes. *J Biol Chem* 266: 22459–22464

278 Olofsson A, Hellman U, Ten Dijke P, Grimsby S, Ichijo H, Morén A, Miyazono K, Heldin CH (1997) Latent transforming growth factor-beta complex in Chinese hamster ovary cells contains the multifunctional cysteine-rich fibroblast growth factor receptor, also termed E-selectin-ligand or MG-160. *Biochem J* 324: 427–434

279 Hirai R, Kaji K (1992) Transforming growth factor beta 1-specific binding proteins on human vascular endothelial cells. *Exp Cell Res* 201: 119–125

280 MacKay K, Danielpour D (1991) Novel 150- and 180-kDa glycoproteins that bind transforming growth factor (TGF)-beta 1 but not TGF-beta 2 are present in several cell lines. *J Biol Chem* 266: 9907–9911

281 MacKay K (1993) Homodimers of the 60 kDa phosphatidylinositol-anchored transforming growth factor-beta 2 binding proteins in FBHEC and MG-63 cells. *Growth Factors* 8: 187–195

282 Cheifetz S, Massagué J (1991) Isoform-specific transforming growth factor-beta binding proteins with membrane attachments sensitive to phosphatidylinositol-specific phospholipase C. *J Biol Chem* 266: 20767–20772

283 Munger JS, Harpel JG, Giancotti FG, Rifkin DB (1998) Interactions between growth factors and integrins: latent forms of transforming growth factor-beta are ligands for the integrin alphavbeta1. *Mol Biol Cell* 9: 2627–2638

284 Munger JS, Huang X, Kawakatsu H, Griffiths MJ, Dalton SL, Wu J, Pittet JF, Kaminski N, Garat C, Matthay MA et al (1999) The integrin alpha v beta 6 binds and activates latent TGF beta 1: a mechanism for regulating pulmonary inflammation and fibrosis. *Cell* 96: 319–328

285 Takeuchi Y, Kodama Y, Matsumoto T (1994) Bone matrix decorin binds transforming growth factor-beta and enhances its bioactivity. *J Biol Chem* 269: 32634–32638

286 Mooradian DL, Lucas RC, Weatherbee JA, Furcht LT (1989) Transforming growth factor-beta 1 binds to immobilized fibronectin. *J Cell Biochem* 41: 189–200

287 Ichijo H, Hellman U, Wernstedt C, Gonez LJ, Claesson-Welsh L, Heldin CH, Miyazono K (1993) Molecular cloning and characterization of ficolin, a multimeric protein with fibrinogen- and collagen-like domains. *J Biol Chem* 268: 14505–14513

288 Huang SS, O'Grady P, Huang JS (1988) Human transforming growth factor beta.alpha

2-macroglobulin complex is a latent form of transforming growth factor beta. *J Biol Chem* 263: 1535–1541

289 McCaffrey TA, Falcone DJ, Du B (1992) Transforming growth factor-beta 1 is a heparin-binding protein: identification of putative heparin-binding regions and isolation of heparins with varying affinity for TGF-beta 1. *J Cell Physiol* 152: 430–440

290 Murphy-Ullrich JE, Schultz-Cherry S, Hook M (1992) Transforming growth factor-beta complexes with thrombospondin. *Mol Biol Cell* 3: 181–188

291 Philip A, Bostedt L, Stigbrand T, O'Connor-McCourt MD (1994) Binding of transforming growth factor-beta (TGF-beta) to pregnancy zone protein (PZP). Comparison to the TGF-beta-alpha 2-macroglobulin interaction. *Eur J Biochem* 221: 687–693

292 Bodmer S, Podlisny MB, Selkoe DJ, Heid I, Fontana A (1990) Transforming growth factor-beta bound to soluble derivatives of the beta amyloid precursor protein of Alzheimer's disease. *Biochem Biophys Res Commun* 171: 890–897

293 MacKay K, Robbins AR, Bruce MD, Danielpour D (1990) Identification of disulfide-linked transforming growth factor-beta 1-specific binding proteins in rat glomeruli. *J Biol Chem* 265: 9351–9356

294 Olofsson A, Miyazono K, Kanzaki T, Colosetti P, Engström U, Heldin CH (1992) Transforming growth factor-beta 1, -beta 2, and -beta 3 secreted by a human glioblastoma cell line. Identification of small and different forms of large latent complexes. *J Biol Chem* 267: 19482–19488

# Bone morphogenetic proteins and related cytokines

*A. Hari Reddi*

Center for Tissue Regeneration and Repair, and Department of Orthopaedic Surgery, University of California, Davis, Medical Center, Research Bldg. I, Rm. 2000, 4635 Second Avenue, Sacramento, CA 95817, USA

## Introduction

Morphogenesis is the developmental cascade of pattern formation, body plan establishment and interpretation and differentiation of the pattern. Morphogenesis is induced by morphogens. Morphogens are generally first identified in fly and frog embryos by genetic approaches, differential displays, substractive hybridization, expression cloning, and this information is then extended to mice and men. This article will demonstrate an alternative biochemical approach based on the regenerative potential of adult mammalian bone. The principles gleaned from bone induction and bone morphogenetic proteins (BMPs) has been extended to frog mesoderm induction and chick and mouse limb morphogenesis. This accrued knowledge can now be applied in dental surgery and orthopaedic surgery.

Bone grafts have been used by orthopaedic surgeons to aid in the recalcitrant bone repair for many years. Decalcified bone implants have been used to treat patients with osteomyelitis [1]. Lacroix hypothesized that bone contains a substance, osteogenin, that initiates bone growth [2]. Urist made the key discovery that demineralized, lyophilized, segments of rabbit bone when implanted intramuscularly induced new bone formation [3]. Bone induction is a sequential multistep cascade [4–6] that mimics embryonic bone morphogenesis. The key steps in this cascade are chemotaxis, mitosis, and differentiation. Chemotaxis is the directed migration of cells in response to a chemical gradient of signals released from the insoluble demineralized bone matrix. The demineralized bone matrix is predominantly composed of type I insoluble collagen and it binds plasma fibronectin [7]. Fibronectin has domains for binding to collagen, fibrin, and heparin. The responding mesenchymal cells attached to the collagenous matrix and proliferated as indicated by [³H] thymidine autoradiography and incorporation into acid-precipitable DNA [8] on day 3. Chondroblast differentiation was evident on day 5, chondrocytes on days 7–8, and cartilage hypertrophy on day 9. There was concomitant vascular invasion on day 9 with osteoblast differentiation. On days 10–12 alkaline phosphatase was maximal.

TGF-β and Related Cytokines in Inflammation, edited by Samuel N. Breit and Sharon M. Wahl

Osteocalcin, bone γ carboxyglutamic acid containing gla protein (BGP), increased on day 28. Hematopoietic marrow differentiated in the ossicle and was maximal by day 21 (Fig. 1). This entire sequential bone development cascade is reminiscent of cartilage and bone morphogenesis in the limb bud [5, 8]. Hence, it has immense implications for the isolation of inductive signals initiating cartilage and bone morphogenesis. In fact, a systematic investigation of the chemical components responsible for bone induction was undertaken and inductive signals were identified and successfully isolated.

## Isolation of bone morphogenetic proteins

The above account of the demineralized bone matrix-induced bone morphogenesis in extraskeletal sites demonstrated the possible presence of morphogens in the bone matrix. Thus a systematic study of the isolation of putative morphogenetic proteins was initiated. A prerequisite for any quest for novel morphogens is the establishment of a battery of bioassays for bone formation. A panel of *in vitro* assays were established for chemotaxis, mitogenesis, and chondrogenesis, and an *in vivo* assay for osteogenesis. Although the *in vitro* assays are expedient, we monitored routinely a labor-intensive *in vivo* bioassay. It is furthermore the only bona fide bone induction assay.

A major stumbling-block in the approach was that the demineralized bone matrix is insoluble. In view of this, dissociative extractants such as 4 M guanidine HCl or 8 M urea as 1% sodium dodecyl sulfate (SDS) solutions at pH 7.4 were used [9]. Approximately 3% of the proteins were solubilized from demineralized bone matrix, and the remaining residue was mainly insoluble type I bone collagen. The soluble extract alone, or the insoluble residue alone, were incapable of new bone induction. However, addition of the extract to the residue (insoluble collagen) and then implantation in a subcutaneous site resulted in bone induction. Thus, it would appear that for optimal osteogenic activity there was a collaboration between soluble extract and the insoluble collagenous substratum [9]. This bioassay was a useful advance in the final purification of bone morphogenetic proteins (BMPs) and led to determination of limited tryptic peptide sequences leading to the eventual cloning of BMPs [10–12].

In order to scale the procedure up, a switch was made to bovine bone. Demineralized bovine bone was not osteoinductive in rats and the results variable. However, when the guanidine extracts of demineralized bovine bone were fractionated on a S-200 molecular sieve column, fractions containing proteins less than 50 kDa were consistently osteogenic when bioassayed after reconstitution with allogeneic insoluble collagen [13, 14]. Thus, fractions inducing bone are not species-specific and are homologous among mammals. It is likely that larger molecular mass fractions and/or the insoluble xenogeneic (bovine and human) collagens were inhibito-

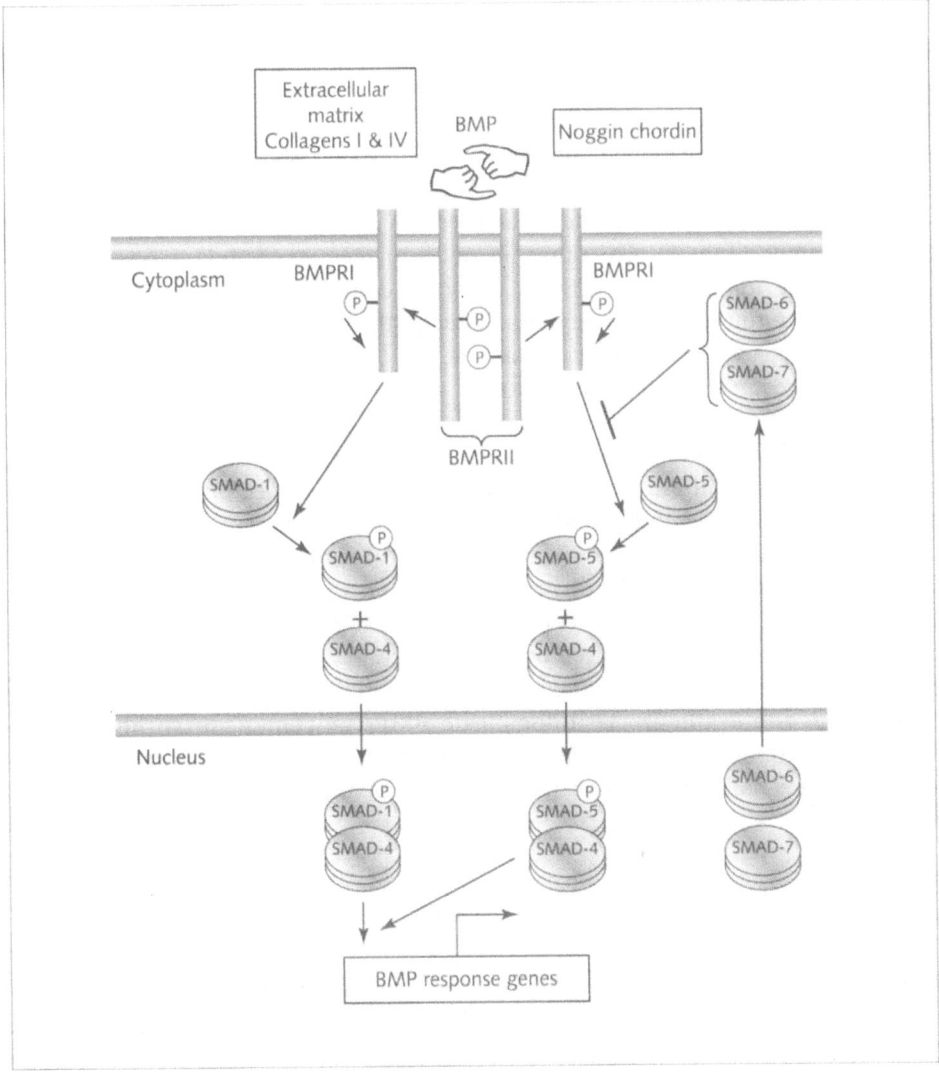

*Figure 1*

*BMP receptors and signalling cascades. BMPs are dimeric signals. Each monomer has two β sheets as in two pointed fingers. BMPs interact with type I and II receptors (BMPR I and II). The oligomeric complex of the BMP receptor is critical for signal transduction. The GS domain of BMPRI is phosphorylated by BMPRII. The activated type I receptor serine/threonine kinase phosphorylates signaling substrates R-Smads 1, 5 or 8. Phosphorylated Smads interact with co-Smad 4 and is translocated from cytoplasm to the nucleus and initiates the transcription BMP-response genes. Inhibitory Smad 6 and 7 inhibit type I receptor mediated phosphorylation of R-Smads 1, 5 and 8.*

ry or immunogenic. Initial estimates revealed that 1 µg of active osteogenic fraction is present in a kilogram of bone. Hence, over a ton of bovine bone was processed to yield optimal amounts for animo acid sequence determination. The amino acid sequences revealed homology to transforming growth factor $\beta_1$ (TGF-$\beta_1$) [14]. The incisive work of Wozney and colleagues cloned BMP-2, BMP-2B (now called BMP-4) and BMP-3 (also called osteogenin). Osteogenic protein-1 and 2 (OP-1 and OP-2) were cloned by Ozkaynak and colleagues [12]. There are nearly 15 members of the BMP family (Tab. 1). The other members of the extended TGF-$\beta$/BMP super-family include inhibins and activins (implicated in follicle stimulating hormone release from pituitary and mesoderm induction), Müllerian duct inhibitory substance (MIS), growth/differentiation factors (GDFs), and nodal [14].

BMPs are dimeric molecules and the conformation is critical for biological actions. Reduction of the single intermolecular disulfide bond resulted in the loss of biological activity. The mature monomer of BMPs consists of about 120 amino acids, with seven canonical cysteine residues. There are three intrachain disulfides and one interchain disulfide bond. The cysteine knot is the critical central core of the BMP molecule. The crystal structure of BMP-7 has been determined [15]. The BMP-7 monomer has $\beta$-pleated sheets in the form of two pointed fingers. In the dimer the pointed fingers are oriented in opposite directions. It is a good possibility that in the very near future, based on ligand-receptor co-crystallography, the receptor contact domains will be defined. Such information will speed up the approaches to design and synthesize peptidomimetic BMPs by combinatorial library techniques using robotic, high-throughput assays. Other innovative approaches include screening for small molecules in natural products and biomimetics and receptor-based assays.

## Cartilage-derived morphogenetic proteins

Morphogenesis of the cartilage is the key rate-limiting step in the dynamics of bone development. Cartilage is the initial model for the architecture of bones. Bone can form either directly from mesenchyme as in intramembranous bone formation observed in limited craniofacial bones or with an intervening cartilage stage as in endochondral bone development [5]. All BMPs first induce the cascade of chondrogenesis, and therefore are cartilage morphogenetic proteins. The hypertrophic chondrocytes in the epiphyseal growth plate mineralize and serves as a template for appositional bone morphogenesis. Cartilage morphogenesis is critical for both bone and joint morphogenesis. The two lineages of cartilage are clear-cut. The first, at the ends of bone, forms articulating articular cartilage. The second is the growth plate chondrocytes which proliferate, mature and hypertrophy, to synthesize cartilage matrix. This is destined to calcify prior to acting as a nidus for replacement by bone and are the "organizer" centers of longitudinal and circumferential growth of carti-

*Table 1 - The BMP family in humans and chromosome location*

| BMP subfamily | Generic name | BMP designation | Chromosome location |
|---|---|---|---|
| BMP 2/4 | BMP-2A | BMP-2 | 20 |
| | BMP-2B | BMP-4 | 14 |
| BMP 3 | Osteogenin | BMP-3 | 4 |
| | Growth/differentiation factor-10 (GDF-10) | BMP-3B | 10 |
| OP-1/BMP7 | BMP-5 | BMP-5 | 6 |
| | Vegetal related-1 (Vgr-1) | BMP-6 | 6 |
| | Osteogenic protein-1 (OP-1) | BMP-7 | 20 |
| | Osteogenic protein-2 (OP-2) | BMP-8 | – |
| | Osteogenic protein-3 (OP-3) | BMP-8B | – |
| Others | BMP-9 | BMP-9 | |
| | BMP-10 | BMP-10 | |
| | Growth/differentiation factor-11 (GDF-11) | BMP-11 | |
| CDMP | Cartilage-derived morphogenetic protein-1 (CDMP-1) | | |
| | Growth/differentiation Factor-5 (GDF-5) | BMP-14 | 20 |
| | Cartilage-derived morphogenetic protein-2 (CDMP-2) | | |
| | Growth/differentiation factor-6 (GDF-6) | BMP-13 | – |
| | Cartilage-derived morphogenetic protein-3 (CDMP-3) | | |
| | Growth/differentiation factor-7 (GDF-7) | BMP-12 | – |
| | BMP-15 | BMP-15 | |

*\*BMP-1 is not a BMP family member with seven canonical cysteines. It is a procollagen-C proteinase related to Drosophila Tolloid and may play a role in modulating BMP actions by proteolysis of BMP antagonists/binding proteins, such as noggin, chordin, and gremlin.*

lage setting into motion the orderly developmental program of endochondral bone formation [5]. The phenotypic stability of the articular (permanent) cartilage is at the crux of the osteoarthritis problem. The "maintenance" factors for articular chondrocytes include TGF-β isoforms and the BMP isoforms.

An *in vivo* chondrogenic bioassay with soluble purified proteins and insoluble collagen identified a chondrogenic fraction in articular cartilage [10]. A concurrent RT-PCR approach with degenerate oligonucleotide primers was undertaken. Two novel genes for cartilage-derived morphogenetic proteins (CDMPs) 1 and 2 were identified and cloned [16]. CDMPs 1 and 2 are also called GDF-5 and GDF-6 (GDF = growth/differentiation factor) [17] and may play a critical role in initiation and maintenance of articular cartilage and joint morphogenesis [16, 17].

## BMPs: pleiotropy and thresholds

Morphogenesis is a sequential multistep cascade. BMPs regulate each of the key steps: chemotaxis, mitosis, and differentiation of cartilage and bone. BMPs initiate chondrogenesis in the limb [18]. The apical ectodermal ridge is the source of BMPs in the developing limb bud. The intricate dynamic, reciprocal interactions between the epithelium and mesenchyme sets into motion the train of events culminating in the pattern formation of digits, radius/ulna and the humerus in the forelimbs.

The chemotaxis of human monocytes is optimal at femtomolar concentration [19]. The apparent affinity was 100–200 pM. The mitogenic response was optimal in the 100 pM range. The initiation of differentiation was in the nanomolar range in solution. However, caution should be exercised as BMPs may be sequestered by extracellular matrix components and the local concentration may be higher when BMPs are bound on the extracellular matrix. Thus, BMPs are pleiotropic regulators that act in a concentration-dependent threshold.

## BMPs bind to extracellular matrix

It is well known that extracellular matrix components play a critical role in morphogenesis. The structural macromolecules and their supramolecular assembly in the extracellular matrix does not explain their role in epithelial-mesenchymal interaction and morphogenesis. This riddle can now be explained by the binding of bone morphogenetic proteins (BMPs) to heparan sulfate, heparin, and type IV collagen [20] of the basement membranes. In fact, this might explain in part the necessity for angiogenesis and vascular invasion into cartilage prior to osteogenesis during development. Dorsal mesoderm induction is modified to neuralization by binding and termination of activin action by follistatin [21]. Similarly, Chordin and Noggin from the Spemann organizer induces neuralization by binding and inactivation of BMP-4. Thus, neural induction is likely to be a default pathway when BMP-4 is rendered non-functional [22, 23]. Hence, an emerging principle in development and morphogenesis is that binding proteins can terminate a dominant morphogen's action and initiate a default developmental pathway. Further, the binding of a soluble morphogen to extracellular matrix (ECM) converts it into an insoluble matrix-bound morphogen which acts locally in the solid state [20] and may protect it from proteolysis and prolong its half-life. In this sense, extracellular matrix is both a structural and functional delivery system for morphogens.

## BMPs: actions beyond bone

Although BMPs were isolated and cloned from bone, recent work with gene knock-outs in mice have revealed a plethora of actions beyond bone. Mice with targeted disruption of BMP-2 caused embryonic lethality. The heart development is abnormal indicating a need for BMP-2 in heart development [24]. BMP-4 "knockouts" exhibit no mesoderm induction and gastrulation is impaired [25]. The targeted deletion of BMP-7 revealed the critical role of this molecule in kidney and eye development [26, 27]. Thus, the BMPs are really true morphogens for such disparate tissues as skin, heart, kidney and eye.

## BMP actions: receptor

Recombinant human BMP-4 binds to two type I receptors, BMPR-IA and BMPR-IB called ALK-3 and ALK-6 (ALK = activin receptor like kinase), respectively [28]. BMP-2, BMP-7 and CDMP-1 (GDF-5) bind to both BMPR-IA and IB. There are two types of BMP receptors, types I and II. Both the receptors are membrane-bound serine/threonine kinases. The type II receptors phosphorylate the type I receptor. The BMP type I receptor kinases phosphorylate the Smads [29]. Smads are related to the *Drosophila Mad (mothers against dpp)* gene and three related nematode genes, *Sma 2, 3* and *4*. The terms Sma and Mad have been fused as Smad to unify the nomenclature. There are eight members in the Smad family and growing. Phosphorylated Smads 1, 5 and 8 are functional mediators of BMP family signaling in partnership with Smad 4. Smads 2 and 3 are signal transducers for the actions of TGF-β and activins. Smad 6 and Smad 7 function as antagonists to inhibit TGF-β/BMP superfamily signaling. The phosphorylated Smad 1 enters as a heteromeric complex with Smad 4 into the nucleus and activates transcription of early response genes [30, 31].

## BMPS: clinical applications

Recombinant human BMP-7 can induce complete regeneration of calvarial bone in baboon, a subhuman primate [32]. Similarly, recombinant human BMP-2 is effective in bone regeneration in an ulnas nonunion model in rabbits [33, 34]. The emerging knowledge in bone morphogenetic proteins has profound impact on the emerging field of tissue engineering, the science of manufacturing spare parts for the human body based on morphogenetic cytokines, extracellular matrix scaffolding and responding stem cells [35]. A prototype paradigm has demonstrated the principle of tissue transformation *in vivo* with applications in orthopaedic, oral and plastic and reconstructive surgery [36].

*Acknolwdgements*
This work is supported by the Lawrence Ellison Chair in Musculoskeletal Molecular Biology. I thank Mrs. Rita Rowlands for her enthusiastic help.

# References

1 Senn N (1889) On the healing of aseptic bone cavities by implantation of antiseptic decalcified bone. *Am J Med Sci* 98: 219–240

2 Lacroix P (1945) Recent investigations on the growth of bone. *Nature* 156: 576

3 Urist MR (1965) Bone: Formation by autoinduction. *Science* 150: 893–899

4 Reddi AH, Huggins CB (1972) Biochemical sequences in the transformation of normal fibroblasts in adolescent rat. *Proc Natl Acad Sci USA* 69: 1601–1605

5 Reddi AH (1981) Cell biology and biochemistry of endochondral bone development. *Collagen Rel Res* 1: 209–226

6 Reddi AH (1984) Extracellular matrix and development, in: KA Piez, AH Reddi (eds): *Extracellular matrix biochemistry*. Elsevier, New York, 247–291

7 Weiss RE, Reddi AH (1980) Synthesis and localization of fibronectin during collagenous matrix mesenchymal cell interaction and differentiation of cartilage and bone *in vivo*. *Proc Natl Acad Sci USA* 77: 2074–2078

8 Reddi AH, Anderson WA (1976) Collagenous bone matrix-induced endochondral ossification and hemopoiesis. *J Cell Biol* 69: 557–572

9 Sampath TK, Reddi AH (1981) Dissociative extraction and reconstitution of bone matrix components involved in local bone differentiation. *Proc Natl Acad Sci USA* 78: 7599–7603

10 Wozney JM, Rosen V, Celeste AJ, Mitsock LM, Whittiers M, Kriz WR, Heweick RM, Wang EA (1988) Novel regulators of bone formation: molecular clones and activities. *Science* 242: 1528–1534

11 Luyten F, Cunningham NS, Ma S, Muthukumaran S, Hammonds RG, Nevins,WB, Wood WI, Reddi AH (1989) Purification and partial amino acid sequence of osteogenin, a protein initiating bone differentiation. *J Biol Chem* 265: 13377–13380

12 Ozkaynak E, Rueger DC, Drier EA, Corbett C, Ridge RJ, Sampath TK, Opperman H (1990) OP-1 cDNA encodes an osteogenic protein in the TGF-β family. *EMBO J* 9: 2085–2093

13 Sampath TK, Reddi AH (1983) Homology of bone inductive proteins from human, monkey, bovine, and rat extracellular matrix. *Proc Natl Acad Sci USA* 80: 6591–6595

14 Reddi AH (1994 Bone and cartilage differentiation. *Curr Opinion Gen Dev* 4: 937–944

15 Griffith DL, Keck PC, Sampath TK, Rueger DC, Carlson WD (1996) Three-dimensional structure of recombinant human osteogenic protein-1: structural paradigm for the transforming growth factor-β superfamily. *Proc Natl Acad Sci USA* 93: 878–883

16 Chang SC, Hoang B, Thomas JT, Vukicevic S, Luyten FP, Ryba NJP, Kozak CA, Reddi

AH, Moos M Jr (1994) Cartilage-derived morphogenetic proteins. *J Biol Chem* 269: 28227–28234

17  Storm EE, Huynh TV, Copeland NG, Jenkins NA, Kingsley DM, Lee S-J (1994) Limb alterations in brachypodism mice due to mutations in a new member of TGF-β super-family. *Nature* 368: 639–642

18  Chen P, Carrington JL, Hammonds RG, Reddi AH (1991) Stimulation of chondrogene-sis in limb bud mesodermal cells by recombinant human BMP-2B and modulation by TGF-β₁ and TGF-β₂. *Exp Cell Res* 195: 509–515

19  Cunningham NS, Paralkar V, Reddi AH (1992) Osteogenin and recombinant bone mor-phogenetic protein-2B are chemotactic for human monocytes and stimulate transform-ing growth factor-β₁ mRNA expression. *Proc Natl Acad Sci USA* 89: 11740–11744

20  Paralkar VM, Nandedkar AKN, Pointers RH, Kleinman HK, Reddi AH (1990) Inter-action of osteogenin, a heparin binding bone morphogenetic protein, with type IV col-lagen. *J Biol Chem* 265: 17281–17284

21  Hemmati-Brivanlou A, Kelly OG, Melton DA (1994) Follistatin an antagonist of activin is expressed in the Spemann organizer and displays direct neuralizing activity. *Cell* 77: 283–295

22  Piccolo S, Sasai Y, Lu B, De Robertis EM (1996) Dorsoventral patterning in *Xenopus*: inhibition of ventral signals by direct binding of chordin to BMP-4. *Cell* 86: 589–598

23  Zimmerman LB, Jesus-Escobar JM, Harland RM (1996) The Spemann organizer signal Noggin binds and inactivates bone morphogenetic protein-4. *Cell* 86: 599–606

24  Zhang H, Bradley A (1996) Mice deficient of BMP-2 are nonviable and have defects in amnion/chorion and cardiac development. *Development* 122: 2977–2986

25  Winnier G, Blessing M, Labosky PA, Hogan BLM (1996) Bone morphogenetic protein-4 is required for mesoderm formation and patterning in the mouse. *Genes Devel* 9: 2105–2116

26  Dudley AT, Lyons KM, Robertson EJ (1995) A requirement for bone morphogenetic protein-7 during development of the mammalian kidney and eye. *Genes Devel* 9: 2795–2807

27  Luo G, Hoffman M, Bronckers ALJ, Sohuki M, Bradley A, Karsenty G (1995) BMP-7 is an inducer of nephrogenesis and is also required for eye development, and skeletal patterning. *Genes Devel* 9: 2808–2820

28  ten Dijke P, Yamashita H, Sampath TK, Reddi AH, Riddle D, Heldin CH, Miyazono K (1994) Identification of type I receptors for OP-1 and BMP-4. *J Biol Chem* 269: 16986–16988

29  Graff JM, Bansal A, Melton DA (1996) *Xenopus Mad* proteins transduce distinct sub-set of signals for the TGF-β superfamily. *Cell* 85: 479–487

30  Chen S, Rubbock MJ, Whitman M (1996) A transcriptional partner for Mad proteins in TGF-β signalling. *Nature* 383: 691–696

31  Heldin CH, Miyazono K, ten Dijke P (1997) TGFβ signaling from cell membrane to nucleus through Smad proteins. *Nature* 390: 465–471

32  Ripamonti U, Van den Heever B, Sampath TK, Tucker MM, Rueger DC, Reddi AH

(1996) Complete regeneration of bone in the baboon by recombinant human osteogenic protein-1 (hOP-1, bone morphogenetic protein-7). *Growth Factors* 12: 273–289

33  Hollinger J, Mayer M, Buck D, Zegzula H, Ron E, Smith J, Jin L, Wozney J (1996) Poly (α-hydroxy acid) carrier for delivering recombinant human bone morphogenetic protein-2 for bone regeneration. *J Controlled Release* 39: 287–304

34  Bostrom M, Lane JM, Tomin E, Browne M, Berbian W, Turek T, Smith J, Wozney J, Schildhauer T (1996) Use of bone morphogenetic protein-2 in the rabbit ulnar nonunion model. *Clin Orthop Rel Res* 327: 272–282

35  Reddi AH (1998) Role of morphogenetic proteins in skeletal tissue engineering and regeneration. *Nature Biotech* 16: 247–252

36  Khouri RK, Koudsi B, Reddi AH (1991 Tissue transformation into bone *in vivo*. *JAMA* 266: 1953–1955

# Biology of glial cell-line derived neurotrophic factor

*Navin Maswood and Don M. Gash*

Department of Anatomy and Neurobiology, University of Kentucky Medical Center, 800 Rose Street, MN 224, Lexington, KY 40536-0298, USA

## Introduction

Neurotrophic factors are cytokines that promote the differentiation, development, growth, maintenance and regeneration of neurons. In 1993, glial cell line-derived-neurotrophic factor (GDNF) was identified as the first member of a new family of cytokines in the transforming growth factor β (TGF-β) superfamily [1]. Over the past five years, three additional members of the GDNF family have been isolated, cloned and sequenced: neuturin [2], persephin [3] and artemin [4]. The present review will concentrate on GDNF, the most extensively studied of the four proteins. The known properties of the other three trophic factors and their comparison to GDNF will be discussed at the end of the chapter.

GDNF was isolated and purified from the conditioned medium of cultured rat B-49 glial cells, using the survival of fetal rat mesencephalic dopamine neurons as a bioassay [1]. While the monomeric form of GDNF consists of 134 amino acids, the biologically active form is a glycoslyated homodimer that migrates in gels with an apparent molecular weight in the 33–45 kDa range [1, 5]. There is a 93% homology between the amino acid sequences of rat and the human GDNF [6]. While GDNF is structurally related to members of the TGF-β superfamily, it shares less than a 20% homology with any of the known TGF-β proteins. However, similar to other members of the TGF-β family, GDNF contains seven conserved cysteine residues [6]. While not closely related, GDNF and TGF-β have been shown to exert synergistic effects on the survival of neuronal populations *in vitro* and *in vivo*, suggesting a role for TGF-β in eliciting the trophic effects of GDNF [7, 8].

## Sites of GDNF expression in the body

GDNF mapping studies initially focused on the nigrostriatal dopaminergic pathway, where GDNF mRNA expression was detected in the embryonic, newborn and adult striatum [9–12]. In addition, GDNF message expression has been detected in the hippocampus, cerebellum, cortex, and spinal cord of embryonic, newborn and adult rats and adult humans [9–10]. Though it was not possible to unequivocally identify all the cells synthesizing GDNF in the *in vivo* studies, Schaar et al. [13] reported GDNF mRNA expression in cultures of cortical astrocytes, basal forebrain astrocytes and fetal mesencephalic neurons. GDNF mRNA expression has also been reported in activated macrophages and microglia in the brain around striatal injury sites [14].

Outside of the CNS, GDNF mRNA is widely expressed in peripheral organs of developing rats, including the kidneys, lungs, gonads and digestive system [10, 15, 16]. The other peripheral organs showing GDNF expression include the bone, liver, heart, blood, skeletal muscles and adrenal glands [15–19].

## GDNF receptors

The cellular responses to the GDNF protein family are mediated *via* a multicomponent receptor complex consisting of (a) one of four identified ligand binding glycoproteins, plus (b) the transmembrane tyrosine kinase protein, cRet. The four glycoproteins are by convention called the GDNF family receptors, alpha 1–4 (GFRα-1–4) [4, 20]. All α subunits are glycosylphosphatidylinositol (GPI) linked glycoproteins with 3–6 glycosylation sites and have an N-terminal hydrophobic putative signal peptide for secretion. The C-terminal has another hydrophobic domain separated by a hydrophilic linker region. All four glycoproteins lack intracellular domains and thus, are unable to transmit signals by themselves. The best evidence to date is that all function through interacting with the cRet receptor.

### GFRα-1

Treanor et al. [21] identified and sequenced the GFRα-1 receptor, demonstrating that GDNF promotes the formation of a physical complex between GFRα-1 and the tyrosine kinase receptor cRet. GFRα-1 is a 468 amino acid protein with a signal peptide for secretion at the amino-terminus, a stretch of 23 hydrophobic amino acids at the carboxy terminus, three glycosylation sites and 30 cysteine residues which appears to have a similar topology to those present in many cytokine receptors [21]. The hydrophobic cluster at the C-terminus is preceded by a group of three small amino acids (Ala Ser Ser), defining a cleavage/binding site for the GPI linkage. Thus, GFRα-1 is an extracellular glycoprotein that is attached to the outer cell membrane. It also has the highest binding affinity for GDNF [20, 22] relative to the other GFRα receptors that have been identified. GFRα-1-deficient mice are unable to respond to either GDNF or neuturin, but regain responsiveness when exposed to GDNF or neuturin in the presence of soluble GFRα-1 protein [23]. GFRα-1-deficient mice display deficits in the kidneys, enteric nervous system, spinal motor and sensory neurons, thus indicating the essential role of this receptor in the development of these systems [23].

## GFRα-2

This is another polypeptide of about 464 amino acids, showing a 63% similarity and 43% identity to rat GFRα-1 subtype. The predicted sequence of the rat GFRα-2 is 97% and 94% identical, respectively, to mouse and human GFRα-2 cloned receptors. It has six potential N-terminus glycosylation sites [20]. Baloh et al. [4] and Buj-Bello et al. [22] have reported GFRα-2 to have a higher binding affinity to neuturin. However, Sanicola et al. [24] observed GDNF binding to soluble GFRα-2 in the presence of the soluble cRet extracellular domain. By using chemical cross linking, Trupp et al. [20] demonstrated specific and direct interactions between GDNF and GFRα-2 in intact cells in the absence of cRet, suggesting that localization of GFRα-2 on the cell membrane may be important for ligand binding.

## GRFα-3

Almost simultaneously in 1998, three separate groups [25–27] identified the GFRα-3 receptor subtype based on sequence homology with the GFRα-1 and GFRα-2 receptors. The GFRα-3 sequence which was identified displayed a 32% and 37% amino acid identity with GFRα-1 and GFRα-2, respectively. All 28 cysteines in the GFRα-3 sequence were found to be conserved in GFRα-1 and GFRα-2. Masure et al. [28] also cloned GFRα-3 receptor and reported that the gene for the GFRα-3 receptor was mapped to human chromosome 5 in a region (q31.1–q31.3) where several disease loci, growth factor and growth factor receptor genes have been localized. The GFRα-3 is composed of 397 amino acids and contains a signal sequence, three potential glycosylation sites and a putative GPI-linked hydrophobic C-terminus [4, 20, 25]. Compared to the first two receptors, it lacks a relatively large region at the C-terminus just before the GPI direction site and the hydrophobic terminus. The sequence homology between GFRα-3 and the first two a-receptors is also low in this region, making it the most variable segment of this receptor subtype [20]. In one study, while GRFα-3 was not seen to bind GDNF directly, it still was able to mediate crosslinking of GDNF to cRet when both receptors were co-expressed in COS cells [20]. Baloh et al. [4] have recently reported that GFRα-3 has the highest binding affinity for artemin, the most recently identified GDNF-related cytokine.

The GFRα-3 receptor subtype is robustly expressed in the developing and adult peripheral nervous system, and more moderately expressed in spinal cord and cerebellum [28]. High expression of GFRα-3 is seen in developing peripheral and cranial nerves, including dorsal root ganglia and trigeminal neurons [26, 27]. The receptor is widely distributed in non-neural tissues, such as the stomach, small intestine, pancreas, appendix, testis, heart, kidneys and glandular cells [4, 25, 28].

Studies conducted by Trupp et al. [20] suggested a graded response of GF receptors to GDNF (GFRα-1 > GFRα-2 > GFRα-3). Thus, GFRα-1 may mediate responses to low GDNF concentrations, whereas the activation of GFRα-2 and GFRα-3 may require higher levels of ligand and/ or cRet co-expression. However, the same ligand can bind to more than one alpha receptor subtype. For example, although GDNF has the highest affinity for GFRα-1 receptor subtype but it can also bind to GFRα-2 receptors, while neuturin has the highest affinity for the GFRα-2 receptor subtype but it can also bind to the GFRα-1 receptor subtype [4].

## GFRα-4

In 1998, Thompson et al. [29] isolated a cDNA encoding the fourth receptor of the α family, designated as GFRα-4, from screening an E-10 chicken brain cDNA library with a mouse GFRα-1 probe. GFRα-4 is a polypeptide containing 431 amino acids, and is more closely related to GFRα-1 and GFRα-2 than GFRα-3. It has about 40% amino acid identity with both mouse and chicken GFRα-1 and GFRα-2 and 27% identity with mouse GFRα-3. Of the 30 cysteine residues which are conserved between GFRα-1 and GFRα-2, 28 are conserved in GFRα-4. GFRα-4 mRNA expression has been detected in the chicken embryo during development of the skin, skeletal muscles, kidney, intestine and lung. Within the CNS, spinal cord expressed the highest levels of GFRα-4, while lower levels were seen in the medulla, pons, cerebellum and midbrain. The lowest levels were found in the forebrain region [29]. Enokido et al. [30] have demonstrated that GRFα-4 has the highest affinity for persephin as its ligand and requires cRet as its signaling subunit.

## cRet, the signaling subunit

Known as the β subunit, the signaling protein is encoded by the cRet proto-oncogene. cRet is highly expressed in the developing central and peripheral nervous system and in the excretory system of the embryonic mouse [31]. The initial clue that cRet was a biologically important receptor for GDNF came from observing that both the cRet knockout mouse and GDNF knockout mouse displayed serious defects in kidney and enteric nervous system development [32].

cRet is a member of the receptor tyrosine kinase superfamily and is activated by the autophosphorylation of tyrosine residues at the C-terminus. Binding of GDNF ligands to the α-subunit may be necessary for the activation of cRet [21, 33]. Studies by Jing et al. [33] have shown that cRet tyrosine kinase is efficiently activated by

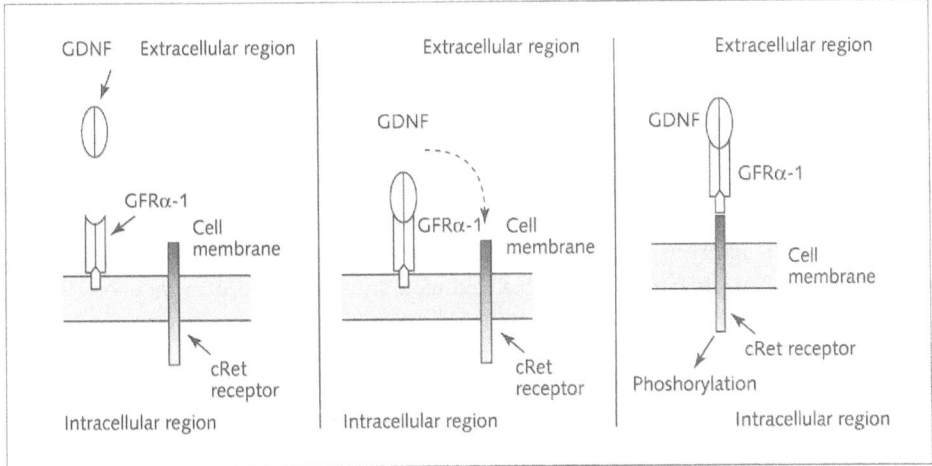

*Figure 1*
*The signaling mechanism of GDNF.*
*The homodimer GDNF binds to the ligand binding subunits, the GFR-α receptors, on the cell surface. The GDNF/GFR-α complex then interacts with the c-Ret tyrosine kinase receptor. The c-Ret tyrosine kinase is the signaling subunit, which has both an extracellular (ligand binding) and an intracellular domain (signaling). c-Ret tyrosine kinase undergoes autophosphorylation when bound by the GDNF/GDNF-α1 complex, activating second messenger cascades in the intracellular region.*

either GDNF or neuturin, when the GFRα receptors are co-expressed with cRet in the same cell, indicating a functional cis-interaction. Thus, c-Ret may interact with the a receptors in many cell populations where both proteins are expressed together. However, in many cells, c-Ret and the a receptors are not co-expressed. In those cases c-Ret may interact with the a receptors localized in the target neurons (an interaction termed "in trans"). In fact, Tian et al. [34] provided evidence that c-Ret activation by GDNF or neuturin can occur "in trans", suggesting a role in neuron-target interaction. However, Trupp et al. [20] also suggested that GDNF might stabilize preformed complexes between cRet and GPI-anchored GDNF receptors at the cell membrane. Thus, both ligand-dependent as well as ligand-independent interactions between GFRα receptors and cRet have been suggested (Fig. 1).

Trupp et al. [35] reported high levels of cRet mRNA expression in dopamine neurons in the adult brain substantia nigra, where exogenously administered GDNF protected cRet positive neurons from 6-hydroxydopamine (6-OHDA)-induced cell death. This evidence indirectly supports the concept that cRet acts as a functional receptor of GDNF and mediates the neurotrophic effects of GDNF.

## Essential functions of GDNF

While GDNF is found in many sites in the nervous system and body, other cytokines are able to compensate for GDNF deficiencies in a number of instances. However, there are some exceptions where either the absence of GDNF or low levels result in cell loss. Motor neurons are an example. Multiple studies have described the potent effects of GDNF on embryonic chicken and rat motoneurons in culture [36] and lesioned motor neurons *in vivo* [37–39]. Two different GDNF-deficient mouse strains have been reported to have a reduced number of motor neurons in the trigeminal ganglion and spinal cord [40, 41].

In addition to motor neurons, mice in whom the GDNF gene has been disrupted display deficits in primary sensory neurons and sympathetic neurons. Also, the metanephric kidneys, ureters and most of the enteric nervous system fail to develop in GNDF knockout mice [40–42]. It is important to realize that these animals provide only a partial picture of the effects of GDNF deficiencies, as they die shortly after birth because of the lack of renal function and their inability to consume milk [23]. Thus, the essential functions of GDNF in later development and maturation can not be ascertained. Therefore, the observation that CNS deficits in GDNF knockout mice are subtle, and even midbrain dopamine neurons appear normal, has to be viewed cautiously.

While not essential for early CNS development, GDNF acts as a survival factor for a number of CNS neurons in various culture and lesion paradigms. The list includes dopamine neurons [43], motor neurons [36], locus coeruleus noradrenergic neurons [44], basal forebrain cholinergic neurons [45], cerebellar Purkinje cells [46], serotonin neurons of the dorsal raphe [47] and thalamic neurons [48]. In addition, pretreatment with GDNF has been shown to protect against apoptotic cell death induced by brain ischemia in the hippocampal CAI region [49]. In the PNS, GDNF has been shown to support the survival of subpopulations of peripheral sympathetic, parasympathetic and autonomic ganglia such as dorsal root ganglia, superior cervical, trigeminal and nodose ganglia [2, 50, 51].

## Antiparkinsonian actions of GDNF

Parkinson's disease results from the progressive degeneration of dopamine neurons in the substantia nigra that send afferents to the caudate nucleus and putamen [52–55]. Whenever the striatal levels of dopamine fall below a critical level, often considered to be ≥95% of age-matched controls, the characteristic features of parkinsonism are expressed: bradykinesia, rigidity, resting tremor and balance and gait abnormalities [67]. As the disease progresses, the continuing loss of dopamine terminals in the striatum reduces the capacity for dopamine uptake, storage and release at the synaptic level [56].

GDNF was initially identified as a dopaminergic trophic factor and many subsequent studies have focused on its potential application in treating Parkinson's disease. Both protective and regenerative trophic actions have been consistently reported for GDNF on midbrain dopamine neurons in cell culture. GDNF increases embryonic dopamine neuron survival as measured by cell counts and functional development as measured by increases in high affinity dopamine uptake [1]. It inhibits the apoptotic death of postnatal substantia nigra dopamine neurons in primary culture [57]. Also, GDNF supports the survival and neuritic growth of cultured dopaminergic neurons injured by the neurotoxin, 1-methyl-4-phenylpyridinium [58].

A number of groups have also shown neuroprotective and regenerative effects of GDNF in animal models of Parkinson's disease [59]. The paradigm for evaluating neuroprotection involves administering GDNF prior to a neurotoxic challenge. As GDNF does not pass through the blood-brain barrier, it is necessary to deliver the trophic factor directly into either the cerebroventricular system or the brain parenchyma. The timing of pre-administration of GDNF is critical; Kearns et al. [60] found that optimal protection against 6-hydroxydopamine (6-OHDA) lesions in the rat were provided by direct GDNF injections into the substantia nigra 6 h prior to exposure to the toxin. Pre-administrations of GDNF have also been found to be effective as early as 24 h prior to 1-methyl-4-phenyl-1,2,3,6-tetrahydropyridine (MPTP) exposure in the mouse [43] and 6-OHDA treatment in the rat [61].

Most studies in animal models have focused on the regenerative effects of GDNF following injuries to dopamine neurons. GDNF administration into the brain parenchyma or ventricles of the rat in the weeks following a unilateral 6-OHDA lesion promotes the recovery of a number of morphological and functional features of CNS dopamine neurons [19, 62, 63]. Drug-induced rotation behavior, a crude index of functional deficiencies in the nigrostriatal dopamine pathway, is reduced by a single injection of GDNF [62]. The functional improvements are concomitant with increases in the number of midbrain dopamine neurons expressing tyrosine hydroxylase (the rate limiting enzyme for dopamine synthesis) and increased levels of tyrosine hydroxylase (TH) activity [19, 63]. Similar morphological and functional improvements have been seen in mice receiving GDNF following MPTP lesions [43].

Studies in non-human primates provide further evidence that GDNF could prove useful as a therapy for Parkinson's disease. Our group has carried out a series of experiments evaluating the efficacy of intracerebrally administered GDNF in rhesus monkeys with hemiparkinsonian features induced by MPTP [64–66]. Three sites of administration have been tested: caudate nucleus, substantia nigra, and lateral ventricle. Functional improvements in parkinsonian features were seen following a single injection into any of the three targets, indicating that GDNF is relatively mobile in the primate brain [64]. Along with improved motor functions, increased levels of dopamine were measured in the substantia nigra and the adjacent ventral tegmental area and globus pallidus. The restorative effects of GDNF were evident on neuronal morphology; midbrain dopamine neurons showed recovery of normal perikaryal cell size and the number of neurons and neuronal processes expressing tyrosine hydroxylase was significantly increased.

Subsequent studies have demonstrated that parkinsonian monkeys display dose-dependent improvements in movement functions in response to GDNF [66]. While some animals responded to monthly injections into the lateral ventricle of as little as 30 µg per month, more consistent responses were seen in monkeys in the 100–1000 µg treatment groups. GDNF can be administered in conjunction with levodopa, the current "gold standard" treatment for Parkinson's disease [65]. Combined GDNF-levodopa treatment results in significantly enhanced functional improvements compared to either drug given separately and a reduction in levodopa-induced side effects (e.g. vomiting and dyskinesias).

One of the consistent observations in studies on rodents and non-human primates has been that a single intracerebral injection of GDNF induces changes in dopamine neurons, which can be measured for days to weeks. For instance, the significant reductions in drug-induced rotation behavior by GDNF in rats with 6-OHDA lesions is not evident until one week after trophic factor administration [62]. In addition, it is not until approximately five weeks after GDNF treatment that dopamine levels in the substantia nigra are restored to normal levels [62, 67]. It takes 1–2 weeks for functional improvements in parkinsonian rhesus monkeys to reach statistical significance [64]. Some improvements in motor functions can be measured for as long as four months following the last GDNF treatment in rhesus monkeys [66], but most monkeys have returned to their pre-treatment baseline after six months of drug washout (Gash and Zhang, unpublished observations).

## GDNF delivery into the CNS

As mentioned earlier, GDNF is like other trophic factors in that the molecule is too large to pass through the blood-brain barrier. While direct injection into the brain is a feasible experimental procedure, better methods are needed if trophic factors are to be utilized for clinical treatments. Our group is testing programmable pumps that can chronically deliver small quantities of GDNF into specific sites in either the brain or intrathecal space of the spinal cord. One series of experiments has used parkinsonian rhesus monkeys with a catheter surgically implanted into the right lateral ventricle *via* MRI-guided stereotaxic procedure [68]. In addition, the animals have a titanium-encased SynchroMed® pump (Medtronics, Minneapolis, MN) implanted subcutaneously in the abdominal region and connected by tubing to the catheter. In the first three animals tested, the daily infusion of 300 µl of vehicle (citrate buffer) had no effect on parkinsonian features. However, within three weeks of beginning infusions of 7.5 µg of GDNF a day, significant improvements in motor functions were measured in all three monkeys.

When large subcutaneous pockets were made to house the pumps, they were well tolerated by the monkeys over the three-month test period. The titanium casing did not elicit a host response. As the solutions in the pump reservoir can be changed by injections through the skin and the rate and mode (e.g. continuous or bolus) of delivery is easily reprogrammed through an external computer, the SynchroMed® pumps offer both flexibility and control in delivering trophic factors into specific CNS sites.

Another approach for delivering trophic factors into the brain has been to utilize adenovirus vectors to transfect cells in adult rodents to produce GDNF [69]. One demonstration that transfected cells produce biologically active trophic factor came from the report by Choi-Lundberg et al. [70] (see also Bilang et al. [71] and Bohn [72]) showing that replication-defective adenoviral vector encoding human GDNF injected near the rat substantia nigra protected dopamine neurons from the progressive degeneration induced by the neurotoxin 6-OHDA. Similar protective effects have been observed in MPTP-lesioned mice nigrostriatal neurons transfected with viral encoded human GDNF gene [73]. In a similar vein, Ribotta et al. [74] have reported pretreatment with adenoviral vector encoding GDNF significantly increased the survival of rat neonatal motoneurons following axotomy.

## Other members of the GDNF family

Neuturin, the second member of the GDNF family, was identified from its survival-promoting properties of superior cervical ganglion neurons in culture by Kotzbauer et al. [2]. Mature neuturin shows an approximate 42% amino acid similarity with mature GDNF [2]. Creedon et al. [75] have demonstrated that neuturin induces cRet phosphorylation in primary cultures of rat superior cervical ganglion neurons and also in fibroblast cells transfected with cRet and GFRα-1, but not cRet alone. In vitro experiments have shown that GFRα-2 is the preferred GPI receptor for neuturin [4]. The signaling pathways activated by neuturin include mitogen-activated protein kinase (MAP-K) and phosphatidyl-inositol-3 kinase (PI-3-K) [75].

Persephin, the third member of the GDNF family, was identified as a result of its homology with GDNF and neuturin by Milbrandt et al. [3]. Persephin shares about a 40% amino acid identity with GDNF and neuturin. Like GDNF and neuturin, persephin has been shown to promote the survival of ventral midbrain dopaminergic neurons and motor neurons in culture. The GPI receptor for persephin is GFRα-4 in combination with cRet [30]. Studies to date indicate that persephin does not bind to either GFRα-1 or GFRα-2 GPI receptors [3].

Artemin, the most recently identified member of the GDNF family, is more similar to neuturin and persephin (~45% identity), and has only ~35% identity with GDNF. Artemin acts as a survival factor for sensory and sympathetic neurons in cul-

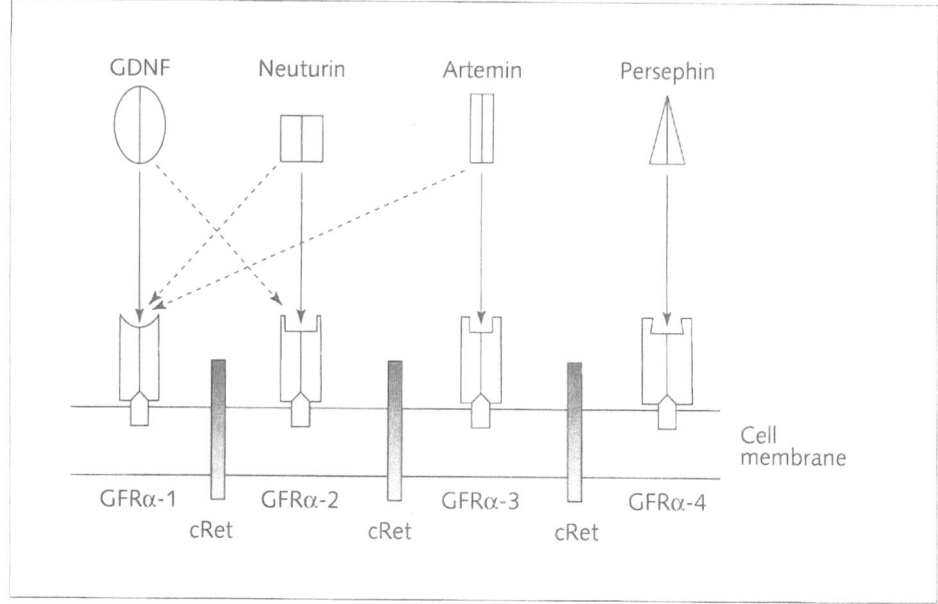

*Figure 2*
*The signaling mechanism of GDNF and its family members.*
*The solid arrows indicate preferred ligand-receptor interactions between GDNF and the other members of its family with the various ligand-binding α subunits; dotted arrows indicate alternate receptor-ligand interaction. At present, c-Ret tyrosine kinase receptor is the only known common signaling subunit for all four types of α subunits.*

ture and also acts as a survival factor for midbrain dopaminergic neurons in culture. Artemin has preferred affinity for GFRα-3-RET complex, but it can also activate the GFRα-1 + cRET complex [4] (Fig. 2).

## Conclusion

Glial cell line-derived-neurotrophic factor (GDNF), along with other members of its family (neuturin, persephin and artemin) play important roles in the growth and development of various central and peripheral neuronal populations. GDNF has been reported to be essential for maintaining the number of motoneurons and for the development of the metanephric kidneys and most of the enteric nervous system. Although not essential, GDNF acts as a survival factor for various CNS neurons, including dopaminergic, noradrenergic, cholinergic, serotonergic and thalamic neurons. Multiple studies in rodents and non-human primates have provided evidence that GDNF could prove useful as a therapy for Parkinson's disease.

The cellular responses to the GDNF protein family are mediated *via* a multi-component receptor complex consisting of the ligand-binding α subunits and the signaling transmembrane subunit, c-Ret. As GDNF does not cross the blood-brain barrier, methods of delivering GDNF into the brain have had to be developed. In addition to the most commonly utilized method of direct intracranial infusions of GDNF into a specific brain region, programmable pumps are being tested that can chronically deliver small quantities of GDNF into specific sites in the brain or the intrathecal space of the spinal cord. Another approach for delivering GDNF into the brain has been to utilize adenovirus vectors to transfect cells in adult rodents to produce GDNF.

In conclusion, since its discovery in 1993, GDNF has been found to be an important cytokine synthesized by many central and peripheral cells. Its potent trophic actions make it a candidate for treating a variety of injuries and diseases affecting man. The initial focus has been on Parkinson's disease where pronounced protective and regenerative effects on dopamine neurons in animal models have been demonstrated.

## Acknowledgement

The authors are grateful to Ms. Susan Tucker for the illustrations used in this chapter.

## References

1   Lin L-FH, Doherty DH, Lile JD, Bektesh S, Collins F (1993) GDNF: a glial cell line-derived neurotrophic factor for midbrain dopaminergic neurons. *Science* 260: 1130–1132

2   Kotzbauer PT, Lampe PA, Heuckeroth RO, Golden JP, Creedon DJ, Johnson EM Jr, Milbrandt J (1996) Neuturin, a relative of glial cell-line-derived neurotrophic factor. *Nature* 384: 467–470

3   Milbrandt J, de Sauvage FJ, Fahrner TJ, Baloh RH, Leitner ML, Tansey MG, Lampe PA, Heuckeroth RO, Kotzbauer PT, Simburger KS et al (1998) Persephin, a novel neurotrophic factor related to GDNF and neuturin. *Neuron* 20: 245–253

4   Baloh RH, Tansey MG, Lampe PA, Fahrner TJ, Enomoto H, Simburger KS, Leitner ML, Toshiyuki A, Johnson EM Jr, Milbrandt J (1998) Artemin, a novel member of the GDNF ligand family, supports peripheral and central neurons and signals through the GFRα3-Ret receptor complex. *Neuron* 21: 1291–1302

5   Lin L-FH, Zhang TJ, Collins F, Armes LG (1994) Purification and initial characterization of rat B49 glial cell-derived neurotrophic factor. *J Neurochem* 63: 758–768

6   Unsicker K (1996) GDNF: A cytokine at the interface of TGF betas and neurotrophins. *Cell Tissue Res* 286: 175–178

7   Krieglstein, K, Henheik P, Farkas L, Jaszai J, Galter D, Krohn K, Unsicker K (1998) Glial cell line-derived neurotrophic factor requires transforming growth factor-β for exerting its full neurotrophic potential on peripheral and CNS neurons. *J Neurosci* 18 (23): 9822–9834

8   Schober A, Hertel R, Arumae U, Farkas L, Jaszai J, Krieglestein K, Saarma M, Unsicker K (1999) Glial cell line-derived neurotrophic factor rescues target deprived sympathetic spinal cord neurons but requires transforming growth factor β as cofactor *in vivo*. *J Neurosci* 19 (6): 2008–2018

9   Stromberg I, Bjorklund L, Johansson M, Tomac A, Collins F, Olson L, Hoffer B, Humpel C (1993) Glial cell line derived neurotrophic factor is in the developing but not adult stratum and stimulates developing dopamine neurons *in vivo*. *Exp Neurol* 124: 401–412

10  Choi-Lundberg DL, Bohn MC (1995) Ontogeny and distribution of glial cell line-derived neurotrophic factor (GDNF) mRNA in rat. *Dev Brain Res* 85: 80–88

11  Springer JE, Mu X, Bergmann LW, Trojanoski JQ (1994) Expression of GDNF mRNA in rat and human nervous tissue. *Exp Neurol* 127: 167–170

12  Springer JE, Seeburger JL, He J, Gabrea A, Blankenhorn EP, Bergman LW (1995) cDNA sequence and differentiatial mRNA regulation of two forms of glial cell line-derived neurotrophic factor in schwaan cells and rat skeletal muscles. *Exp Neurol* 131: 47–52

13  Schaar DG, Sieber BA, Dreyfus CG, Black IB (1993) Regional and cell specific expression of GDNF in rat brain. *Exp Neurol* 124 (2): 368–371

14  Batchelor PE, Liberatore GT, Wong JYF, Porritt MJ, Frerichs F, Donnan GA, Howells DW (1999) Activated macrophages and microglia induce dopaminergic sprouting in the injured striatum and express brain-derived neurotrophic factor and glial cell line-derived neurotrophic factor. *J Neurosci* 19(5): 1708–1719

15  Suter-Crazzolara C, Unsicker K (1994) GDNF is expressed in two forms in many tissues outside the CNS. *Neuroreport* 5: 2486–2488

16  Trupp M, Ryden M, Jornavall FH, Timmusk T, Arenas E, Ibanez CF (1995) Peripheral expression and biological activities of GDNF, a new neurotrophic factor for avian and mammalian peripheral neurons. *J Cell Biol* 130: 137–148

17  Grondin R, Gash DM (1998) Glial cell line-derived neurotrophic factor (GDNF): a drug candidate for treatment of Parkinson's disease. *J Neurol* 245 (suppl 3): 35–42

18  Lapchak PA, Jiao SS, Miller PJ, Williams LR, Cummins V, Inouye G, Matheson CR, Yan Q (1996) Pharmacological characterization of glial cell line-derived neurotrophic factor: Implications for GDNF as a therapeutic molecule to treat neurodegenerative diseases. *Cell Tissue Res* 286: 179–189

19  Lapchak PA, Gash DM, Jiao S, Miller PJ, Hilt D (1997) Glial cell line-derived neurotrophic factor: a novel therapeutic approach to treat motor dysfunctions in Parkinson's disease. *Exp Neurol* 144: 29–34

20  Trupp M, Raynoschek C, Belluardo N, Ibanez CF (1998) Multiple GPI-anchored recep-

tors control GDNF-dependent and independent activation of c-Ret receptor tyrosine kinase. *Mol Cell Neurosci* 11: 47–63

21  Treanor JJS, Goodman L, Sauvage F de, Stone DM, Poulsen KT, Beck CD, Gray C, Armanini MP, Pollock RA, Hefti F et al (1996) Characterization of a multicomponent receptor for GDNF. *Nature* 382: 80–83

22  Buj-Bello A, Adu J, Pinon LGP, Horton A, Thompson J, Rosenthal A, Chinchetru M, Buchman V, Davies AM (1997) Neuturin responsiveness requires a GPI-linked receptor and the ret receptor tyrosine kinase. *Nature* 387: 721–724

23  Cacalano G, Farinas I, Wang Li-C, Hagler K, Forgie A, Moore M, Armanini M, Phillips H, Ryan AM, Reichardt LF et al (1998) GFRα1 is an essential receptor component for GDNF in the developing nervous system and kidney. *Neuron* 21: 53–62

24  Sanicola M, Hession C, Worley D, Carmillo P, Ehrenfels C, Walus L, Robinson S, Jawarski G, Wei H, Tizard R et al (1997) Glial cell-line-derived neurotrophic factor-dependent Ret activation can be mediated by two different cell surface accessory proteins. *Proc Natl Acad Sci USA* 94: 6238–6243

25  Naveilhan P, Baudet C, Mikaels A, Shen L, Westphal H, Ernfors P (1998). Expression and regulation of GFRα3 a glial cell line-derived neurotrophic factor family receptor. *Proc Natl Acad Sci USA* 95: 1295–1300

26  Widenfalk J, Tomac A, Lindqvist E, Hoffer B, Olson L (1998) GFRα-3, a protein related to GFRα-1, is expressed in developing peripheral neurons and ensheathing cells. *Eur J Neurosci* 10: 1508–1517

27  Worby CA, Vega QC, Chao HHJ, Seasholtz AF, Thompson RC, Dixon JE (1998) Identification and characterization of GFRα-3, a novel co-receptor belonging to the glial cell line-derived neurotrophic receptor family. *J Biol Chem* 273 (6): 3502–3508

28  Masure S, Miroslav CIK, Pangalos MN, Bonaventure P, Verhasselt P, Anne S, Lesage J, Leysen JE, Gordon RD (1998) Molecular cloning, expression and tissue distribution of glial-cell-derived neurotrophic factor family receptor α-3 (GFRα-3). *Eur J Biochem* 251: 622–630

29  Thompson J, Doxakis E, Pinon LGP, Strachan P, Buj-Bello A, Wyatt S, Buchman VL, Davies AM (1998) GFRFα-4, a new GDNF family receptor. *Mol Cell Neurosci* 11: 117–126

30  Enokido Y, de Sauvage F, Hongo JA, Ninkina N, Rosenthal A, Buchman VL, Davies AM (1998) GFRα-4 and the tyrosine kinase Ret form a functional receptor complex for persephin. *Curr Biol* 8: 1019–1022.

31  Tsuzuki T, Takahashi M, Asai N, Iwashita T, Matsuyama M, Asai J (1995) Spatial and temporal expression of the ret proto-oncogene product in embryonic, infant and adult rat tissues. *Oncogene* 10: 191–198

32  Schuchardt A, D'Agati V, Larsson-Blomberg L, Costantini F, Pachnis V (1994) Defects in the kidneys and the enteric nervous system of mice lacking the tyrosine kinase receptor Ret. *Nature* 367: 380–383

33  Jing S, Wen D, Yu Y, Holst PL, Luo Y, Fang M, Tamir R, Antonio L, Hu Z, Cupples R

et al (1996) GDNF-induced activation of the Ret protein tyrosine kinase is mediated by GDNFα, a novel receptor for GDNF. *Cell* 15: 1113–1124

34  Tian Y, Scully S, Yu Y, Fox GM, Jing S, Zhou R (1998) Expression of GDNF family receptor components during development: Implications in the mechanisms of interaction. *J Neurosci* 18(12): 4684– 4686

35  Trupp M, Arenas E, Fainzilber M, Nilsson A-S, Sieber B-A, Grigoriou M, Kilkenny C, Salazar-Grueso E, Pachnis V, Arumae U et al (1996) Functional receptor for GDNF encoded by the c-Ret protooncogene. *Nature* 381: 785–789

36  Henderson CE, Phillips HS, Pollock RA, Davies AM, Lemeulle C, Armani M, Simpson LC, Moffet B, Vandlen RA, Koliatos VE et al (1994) GDNF: a potent survival factor for motoneurons present in peripheral nerve and muscle. *Science* 266: 1062–1064

37  Li L, WU W, Lin L-F, Lei M, Oppenheim RO, Houenou LJ (1995) Rescue of adult mouse motoneurons from injury-induced cell death by glial cell line-derived neurotrophic factor. *Proc Natl Acad Sci USA* 92: 9771–9775

38  Oppenheim RW, Houenou LJ, Johnson JE, Lin L-FH, Li L, Lo AC, Newsom AL, Prevette DM, Wang S (1995) Developing motor neurons rescued from programmed and axotomy-induced cell death by GDNF. *Nature* 373: 344–346

39  Yan Q, Matheson C, Lopez OT (1995) *In vivo* neurotrophic effects of GDNF on neonatal and adult facial neurons. *Nature* 373: 341–342

40  Moore MW, Klein RD, Farinas I, Sauer H, Armanini M, Phillips HS, Reichardt LF, Ryans AM, Carver-Moore K, Rosenthal A (1996) Renal and neuronal abnormalities in mice lacking GDNF. *Nature* 382: 76–79

41  Sanchez MP, Silos-Santiago I, Frisen J, He B, Lira SA, Barbacid M (1996) Renal agenesis and the absence of enteric neurons in mice lacking GDNF. *Nature* 382: 70–73

42  Pichel JG, Shen L, Sheng HZ, Grandholm A-C, Drago J, Grindberg A, Lee EJ, Huang SP, Saarma M, Hoffer BJ et al (1996) Defects in enteric innervation and kidney development in mice lacking GDNF. *Nature* 382: 73–76.

43  Tomac A, Lindqvist E, Lin L-FH, Ogren SO, Young D, Hoffer BJ, Olson L (1995) Protection and repair of the nigrostrisatal dopaminergic system by GDNF *in vivo*. *Nature* 373: 335–339

44  Arenas E, Trupp M, Akerud P, Ibanez CF (1995) GDNF prevents degeneration and promotes the phenotype of brain noradrenergic neurons *in vivo*. *Neuron* 15: 1465–1473

45  Williams LR, Inouye G, Cummins V, Pelleymounter M-A (1996) Glial cell line-derived neurotrophic factor sustained axotomized basal forebrain cholinergic neurons *in vivo*: dose-response comparison to nerve growth-factor and brain-derived neurotrophic factor. *J Pharmacol Exp Ther* 277: 1140–1151

46  Mount HTJ, Dean DO, Alberch J, Dreyfus CF, Black IB (1995) Glial cell line-derived neurotrophic factor promotes the survival and morphological differentiation of Purkinje cells. *Proc Natl Acad Sci USA* 92: 9092–9096

47  Trupp M, Belluardo N, Funakoshi H, Ibanez CF (1997) Complementary and overlapping expression of glial cell-line-derived neurotrophic factor (GDNF), c-Ret proto-onco-

gene, and GDNF receptor -alpha indicates multiple mechanisms of trophic actions in the adult rat CNS. *J Neurosci* 17: 3554–3567

48    Martin D, Miller G, Rosendhal M, Russel D A (1995) Potent inhibitory effects of glial-derived neurotrophic factor against kainic acid mediated seizures in the rat. *Brain Res* 683: 172–178

49    Miyazaki H, Okuma Y, Fujii Y, Nagashima K, Nomura Y (1999) Glial cell line-derived neurotrophic factor protects against delayed neuronal death after transient forebrain ischemia in rats. *Neurosci Lett* 89(3): 643–647

50    Trupp M, Ryden M, Jornavall FH, Timmusk T, Arenas E, Ibanez CF (1995) Peripheral expression and biological activities of GDNF, a new neurotrophic factor for avian and mammalian peripheral neurons. *J Cell Biol* 130: 137–148.

51    Buj-Bello A, Buchmam VL, Horton A, Rosenthal A, Davies AM (1995) GDNF is an age-specific survival factor for sensory and autonomic neurons. *Neuron* 15: 821–828

52    Hornykiewicz O, Kish SJ (1987) Biochemical pathophysiology of Parkinson's disease. *Adv Neurol* 45: 19–34

53    Graybiel AM, Hirsch EC, Agid Y (1990) The nigrostriatal system in Parkinson's disease. [Review]. *Ad Neurol* 53: 17–29

54    Long AE, Lozano AM (1998) Parkinson's disease. First of two parts. *N Engl J Med* 339 (15): 1044–1053

55    Long AE, Lozano AM (1998) Parkinson's disease. Second of two parts. *N Engl J Med* 339 (16): 1130–1143

56    Mouradian MM, Chase TN (1988) Central mechanisms and Levodopa response fluctuations in Parkinson's disease. *Clin Neuropharmacol* 11: 378–385

57    Burke RB, Antonelli M, Sulzer D (1998) Glial cell line-derived neurotrophic factor inhibits apoptotic death of postnatal substantia nigra dopamine neurons in primary culture. *J Neurochem* 71: 517–525

58    Hou J-GG, Lin L-FH, Mytilinenou C (1996) Glial cell line-derived neurotrophic factor exerts neurotrophic effects on dopaminergic neurons *in vitro* and promotes their survival a nd regrowth after damage by 1-methyl-4-phenylpyridinium. *J Neurochem* 66: 74–82

59    Gash DM, Zhang Z, Gerhardt GA (1998) Neuroprotective and neurorestorative properties of GDNF. *Ann Neurol* 44: 121–125

60    Kearns C, Cass WA, Smoot K, Kryscio R, Gash DM (1997) GDNF protection against 6-OHDA: Time dependence and requirement for protein synthesis. *J Neurosci* 17: 7111–7118

61    Kearns C, Gash DM (1995) GDNF protects nigral dopamine neurons against 6-hydroxydopamine *in vivo*. Brain Res 672: 104–111

62    Hoffer BJ, Hoffman A, Bowenkamp K, Huettl P, Hudson, J, Martin D, Lin L-FH, Gerhardt GA (1994) Glial cell line-derived neurotrophic factor reverses toxin-induced injury to midbrain dopaminergic neurons *in vivo*. *Neurosci Lett* 182: 107–111

63    Bowenkamp KE, Hoffman AF, Gerhardt GA, Henry MA, Biddle PT, Hoffer BJ,

Granholm AC (1995) Glial cell line-derived neurotrophic factor supports survival of injured midbrain dopaminergic neurons. *J Comp Neurol* 355: 479–489

64  Gash DM, Zhang Z, Ovadia A, Cass WA, YI A, Simmerman L, Russel D, Martin D, Lapchak PA, Collins F et al (1996) Functional recovery in Parkinsonian monkeys treated with GDNF. *Nature* 380: 252–255

65  Miyoshi Y, Zhang Z, Ovadia A, Lapchak PA, Collins F, Hilt D, Lebel C, Kryscio R, Gash DM (1997) Glial cell line-derived neurotrophic factor-levodopa interactions and reduction of side effects in parkinsonian monkeys. *Ann Neurol* 42: 208–214

66  Zhang Z, Miyoshi Y, Lapchak PA, Collins F, Hilt D, Lebel C, Kryscio R, Gash DM (1997) Dose response to intraventricular glial cell line-derived neurotrophic factor administration in parkinsonian monkeys. *J Pharmacol Exp Ther* 282: 1396–1401

67  Hoffman AF, Herbert MA, Hoffer BJ, Zhang Z, Cass WA, Gash DM, Gerhardt GA (1998) Functional effects of GDNF on dopamine neurons in animal models of Parkinson's disease. In: A Fisher, I Hanin, M Yoshida (eds): *Progress in Alzheimer's and Parkinson's diseases*. Plenum Press, New York, 607–614

68  Grondin R, Zhang Z, Beck K, Hilt D, Elsberry D, Gash DM (1998) Chronic intracerebral infusion of glial cell line-derived neurotrophic factor (GDNF) in parkinsonian Rhesus monkeys. *Soc Neurosci Abstr* 24: 42

69  Davidson BL, Bohn MC (1997) Recombinant adenovirus. A gene transfer vector for study and treatment of CNS diseases. *Exp Neurol* 144: 125–130

70  Choi-Lundberg, Lin Q, Mohajeri H, Chang YN, Chiang YL, Hay CM, Davidson BL, Bohn MC, (1997) Dopaminergic neurons protected from degeneration by GDNF gene therapy. *Science* 275: 838–841

71  Bilang-Bleuel A, Revah F, Colin P, Locquet I, Robert J-J, Mallet J, Horelou P (1997) Intrastriatal injection of an adenoviral vector expressing glial-cell-line-derived neurotrophic factor prevents dopaminergic neuron degeneration and behavioral impairment in a rat model of Parkinson's disease. *Proc Natl Acad Sci USA* 94: 8818–8823

72  Bohn M (1999) A commentary on glial cell line-derived neurotrophic factor (GDNF). *Biochem Pharmacol* 57: 135–142

73  Kojima H, Abiru Y, Sakajiri K, Watabe K, Ohishi N, Takamori M, Hatanaka H, Yagi K (1997) Adenovirus-mediated transduction with human glial cell line-derived neurotrophic factor gene prevents 1-methyl-4-phenyl-1,2,3,6-tetrahydropyridine-induced dopamine depletion in striatum of mouse brain. *Biochem Biophys Res Commun* 238: 569–573

74  Ribotta MG, Revah F, Pradier L, Loquet I, Mallet J, Privat A (1997) Prevention of motoneuron death by adenovirus-mediated neurotrophic factors. *J Neurosci Res* 48: 281–285

75  Creedon DJ, Tansey GM, Baloh HR, Osborne PA, Lampe PA, Fahrner TJ, Heuckeroth RO, Milbrandt J, Johnson EM Jr (1997) Neuturin shares receptors and signal transduction pathways with glial cell line-derived neurotrophic factor in sympathetic neurons. *Neurobiology* 94: 7018–7023

# TGF-β superfamily cytokines in wound healing

*Carola U. Niesler and Mark W.J. Ferguson*

Division of Cells Immunology and Development, School of Biological Sciences, University of Manchester, 3.239 Stopford Building, Oxford Road, Manchester M13 9PT, UK

## Introduction

Scarring and impaired wound repair are major causes of numerous clinical problems. In children the generation of scar tissue can interfere with normal growth and result in various deformities (such as those resulting from cleft lip and palate surgery or severe burns to the limbs and body). Scar tissue also impairs the function of many organs leading to disease processes such as liver cirrhosis, post transplant scarring of kidneys, lungs etc. as well as contributing to the generation of intestinal obstructions, adhesions and strictures, impaired vision and defective hearing. Impaired wound healing on the other hand results in chronic difficulties in treating conditions such as venous ulcers, diabetic ulcers and pressure sores. Finally, scarring often results in undesirable cosmetic abnormalities that have severe and significant psychological consequences.

The TGF-β superfamily is a large family of cytokines shown to be extremely important in the biological processes required for normal wound healing and optimal scar formation. Members of this family regulate a wide range of cellular functions, including proliferation, differentiation, apoptosis, extracellular matrix deposition, adhesion and migration and play a very important role in development [1–3]. This has been elegantly demonstrated in the overall, and also wound healing, phenotype of the numerous TGF-β superfamily knockout animals generated during the last decade. The superfamily currently consists of over 40 members isolated from a variety of species including human, mice, chicken, *Drosophila melanogaster* and *Xenopus laevis* [4–6]. The TGF-β's, bone morphogenetic proteins (BMP's), activins with their negative regulators inihibins, growth and differentiation factors (GDF's) and Mullerian-inhibiting substances (MIS) represent the main members found within this superfamily (reviewed in [7–9]).

TGF-β and Related Cytokines in Inflammation, edited by Samuel N. Breit and Sharon M. Wahl

## TGF-β superfamily members

### TGF-β

To date five isoforms of TGF-β have been isolated. The three mammalian isoforms, TGF-$\beta_1$, TGF-$\beta_2$ and TGF-$\beta_3$ have been extensively studied in various aspects of tissue repair. TGF-$\beta_1$ was originally discovered as a secreted protein that could, together with other growth factors, transform normal cells. We now know that this isoform has many, often opposing effects on numerous cell types. The active 25 kDa TGF-$\beta_1$ molecule consists of two identical polypeptide chains which are linked by disulphide bonds [10]. TGF-$\beta_1$ is secreted from cells and released from platelets as an inactive latent complex that is unable to bind to and activate its receptors. Currently there are two types of latent forms, one termed the small latent complex and the other referred to as the large latent complex (reviewed in [2, 11]). When the active TGF-β moiety is non-covalently bound to the latency associated peptide (LAP) it is known as the small latent complex. LAP and TGF-β are products of one gene. If the small latent complex is covalently bound to a latent TGF-β binding protein (LTBP) the unit is referred to as the large latent complex. The LTBP's are products of different genes and at least three have been identified. Both the LTBP and the LAP must be removed to allow TGF-$\beta_1$ activation, but it is the LAP that confers latency to TGF-β [12, 13]. LTBP may function to enhance the secretion of the complex as well as to promote binding of TGF-β's to the extracellular matrix and aid its activation [14–16]. Active TGF-β can also associate with numerous matrix proteins such as biglycan, decorin, type IV collagen, fibronectin, dermatopontin and thrombospondin as well as $\alpha_2$-macroglobulin [17–19].

The activation of TGF-β is a major point of control in its actions and there are a number of mechanisms involved in the activation of this growth factor. *In vivo*, these include the proteases such as plasmin, calpain and MMP-9, thrombospondin, transglutaminase, the mannose 6-phosphate receptor (M6PR) and integrins (Fig. 1). Control of activity is critically important in wound healing as the initial bolus of TGF-$\beta_1$ present at the wound site arrives within seconds as the latent complex is released from degranulating platelets.

### Proteolytic mechanisms of activation

Of the proteases known to activate latent TGF-$\beta_1$, plasmin was the first to be identified and has been extensively studied [20]. This activation was proposed to occur by proteolytic nicking which leads to disruption of the tertiary structure and non-covalent bonds [20]. Other enzymes such as calpain, furin and substilisin-like endoproteases have now also been shown to be involved in activation of latent TGF-$\beta_1$ [21, 22]. The process of activation involving proteases is most likely to require input

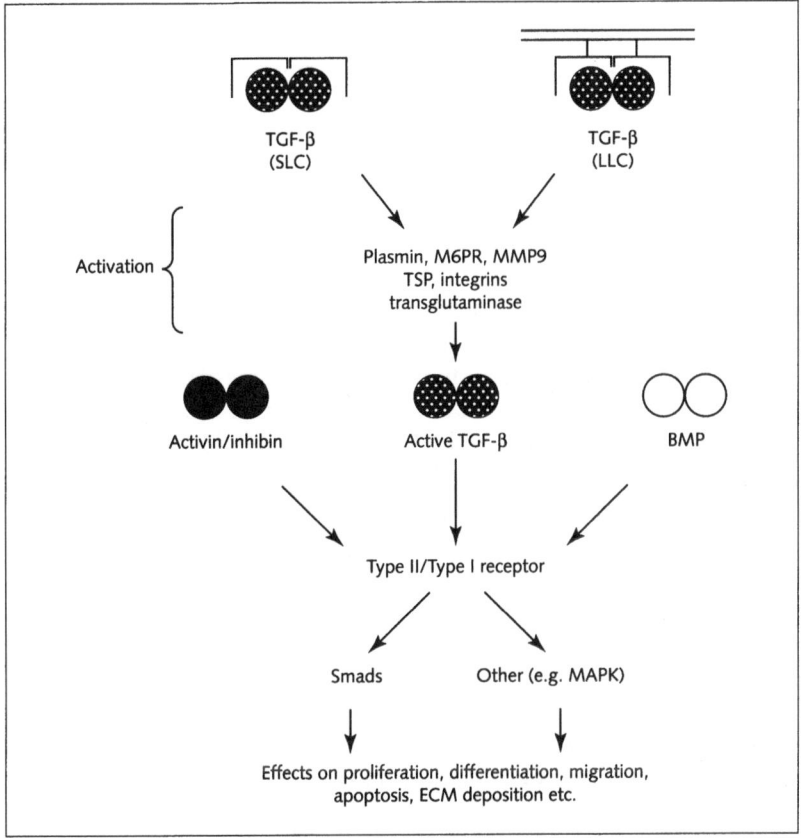

Figure 1
Basic signal transduction pathway pf TGFβ's, activins and BMP's .
LLC, Large latent complex; SLC, small latent complex.

from numerous components, including the M6P receptor and perhaps also transg-lutaminase to link the LAP-TGF-β to the cell surface. The plasminogen and uroki-nase receptors have been reported to occur and interact on the same cell type [23, 24]. In one model of TGF-$\beta_1$ activation the M6PR is proposed to complex both the urokinase plasminogen activator receptor (uPA-R) and plasminogen on human monocytes to bring about activation of latent TGF-$\beta_1$ [25]. The LAP contains man-nose 6-phosphate residues and can thereby bind the small latent complex to the M6PR. Furthermore, the controlled conversion of plasminogen to plasmin by the combined action of the uPA-R and M6PR is required, as addition of plasmin itself to the cells did not bring about the same activation. Cross-linking of the large latent complex to the extracellular matrix by transglutaminase has been proposed to be an early step in the activation of TGF-$\beta_1$ [26]. Covalent interaction of the transglutaminase reactive residues on the amino terminus of LTBP-1 with the extracellular matrix (ECM) may sequester the complex rendering it available for proteolytic degradation and subsequent activation [26, 27].

## Non-proteolytic mechanisms of activation

Non-proteolytic mechanisms are also important for TGF-$\beta_1$ activation. The platelet and matrix protein thrombospondin-1 is an important physiological regulator of TGF-$\beta_1$ activation [28–30]. Studies have shown that a specific KRFK sequence in thrombospondin-1 (TSP-1) interacts with a LSKL sequence near the amino terminus of LAP [31]. Interaction between TSP-1 and LAP-TGF-$\beta_1$ probably results in a conformational change of the small latent complex, which leads to a conversion of the TGF-$\beta_1$ from the inactive to the active TGF-$\beta_1$ form [31]. A number of integrins are able to bind latent TGF-$\beta_1$ *via* the RGD binding site in LAP. These include $\alpha_v\beta_1$, $\alpha_v\beta_6$ and $\alpha_v\beta_5$ [32, 33]. The integrin $\alpha_v\beta_6$ is expressed primarily on epithelial cells and is able to activate latent TGF-$\beta_1$. This requires association of the integrin with the actin cytoskeleton [33]. Reactive oxygen species, which play a pivotal role in wound repair and the development of fibrosis, have also been shown to activate TGF-$\beta_1$ [34–36]. It is suggested that the activation occurs as a result of oxidation of specific amino acids in the latency conferring peptide which leads to a conformational change and resultant release of TGF-$\beta_1$ from the latent complex [34].

## Activins and inhibins

The activins and inhibins were originally identified as gonadal factors that regulate (positively or negatively, respectively) the production of follicle stimulating hormone (FSH) in the pituitary [8, 37]. They are synthesized as pre-propeptides, processed to the active dimer and secreted from the cells. Activins consist of $\beta$A and $\beta$B subunits bound by disulphide bonds to give either homodimeric activin A ($\beta$A$\beta$A), homodimeric activin B ($\beta$B$\beta$B) or heteromeric activin AB ($\beta$A$\beta$B). The inhibins on the other hand are $\alpha$:$\beta$ heterodimers ($\alpha$:$\beta$A and $\alpha$:$\beta$B) ([38], reviewed in [37]). Follistatin is a protein monomer, unrelated to activins and inhibins, which can antagonize the action of activins *in vitro*. *In vivo*, follistatin can bind to heparan sulphate proteoglycans on the cell surface and thereby sequester activins or facilitate their presentation to the activin type II receptors [39]. Mice deficient in follistatin and activin have similar defects supporting the theory that, as with the presentation of TGF-$\beta$ to TGF-$\beta$-receptor (TGF-$\beta$R) type II by betaglycan, activin may be presented to its type II receptor by follistatin [37, 40, 41].

*Table 1 - Receptor subtypes used by the TGF-β superfamily members. As most of the TGF-β type I receptors were discovered at different times a neutral nomenclature: ALK (activin receptor-like kinase) was used until the physiological ligand was discovered. These are shown in brackets. The mammalian ligand for ALK7 is not known and although ALK1 binds to TGF-β$_1$, it does not mediate a response [9].*

| Receptor subtype | TGF-β$_1$ | Activin | BMP |
|---|---|---|---|
| Type 1 | TGF-βRI (ALK5) | ActR-1 (ALK2) | BMPR-1A (ALK3) |
| | | ActR-1B (ALK4) | BMPR-1B (ALK6) |
| | | | ActR-1 (ALK2) |
| Type 2 | TGF-βRII | ActR-II | BMPR-II |
| | | ActR-IIB | ActR-II |
| | | | ActR-IIB |

## Bone morphogenetic proteins

The bone morphogenetic proteins (BMP's: also known as osteogenins, osteogenic proteins (OP's) and dpp-Vg1-related (DVR) factors) were originally purified as factors that induce ectopic bone and cartilage formation when implanted under skin or into the muscle of rats. BMP1–8 have been isolated and subsequently shown to regulate numerous early developmental processes, both in vertebrates and invertebrates (reviewed in [5, 8]). BMP's are synthesized as precursor molecules consisting of a propeptide sequence, amino-terminal signal sequence and the mature protein. The mature proteins assemble as homo- or heterodimers to form the active signaling molecule. Although important in bone formation during embryogenesis, the BMP signaling pathway is also vital for the growth and repair of skeletal tissue after birth. For instance, the so-called short-ear mouse (which is known to have Bmp5 genetic deletions) has numerous skeletal and cartilage defects when born and also problems repairing rib fractures postnatally [5]. The BMP's are also expressed in many soft tissues in higher animals where their physiological role is unclear.

## Receptor signal transduction

The TGF-β superfamily members exert their effects *via* a set of Type II and Type I receptors (Tab. 1) and thereby recruit downstream signaling elements such as the Smads.

Once activated, the TGF-β signal is propagated across the plasma membrane by two structurally similar serine-threonine kinase receptors, TGF-βR type I and type II. Ligand binding to the oligomeric TGF-βRII induces recruitment of the type I receptor and brings about heteromeric oligomerisation together with subsequent transphosphorlyation of TGF-βRI by TGF-βRII. This phosphorylation occurs in the GS domain, a glycine/serine rich region in the juxtamembrane domain, of the type I receptor. The type III TGF-β receptor (betaglycan) is a non-signaling receptor, which functions predominantly to present the TGF-β to the type II receptor. A type V receptor has also been described, however, the exact function of this protein is unclear [42]. Activin signaling occurs *via* heteromeric receptor complexes in a manner similar to that of TGF-β. These complexes consist of type I (Activin RI and Activin RIb) and type II (Activin RII and Activin RIIb) serine/threonine kinase receptors [38]. The BMP receptor system is slightly different to that used by the TGF-b's and activins. The BMP ligand binds to both the type I and type II receptors with low affinity resulting in a high affinity receptor-ligand complex [43]. Furthermore, the BMP's are able to signal *via* the activin receptors, which allows for cross talk between the signaling systems.

## Signaling from the cytoplasm to the nucleus

The activated type I receptor phosphorylates downstream target signaling molecules such as the members of the Smad or MAPK (mitogen activated protein kinase) family. The term "Smad" was coined from "Sma" and "Mad". Mad (*mothers against dpp*) was isolated as a gene in *Drosophila* involved in Dpp (a BMP homologue) signaling. Sma-2, sma-3 and sma-4, genes in *C. elegans*, are homologous to Mad (reviewed in [7, 8]). To date nine Smad genes have been identified in *Xenopus laevis*, mouse and man. These are divided into three classes based on their structure and function and it is only the receptor-regulated Smads that differ between the Activin/ TGF-β and the BMP pathway (Tab. 2).

The type I receptor directly and transiently phosphorylates the receptor-regulated Smads (R-Smads). These Smads contain a critical amino acid sequence, which determines the signaling specificity of Smad 2 and Smad 3 for the Activin/TGF-β pathway as opposed to Smad 1, 5 and 8 for the BMP pathway (Tab. 2) [44]. The phosphorylation of R-Smads induces them to form hetero-oligomers with Smad 4, the only common partner Smad (Co-Smad) identified to date (reviewed in [7, 8]). In response to TGF-β or activin Smad 2, Smad 3 and Smad 4 form a complex, which can then translocate to the nucleus and induce gene transcription. In response to BMP stimulation Smad 4 and Smad 1, and possibly also Smad 5 and Smad 9, associate and move to the nucleus. The inhibitory Smads (I-Smads), Smad 6 and Smad 7 prevent signaling by the TGF-β superfamily members by associating with the type 1 receptor, thereby interfering with the phosphorylation of the R-Smads. The I-

*Table 2 - TGF-β family members and their Smad signaling molecules (adapted from [7, 8]).*

| Smad class | TGF-β pathway | BMP pathway | Activin pathway |
|---|---|---|---|
| Receptor regulated/ | Smad 2 | Smad 1 | Smad 2 |
| Pathway-restricted Smads | Smad 3 | Smad 5 | Smad 3 |
| | | Smad 8 | |
| | | Smad 9? | |
| Common partner Smads | Smad 4 | Smad 4 | Smad 4 |
| Inhibitory Smads | Smad 6 | Smad 6 | Smad 6 |
| | Smad 7 | Smad 7 | Smad 7 |

Smads may therefore act as auto-regulatory negative feedback signals during TGF-β signal transduction (reviewed in [3, 7, 8]).

Non-Smad (such as the MAPK pathway) and non-transcriptional regulation by TGF-β also play a role in TGF-β superfamily signaling. The linker region of Smad 1 can be phosphorylated by MAPK, thereby inhibiting its translocation to the nucleus (reviewed in [3]). Furthermore, TAK1 (TGF-β-activated kinase) is activated in response to BMP and TGF-β and it has been shown that the expression of an inhibitory TAK1 can prevent gene induction in response to BMP, but not activin (reviewed in [3]). Receptor tyrosine kinase signaling pathways therefore play a role in regulating the TGF-β serine/threonine kinase signaling pathway.

## Expression of TGF-β's during wound repair

TGF-β ligand and receptor levels have been analyzed in normal and impaired excisional adult murine wounds as well as ovine incisional and excisional wounds [45–47]. In normal adult murine skin, TGF-β3 was expressed at a much lower level than TGF-$\beta_1$ and TGF-$\beta_2$, and TGF-βRII was expressed at a higher level than the type I receptor. Following wounding TGF-$\beta_1$ mRNA levels increased nine-fold within 24 h and remained elevated for a number of days. TGF-$\beta_2$ mRNA increased 4.5-fold at day 5 and decreased at day 7, whereas TGF-$\beta_3$ mRNA was low during the first three days post-wounding after which it steadily increased reaching a maximal 12-fold increase at seven days post-wounding. The expression levels of both receptors II and I increased at one day post-wounding and remained elevated beyond day 13 when compared with the control skin [45]. In contrast to mRNA expression studies, analysis of TGF-β activity in adult rat skin shows two distinct and prominent peaks of TGF-β activity at one hour and five days post-wounding [48]. TGF-

$\beta_1$ was found to be the prominent isoform at both timepoints. The rapidly accumulating and degranulating platelets at the wound site are probably the major source of the early TGF-$\beta$ activity, whereas the later peak may be derived from infiltrating macrophages, fibroblasts, keratinocytes and endothelial cells [48]. In normal adult ovine skin, TGF-$\beta$ ligand and receptor expression were similar through all layers of the epidermis with the exception of TGF-$\beta_1$, which was expressed mainly in the stratum corneum [46, 47]. TGF-$\beta$RII (ALK5) and TGF-$\beta$RI expression increased at one day post-wounding in the epidermis adjacent to the wound and at five days post-wounding in the dermis, whereas TGF-$\beta$ ligand expression was increased in all skin layers at day 1. ALK1 showed weak staining until day 10 after which it became intense. The migrating epithelium, however, remained completely devoid of receptor and ligand immunoreactivity until re-epithelialisation was complete [46, 47]. Immunoreactivity for the TGF-$\beta$ receptors therefore in general occurs one to five days later than TGF-$\beta$ isoform staining sugesting that the ligands may themselves increase receptor expression. Furthermore, the switch from ALK5 to ALK1 expression may, together with the change in TGF-$\beta$ ligand levels, represent one mechanism whereby TGF-$\beta$ isoforms bring about their distinct effects on wound repair and remodeling (see section on isoform-specific effects). In contrast to murine adult wound healing, no mRNA or protein expression for TGF-$\beta$RI or TGF-$\beta$RII was observed post-wounding in the fetal dermis (A. Cowin, unpublished observations). Furthermore, in comparison to adult skin, there are lower levels of TGF-$\beta$ ligands in both unwounded and wounded fetal skin (A. Cowin unpublished observations; [49, 50]). The expression of TGF-$\beta_1$, but not TGF-$\beta_2$ or TGF-$\beta_3$, in fetal skin is transiently increased following wounding (A. Cowin, unpublished observations; [50]). When compared with other isoforms, strong staining for TGF-$\beta_3$ was observed in the epidermis of fetal skin (A. Cowin, unpublished observations). The differences in the profile of TGF-$\beta$ ligand and receptor expression observed between adult and fetal skin underline the importance of this family in scar-free vs. scar-forming wound repair.

The function of activin, inhibin and BMP's in normal and wounded skin is being elucidated. In healing excisional mouse wounds activin A and activin B mRNA levels increased at one day post-wounding and remained elevated for seven days and 13 days, respectively [51]. Activin receptor and follistatin were expressed in normal and wounded skin, but the levels of expression were unaffected during the repair process. These results suggest that activins may be important in wound repair. The BMP's have been well studied in terms of their role in bone and cartilage repair and less well in cutaneous wound repair. In the unwounded human fetal skin, BMP2 is detected at low levels in the epidermis and developing hair follicles [52]. BMP6 protein is expressed at low levels in unwounded adult murine skin and is upregulated in the epidermis and hair follicles close to the incision at three days post-wounding [53]. BMP-6 remained elevated in the suprabasal levels of the epidermis for 25 days and returned to normal levels by 42 days post-wounding.

*Table 3 - Phenotype of the TGF-β knockout (KO) mice generated to date.*

| TGF-β KO | Phenotype | Defects | Refs. |
|---|---|---|---|
| TGF-β₁ | Initially grossly indistinguishable from wildtype, but then develop wasting syndrome | Wasting phenotype between 15–36 days. Severe weight loss and multifocal organ-dependent mixed inflammatory response. Affects heart, stomach, diaphragm, liver, lung, salivary gland and pancreas. | [55] [54] |
| TGF-β₂ | Perinatal mortality | Series of developmental defects affecting heart, lung, craniofacial area, limbs, spinal column, eye and inner ear. | [58] |
| TGF-β₃ | Die within 20 h of birth | Cleft palate and delayed pulmonary development. Features are unique and consistent. | [59] [63] |
| TGF-βRII | Embryonic lethal (E10.5) | Defects in yolk sac hematopoiesis and vasculogenesis | [101] |

## Knockout and transgenic animal studies

To investigate the importance of TGF-β superfamily members, numerous mice lacking specific components of the signaling pathway have been generated over the last decade. These are outlined in Tables 3–6. Adult wound healing studies have been carried out on a number of these, but as many mice generated are embryonic lethal, only fetal wound healing studies can potentially be carried out on them.

## TGF-β

TGF-β₁ knockout mice are normal during the first two weeks of life. After this they rapidly develop a wasting syndrome and die by 3–4 weeks of age [54, 55]. These mice have mild inflammatory infiltrates in the heart at postnatal day 5, by day 7 this had spread to the lungs, salivary glands and pancreas and to almost all other organs by day 14 [55]. The perinatal survival of the TGF-β₁ knockout mice is probably due to placental transmission of maternal TGF-β₁ [56]. Wound healing studies have been carried out during the first three weeks of life of these TGF-β₁ knockout mice [57].

*Table 4 - Phenotype of activin and inhibin knockout (KO) mice generated to date*

| Activin KO | Phenotype | Defects | Refs. |
|---|---|---|---|
| Activin βA | Die within 24 h of birth | Lack whiskers and incisors<br>Craniofacial abnormalities<br>(e.g. cleft palate) | [40]<br>[102] |
| Activin βB | Viable | Eyelid defects.<br>Female cannot rear offspring | [103] |
| Activin βA/Activin βB (homozygous) | Perinatal death | Sum of defects of both knockouts | [40] |
| ActRIA (ALK2) (E7.5–E9.5) | Embryonic lethal | Gastrulation not completed.<br>Mesoderm formation disrupted<br>Abnormal visceral endoderm morphology. | [104] |
| ActRIIA/ActRIIB (homozygotes) | Resorbed by E8.5 | Growth arrested at egg cylinder stage<br>No mesoderm formation. | [105] |
| ActRcII | 25% die at birth<br>75% are viable | Some have skeletal and facial defects<br>Follicle-stimulating hormone suppressed<br>Reproductive ability abnormal | [106] |
| Follistatin | Die within 24 h of birth | Growth retarded<br>Skeletal defects of hard palate<br>Whiskers are thin and curled | [102]<br>[107] |

| Inhibin KO | | | |
|---|---|---|---|
| α-Inhibin | Begin to die after 7 weeks of age | Gonadal sex-chord stromal tumors<br>in 100% of mice<br>Wasting syndrome and severe<br>weight loss<br>Hepatocellular necrosis and depletion<br>of parietal cells of glandular stomach | [108] |
| α-Inhibin/ActRII (Homozygous mutant) | Embryonic lethal | Gonadal sex-chord stromal tumors<br>Elevated Activin A & B serum levels<br>No weight loss<br>No abnormalities in liver or stomach | [109] |

Early wound healing in these mice proceeds relatively normally, but at ten days post-wounding the knockouts displayed a marked inflammatory cell infiltrate together with a decrease in percentage wound closure and re-epithelialisation, granulation tissue formation, collagen deposition and vasculogenesis [57]. TGF-$\beta_2$ null mice exhib-

*Table 5 - Phenotype of BMP knockout (KO) mice*

| BMP KO | Phenotype | Defects | Refs. |
|---|---|---|---|
| Bmp6 | Viable | No obvious defects | [110] |
| | | Delay in ossification of developing sternum | |
| Bmp2 | Embryonic lethal | Fail to close proamniotic canal | [75] |
| | | Defect in cardiac development | |
| Bmp4/Bmp7 (heterozygotes) | Viable | Minor skeletal defects (ribs and limbs) | [76] |
| Bmp2/Bmp7 (heterzygotes) | Viable | No abnormalities | [76] |
| Bmp5/Bmp7 (heterozygotes) | Viable | No abnormalities | [76] |
| Bmp5/Bmp7 (Double mutant) | Embryonic lethal (E10.5) | | [111] |
| Bmp8a (heterozygous and homozygous) | Viable | Normal embryonic and postnatal development | [112] |
| | | Defects in maintenance of spermatogenesis | |
| | | and integrity of epididymal epithelium | |
| BMP8b | Viable | Germ cell degeneration leading to male | [113] |
| | | infertility | |
| BMP4 | Embryonic lethal | Lens induction absent | [114] |
| | (E6.5) | No primordial germ cells | [115] |
| | | Lack allantois | |
| BMPR (ALK-3) | Embryonic lethal | No mesoderm formation | [116] |
| | (E9.5) | Ectoderm cell proliferation reduced | |

it numerous developmental defects and die during or shortly before or after birth [58]. Developmental processes involving epithelial-mesenchymal interactions, angiogenesis, cell growth, ECM production and tissue remodeling are most routinely affected [58]. Fetal wound healing studies have not been documented in these mice. The TGF-β$_3$ knockout mice die within 20 h of birth due to an extensive cleft palate phenotype [59]. Interestingly, no other craniofacial abnormalities are noted in these knockout mice suggesting a specific role for TGF-β$_3$ in regulating epithelial-mesenchymal interactions in the palate [59]. In our lab, fetal wound healing studies carried out on these mice have revealed an important role for TGF-β$_3$ in the biology of scarless fetal wound repair. Embryos from the TGF-β$_3$ null mouse heal with a scar, whereas wildtype embryos display scarless wound healing [60]. The wound repair process in the knockout animals is characterized by delayed and abnormal re-epithelialisation as well as a decreased fibroblast infiltration into the wound. When com-

*Table 6 - Phenotype of Smad knockout (KO) mice*

| Smad KO | Phenotype | Defects | Refs. |
|---------|-----------|---------|-------|
| Smad2 | Embryonic lethal (E6.5–E8.5) | Severe gastrulation defects | [78] |
| | | Lack mesoderm | [79] |
| | | No organized egg cylinder | |
| Smad5 | Embryonic lethal (E9.5–E11.5) | Disrupted angiogenesis | [81] |
| | | Increased apoptosis in mesenchyme | [117] |
| | | Carniofacial and neural tube abnormalities | [118] |
| | | Defects in left-right patterning | |
| Smad3 | Viable and survive to adulthood | Die between 1–8 months of age | [80] |
| | | Forelimb malformations | [82] |
| | | Mucosal infection | |
| | | Primary defect in immune function | |
| Smad4 (DPC4) | Embryonic lethal (E6.5–E8.5) | Developmentally arrested before gastrulation | [83] |
| | | No egg cylinder formation | [84] |
| | | No mesoderm in embryo | |

pared with wildtype cells, dermal fibroblasts isolated from knockout animals at E17 showed decreased invasiveness into type I collagen gels and an increased rate of proliferation. Exogenous addition of TGF-$\beta_3$, but not TGF-$\beta_1$, partially restored the invasive property of the cells suggesting an isoform-specific effect on cell motility. On the other hand, TGF-$\beta_1$ and TGF-$\beta_3$ were both able to reduce proliferation in the knockout cells indicating a non-isoform specific effect on cell growth. Taken together these results confirm the importance of TGF-$\beta_3$ in normal wound repair and as a potential therapy in the prevention of scarring in humans.

Mice expressing the active portion of porcine TGF-$\beta_1$ cDNA under control of the mouse albumin gene have also been generated [61]. The transgenic line 25, which expresses the highest levels of TGF-$\beta_1$, displays pronounced hepatic fibrosis and apoptosis and 20% of these animals die at 4–6 weeks of age due to renal failure [61]. Surprisingly, however, incisional wounds healed with reduced scarring and were characterized by an increased basket-weave organization of the collagen when compared with the control wounds [62]. These results highlight the difference between wound analyses in transgenic animals versus wound analysis following addition, either topically or systemically, of exogenous agents. In contrast, polyvinyl alcohol (PVA) sponges implanted subcutaneously in these transgenic mice showed an increase in cellularity, granulation tissue formation and collagen synthesis. Furthermore, cutaneous wound tissue stained more intensely for TGF-$\beta_3$ and TGF-$\beta$RII, but less for TGF-$\beta_1$, whereas PVA sponges from transgenic mice stained more intensely for all three TGF-β isoforms as well as both TGF-β receptors. These data underline important differences in host response patterns between these two common wound repair models. High systemic active TGF-$\beta_1$ may downregulate or desensitize TGF-β receptors such that the local TGF-β response to wounding is actually attenuated in the TGF-$\beta_1$ overexpressing mice. Likewise an implanted PVA sponge is more like a model of a perfused foreign body reaction and the higher levels of active TGF-$\beta_1$ in the perfusate probably stimulate extracellular matrix deposition. The increased quality in scarring observed in the cutaneous incisional wounds may also be explained by the knowledge that exogenous addition of TGF-$\beta_3$ or neutralization of TGF-$\beta_1$/TGF-$\beta_2$ has been shown experimentally to markedly improve scarring. There may be some sort of inverse cross-regulation between TGF-$\beta_1$ and TGF-$\beta_3$ during wound healing such that when TGF-$\beta_1$ levels are high, the levels of TGF-$\beta_3$ will be low and vice versa. This theory is further reinforced by the fact that, in transgenic mice heterozygous for the TGF-$\beta_3$ null mutation where the level of TGF-$\beta_3$ is reduced by 50%, TGF-$\beta_1$ levels are increased far more than in the homozygous null mice at one day post-wounding [63].

Wound healing studies have also been carried out in mice lacking mechanisms of TGF-β activation. Mice lacking plasminogen (and therefore also the serine protease plasmin) survive to adulthood but develop multiple spontaneous thrombotic lesions resulting in a high rate of morbidity and mortality at an early age [64]. Wound healing is severely retarded in this knockout. Mice display impaired keratinocyte migration and one third of the wounds have not healed by six weeks post-wounding [64]. When analyzed qualitatively, cell migration and tissue remodeling was not adversely affected. Impaired healing is most likely due to the excess fibrin deposited in the wound and possibly also due to the decreased cleavage of other matrix components by plasmin [64]. Crossing the plasminogen knockout with the fibrinogen knockout ameliorates the adverse affect on wound healing [65]. TSP-1 knockouts display delayed wound organization and prolonged neovascularisation following 3 mm punch biopsies on the dorsal surface [66]. In another study, inhibition of TSP-1 production at the wound site by topical application of antisense TSP-1 oligomers resulted in a delay in re-epithelialisation and dermal organization [67]. In the control animals, the dermis at day 5 contained fibroblasts and monocytes, whereas the wounds in the treated animals were necrotic and populated primarily with neutrophils. TSP-1 has been shown to be required for the recognition of apoptotic neutrophils by phagocytes suggesting a reason for the increased number of neutrophils in the wound [68]. Mice lacking TSP-2 have abnormalities in collagen fibrillogenesis and angiogenesis, particularly in the skin, and also have dermal fibroblasts that are defective in adhesion [69]. Excisional wounds in these mice lost their scab two days earlier than those in the wildtype animals and were also reported to display a more basket-weave pattern of collagen deposition at 14 days post-wounding [70]. No differences in rates of re-epithelialisation were seen, however, as with the TSP-1 knockout, wounds displayed prolonged neovascularisation. Thus, although TSP-1 and TSP-2 adversely affect wound vascularisation, they have differing effects on wound repair. Mice homozygous for a null mutation in the $\beta_5$-integrin display no difference in their wound repair when compared with wildtype animals despite the fact that keratinocytes isolated from the null mice show impaired migration *in vitro* [71].

The insulin-like growth factor 2 (IGF2)/M6PR together with plasmin is important for the activation of TGF-$\beta$ [25]. Mice lacking only the type 2 IGFR die perinatally due to increased IGF2 serum levels which result in multiple defects including overgrowth, organomegaly and heart abnormalities [72]. Deletion of IGF2 ensures the viability of these mice [72]. Studies on wound repair in the IGF2/M6PR null mice have been carried out in our lab. These mice display an early delay in wound healing and a later decrease in the quality of scarring (unpublished observations).

Finally, the expression of transglutaminase following wounding has been analysed in rat skin [73]. These studies showed that 1–5 days post-wounding the level of transglutaminase activity is increased across all layers of the skin. This may be responsible for aiding the activation of the TGF-$\beta$ induced during early wound healing. Furthermore, it has been shown in our lab that topical application of transglutaminase inhibitors improves subsequent scarring (unpublished observations).

## Activins and inhibins

Knockout studies have shown that activins and their receptors are important for embryonic and adult development and are particularly critical for mesoderm induction [4]. Specifically, activin $\beta$A is important for craniofacial develoment whereas activin $\beta$B is critical for normal development and reproduction. Inhibins, on the other hand, are not essential for extra-embryonic or embryonic development, but are required for normal reproductive maturity in adult mice. Activin is expressed strongly following wounding and wound healing studies have been carried out on transgenic mice that over-express the activin $\beta$A chain in the epidermis under the control of the keratin-14 promoter. These mice are significantly smaller than their wildtype counterparts and display a severe thickening of the epidermis. Following injury an increase in granulation tissue formation was observed, the wound repair was enhanced at day 5 and there was a slight increase in the degree of scarring observed [74]. Studies in our lab have shown that exogenous addition of recombinant activin A to rat incisional wounds brings about an increase in the rate of re-epithelialisation and improves the quality of scarring. Activin A has also been shown to be neuroprotective *in vitro* and within six hours of brain injury there is a strong upregulation of activin $\beta$A mRNA [38]. Together these studies suggest that transient increases in activin expression following injury may play a role in the tissue repair process, however prolonged expression may be pro-fibrotic.

## BMP's

BMP2 is critical for normal extra-embryonic and embryonic development [75]. BMP6 null mice are not able to close their proamniotic canal and also display defects in their cardiac development [75]. BMP4 and BMP7 on the other hand play a role in controlling digit number and also in the guidance of ribs toward the sternum [76]. To analyze the effect of BMP2 on full-thickness osteochondral defects, trochlear grooves were made in the right femur of New Zealand White rabbits. Addition of rhBMP2 accelerated the formation of new subchondral bone and enhanced the histological appearance of the overlying articular surface [77]. Signaling *via* the BMP pathway is therefore likely to be important in regulating the processes that result in new bone formation. The role of BMP2 in wound repair has been assessed in fetal lambs [52]. In this model, BMP2-induced extensive epidermal and dermal growth when compared with controls. Treated wounds displayed a 50% increase in the thickness of the dermis and the wounds healed with an adult-like pattern of scar formation. BMP6 expression is upregulated in the murine epidermis near the site of injury and fibroblasts in the wound bed following wounding [53]. In mice overexpressing BMP6 in the epidermis, reepithelialisation and remodeling of granulation tissue of full thickness excisional and incisional wounds is significantly delayed [53]. Transgenic animals required at least 13 days for complete reepithelialisation of incisional wounds, whereas control mice need only seven days. These studies suggest a role for BMP2 and BMP6 as negative regulators of early and late wound repair.

## Smad signaling pathway

Mice null for Smad 3 survive to adulthood, whereas the Smad 2, Smad 4 and Smad 5 knockout mice are embryonic lethal [78–84]. Smad 3 null mice are smaller than their wildtype littermates and display an early phenotype of forelimb malformation, which is similar to that seen in mice expressing a transgenic dominant negative type II TGF-β receptor in bone [85]. Splenocytes isolated from these animals, and stimulated with αCD3, are resistant to anti-proliferative effects of TGF-$\beta_1$ and have a decreased ability to reduce the levels of a number of cytokines [80]. Wound healing experiments have been carried out in the Smad 3 null mice [86]. These mice display an increased rate of wound healing (wound width reduced and re-epithelialisation accelerated) with a decrease in the total number of fibroblasts and inflammatory cells as well as quantities of granulation tissue at the wound site. Topical application of TGF-$\beta_1$ to the wounds increased matrix deposition without increasing fibroblast cell number, but had no effect on re-epithelialisation. Furthermore, mouse embryonic fibroblasts from Smad 3 knockout mice are partially resistant to the anti-proliferative effects of TGF-$\beta_1$ [80]. As a result of these studies,

Massague and Ashcroft et al. have suggested a role for Smad 3 as a negative modulator of keratinocyte proliferation and a role for Smad 2 as a positive regulator of extra-cellular matrix deposition [86, 87]. These distinct roles for Smad family members expose potential new targets for therapeutic intervention during wound healing.

## Isoform specific effects of mammalian TGF-β's

TGF-β's are important in wound repair and scar formation in an isoform-specific manner. In adult rodent incisional wounds, neutralisation of TGF-$\beta_1$ and TGF-$\beta_2$ markedly reduced the influx of inflammatory cells, deposition of fibronectin, collagen 1 and collagen 3 during early wound repair while concomitantly increasing the tensile strength and scar quality of the wound [88, 89]. Furthermore, in these same studies it was shown that addition of TGF-$\beta_3$ had a similar effect. However addition of TGF-$\beta_1$ did not improve the final quality of the scar. These data highlight the distinct differences in the effects of TGF-β isoforms on wound repair and remodeling. Neutralisation of TGF-$\beta_1$ did not have as marked an effect as the combined neutralization of TGF-$\beta_1$ and TGF-$\beta_2$, whereas anti-TGF-$\beta_2$ antibodies had little effect. TGF-$\beta_2$ therefore enhances the action of TGF-$\beta_1$. In rabbits the addition of recombinant human anti-TGF-$\beta_2$ monoclonal antibodies significantly improves conjunctival scarring [90]. In Wistar rats the application of anti-TGF-$\beta_1$ neutralising antibodies resulted in a more regenerative healing pattern in chronic gastric ulcers, whereas addition of TGF-$\beta_1$ itself led to excessive scarring. Interestingly, however, both the neutralising antobodies and the growth factor brought about significant increases in the rate of healing of ulcers [91]. The use of antisense oligodeoxynucleotides to TGF-$\beta_1$ on adult wounds also brought about a marked reduction in the scarring when compared with control wounds [92]. TGF-$\beta_1$ affects scarring in the central nervous system. When TGF-$\beta_1$ is injected into the brains of injured rats the scarring response is dramatically increased, conversely, when a neutralizing antibody to TGF-$\beta_1$ is injected, the scar tissue is attenuated [93]. TGF-$\beta_1$ has also been shown to play a pivotal role in peritoneal healing and fibrous adhesion formation. Addition of anti-TGF-$\beta_1$ antibodies in a model of abdominal adhesions in rats reduced the severity of adhesions, whereas antibodies to TGF-$\beta_2$ had no effect [94]. Fetal wounding studies in the TGF-$\beta_3$ knockout mouse have demonstrated the importance of TGF-$\beta_3$ in the generation of a good quality scar. Early fetal surgical skin wounds heal rapidly without a scar and with a markedly reduced inflammatory response, which in turn generates an altered profile of growth factors [95, 96]. The generation of a scar in the TGF-$\beta_3$ knockout mouse embryos underlines the importance of this molecule in the positive regulation of scarless dermal regeneration.

## Preclinical studies of TGF-β in impaired wound repair

There is a large amount of literature which demonstrates that the addition of TGF-β, both locally or systemically, improves wound healing in various animal models (reviewed in [1, 2]). In summary these studies show that addition of TGF-$\beta_1$ improves wound repair by accelerating reepithelialisation, influx of fibroblasts and macrophages and accumulation of granulation tissue as well as increasing the tensile strength of the wound by increasing the deposition of collagen. Numerous studies have also shown that TGF-$\beta_1$ can accelerate repair in a variety of impaired wound healing models. In these cases very often a single dose of topically applied TGF-$\beta_1$ is able to bring about the necessary improvements. In aged rats as well as glucocorticoid-treated rats TGF-$\beta_1$ increased the breaking strength to levels similar to those seen in normal animals [97, 98]. In animals treated with radiation low doses of TGF-$\beta_1$ improved the wound strength and in steroid-impaired wound healing TGF-$\beta_1$ stimulated healing by increasing reepithelialisation as well as the deposition of granulation tissue [99, 100].

## Clinical applications of TGF-β in wound healing

In humans, impaired wound healing commonly occurs as a result of chemotherapy, metabolic disorders, ageing, vascular disease, pressure or radiation therapy. Despite the wealth of animal data supporting the beneficial effect of TGF-$\beta_1$ on normal and impaired wound healing, no clinical studies have as yet been carried out using this isoform. Early studies using TGF-$\beta_2$ to treat venous stasis ulcers were encouraging, showing a reduction in total ulcer area. However, in subsequent studies the results were not as impressive. The problem with topical application of growth factors to chronic wounds lies in the high levels of proteases found at the wound site. As a result, in the absence of protease inhibitors, this mode of delivery is unlikely to have the desired therapeutic effect. Furthermore, in nearly all clinical trials of chronic wound healing agents there is a significant placebo effect. The control arm in these studies heals well due to the good care experienced by all patients and this therefore makes it difficult to assess the beneficial effects of the exogenous agent. TGF-$\beta_3$ has also been assessed in the treatment of venous stasis ulcers and, as with TGF-$\beta_1$, although early studies were positive, in phase three of the clinical trial TGF-$\beta_3$ was found to have no beneficial effect. In the light of the animal data showing that TGF-$\beta_3$ improves scarring rather than wound repair, it may be more reasonable to test this growth factor as an anti-scarring agent. Such studies have been initiated in man. Neutralizing antibodies to TGF-$\beta_2$ have already been shown to increase the quality of scarring in human glaucoma. In phase two clinical studies, human recombinant phage antibodies to TGF-$\beta_1$ and TGF-$\beta_2$ are about to enter human clinical studies in a variety of scar preventing applications (e.g. dermal scarring). Mannose-6-phosphate, which prevents the activation of TGF-$\beta$, is also under human clinical trial as a scar preventing therapy in the skin.

## Conclusions

Acute wound repair in adults is optimized for speed of healing under dirty conditions and usually results in scarring. Animal studies, both fetal versus adult as well as transgenic and knockout versus wildtype, have provided major insights into the factors and processes regulating wound repair and scar formation. In this regard, the TGF-$\beta$ superfamily, and specifically TGF-$\beta_1$, TGF-$\beta_2$ and TGF-$\beta_3$, have emerged as major players in the control of wound healing and scarring. According to the 1999/2000 Theta and Clinica Reports on Wound Healing, every year in the developing world 35 million people undergo elective surgery that result in a scar, 18.5 million are injured due to trauma, ten million have keloid scars, seven million are injured by burning, five million suffer from chronic pressure sores and four million from venous and diabetic ulcers. These figures highlight the critical need for further advances in the clinical treatment of acute and chronic wounds both to accelerate healing and to reduce scarring. In this respect, modulation of transforming growth factor beta levels shows much promise.

*Acknowledgements*
Original research summarized in this paper was supported by Johnson & Johnson Medical Inc. for which we are grateful.

## References

1   Roberts AB, Sporn MB (1993) Physiological actions and clinical applications of transforming growth factor-$\beta$ (TGF-$\beta$). *Growth Factors* 8: 1–9
2   O'Kane S, Ferguson MWJ (1997) Transforming growth factor $\beta$s and wound healing. *Int J Biochem Cell Biol* 29: 63–78
3   Whitman M (1998) Smads and the early developmental signaling by the TGF$\beta$ superfamily. *Genes Dev* 12: 2445–2462
4   Kingsley DM (1994) The TGF-$\beta$ superfamily: new members, new receptors and new genetic tests of function in different organisms. *Genes Dev* 8: 133–146
5   Kingsley DM (1994) What do BMPs do in mammals? Clues from the short-ear mutation. *Trends Genet* 10: 16–21
6   Meno C, Saijoh Y, Fuji H, Ikeda M, Yokoyama T, Yokoyama M, Toyoda Y, Hamada H

(1996) Left-right assymetric expression of the TGFβ family member lefty in mouse embryos. *Nature* 381: 151–155

7    Heldin C-H, Miyazono K, ten Dijke P (1997) TGF-β signalling from cell membrane to nucleus through smad proteins. *Nature* 390: 465–471

8    Kawabata M, Miyazono K (1999) Signal transduction of the TGFβ superfamily by smad proteins. *J Biochem* 125: 9–16

9    Massagué J (1998) TGF-β signal transduction. *Annu Rev Biochem* 67: 753–791

10   Assoian RK, Komoriya A, Meyers CA, Miller DM, Sporn MB (1983) Transforming growth factor-β in human platelets: identification of a major storage site, purification and characterisation. *J Biol Chem* 258: 7155–7160

11   Miyazono K, Ichijo H, Heldin CH (1993) Transforming growth factor-beta: Latent forms, binding proteins and receptors. *Growth Factors* 8: 11–22

12   Gentry LE, Webb NR, Lim GJ, Brunner AM, Ranchalis JE, Twardzik DR, Lioubin MN, Marquardt H, Purchio AF (1987) Type 1 transforming growth factor beta: amplified expression and secretion of mature and precursor polypeptides in Chinese hamster ovary cells. *Mol Cell Biol* 7: 3418–3427

13   Gentry LE, Nash BW (1990) The pro domain of pre-pro-transforming growth factor beta 1 when independently expressed is a functional binding protein for the mature growth factor. *Biochemistry* 29: 6851–6857

14   Miyazono K, Olofsson A, Colosetti P, Heldin CH (1991) A role of the latent TGF-β1 binding protein in assembly and secretion of TGFβ1. *EMBO J* 10: 1091–1101

15   Taipale J, Maiyazono K, Heldin CH, Keski-Oja J (1994) Latent transforming growth factor-beta 1 associates to fibroblast extracellular matrix *via* latent TGFβ binding protein. *J Cell Biol* 124: 171–181

16   Flaumenhaft R, Abe M, Sato Y, Maiyazono K, Harpel J, Heldin CH, Rifkin DB (1993) Role of the latent TGF-beta binding protein in the activation of latent TGFβ by co-cultures of endothelial and smooth muscle cells. *J Cell Biol* 120: 995–1002

17   Noble NA, Harper JR, Border WA (1992) *In vivo* interactions of TGF-beta and extracellular matrix. *Prog Growth Factor Res* 4: 369–382

18   O'Connor-McCourt MD, Wakefield LM (1987) Latent transforming growth factor-beta in serum. A specific complex with alpha 2-macroglobulin. *J Biol Chem* 262: 14090–14099

19   Okamoto O, Fujiwara S, Abe M, Sato Y (1999) Dermatopontin interacts with transforming growth factor β and enhances its biological activity. *Biochem J* 337: 537–541

20   Lyons RM, Gentry LE, Purchio AF, Moses HL (1990) Mechanism of activation of latent recombinant transforming growth factor β1 by plasmin. *J Cell Biol* 110: 1361–1367

21   Ming Chu T, Kawinski E (1998) Plasmin, substilisin-like endoproteases, tissue plasminogen activator are involved in activation of latent TGF-β1 in human seminal plasma. *Biochem Biophys Res Commun* 253: 128–134

22   Abe M, Oda N, Sato Y (1998) Cell-associated activation of latent transforming growth factor-β by calpain. *J Cell Physiol* 174: 186–193

23   Nykjær A, Christensen EI, Vorum H, Hager H, Peterson CM, Røigaard H, Min HY, Vilhardt F, Møller LB, Kornfeld S et al (1998) Mannose 6-phosphate/Insulin-like growth

factor-II receptor targets the urokinase receptor to lysosomes *via* a novel binding interaction. *J Cell Biol* 141: 815–828

24   Plow EF, Freaney DE, Plescia J, Miles LA (1986) The plasminogen system and cell surfaces: evidence for plasminogen and urokinase receptors on the same cell type. *J Cell Biol* 103: 2411–2420

25   Godár S, Horejsi V, Weidle UH, Binder BR, Hansmann C, Stockinger H (1999) M6P/IGFII-receptor complexes urokinase receptor and plasminogen for activation of transforming growth factor-β1. *Eur J Immunol* 29: 1004–1013

26   Nunes I, Gleizes P-E, Metz CN, Rifkin D (1997) Latent transforming growth factor-β binding protein domains involved in activation and transglutaminase-dependent cross-linking of latent transforming growth factor-β. *J Cell Biol* 136: 1151–1163

27   Kojima S, Kiyomitsu N, Rifkin DB (1993) Requirement for transglutaminase in the activation of latent transforming growth factor-beta in bovine endothelial cells. *J Cell Biol* 121: 439–448

28   Crawford SE, Stellmach V, Murphy-Ullrich JE, Ribeiro SM, Lawler J, Hynes RO, Boivin GP, Bouck N (1998) Thrombospondin-1 is a major activator of TGF-beta1 *in vivo*. *Cell* 93: 1159–1170

29   Schultz-Cherry S, Murphy-Ullrich JE (1993) Thrombospondin causes activation of latent transforming growth factor-β secreted by endothelial cells by a novel mechanism. *J Cell Biol* 122: 923–932

30   Schultz-Cherry S, Ribeiro S, Gentry L, Murphy-Ullrich JE (1994) Thrombospondin binds and activates the small and large forms of latent transforming growth factor-β in a chemically defined system. *J Biol Chem* 269: 26775–26782

31   Ribeiro SMF, Poczatek M, Schultz-Cherry S, Villain M, Murphy-Ullrich JE (1999) The activation sequence of thrombospondin-1 interacts with the latency-associated peptide to regulate activation of latent transforming growth factor-β. *J Biol Chem* 274: 13586–13593

32   Munger JS, Harpel JG, Giancotti FG, Rifkin DB (1997) Interactions between *Growth Factors* and integrins: latent forms of transforming growth factor-β are ligands for the integrin $\alpha_v\beta_1$. *Mol Biol Cell* 9: 2627–2638

33   Munger JS, Huang X, Kawakatsu H, Griffiths MJD, Dalton SL, Wu J, Pittet J-F, Kaminski N, Garat C, Matthay MA et al (1999) The integrin avb6 binds and activates latent TGFβ1: A mechanism for regulating pulmonary inflammation and fibrosis. *Cell* 96: 319–328

34   Barcellos-Hoff MH, Dix TA (1996) Redox-mediated activation of latent transforming growth factor-beta 1. *Mol Endocrinol* 10: 1077–1083

35   Beinert T, Binder D, Stuschke M, Jorres RA, Oehm C, Fleischhacker M, Sezer O, Mergenthaler HG, Werner T, Possinger K (1996) Oxidant-induced lung injury in anticancer therapy. *Eur J Med Res* 4: 43–53

36   Dominguez-Rosales JA, Mavi G, Levenson SM, Rojkind M (2000) H(2)O(2) is an important mediator of physiological and pathological healing responses. *Arch Med Res* 31: 15–20

37    Matzuk MM, Kumar TR, Shou W, Coerver KA, Lau AL, Behringer RR, Finegold MJ
      (1996) Transgenic models to study the roles of inhibins and activins in reproduction,
      oncogenesis, and development. *Recent Prog Horm Res* 51: 123–154

38    Munz B, Hubner G, Tretter Y, Alzheimer C, Werner S (1999) A novel role of activin in
      inflammation and repair. *J Endocrinol* 161: 187–193

39    Nakamura T, Sugino K, Titani K, Sugino H (1991) Follistatin, an activin-binding pro-
      tein, associates with heparan sulfate chains of proteoglycans on follicular granulosa
      cells. *J Biol Chem* 266: 19432–19437

40    Matzuk MM, Kumar TR, Vassalli A, Bickenbach JR, Roop DR, Jaenisch R, Bradley A
      (1995) Functional analysis of activins during mammalian development. *Nature* 374:
      354–356

41    Matzuk MM, Lu N, Vogel H, Sellheyer K, Roop DR, Bradley A (1995) Multiple defects
      and perinatal death in mice deficient in follistatin. *Nature* 374: 360–363

42    O'Grady P, Kuo M-D, Baldassare JJ, Huang SS, Huang JS (1991) Purification of a new
      type of high molecular weight receptor (Type V Receptor) of transforming growth fac-
      tor β (TGF-β) from bovine liver. *J Biol Chem* 266: 8583–8589

43    Rosenzweig BL, Imamura T, Okadome T, Cox GN, Yamashita H, ten Dijk P, Heldin
      CH, Miyazono K (1995) Cloning and characterisation of a human type II receptor for
      bone morphogenetic proteins. *Proc Natl Acad Sci USA* 92: 7632–7636

44    Lo RS, Chen Y-G, Shi Y, Pavletich NP, Massagué J (1998) The L3 loop: a structural
      motif determining specific interactions between SMAD proteins and TGF-β receptor.
      *EMBO J* 17: 996–1005

45    Frank S, Madlener M, Werner S (1996) Transforming growth factor β1, β2, and β3 and
      their receptors are differentially regulated during normal and impaired wound healing.
      *J Biol Chem* 271: 10188–10193

46    Gold LI, Sung JJ, Siebert JW, Longaker MT (1997) Type I (RI) and type II (RII) recep-
      tors for transforming growth factor-β isoforms are expressed subsequent to transform-
      ing growth factor-β ligands during excisional wound repair. *Am J Path* 150: 209–222

47    McMullen H, Longaker MT, Cabrera RC, Sung J, Canete J, Siebert JW, Lorenz P, Gold
      LI (1994) Spatial and temporal expression of transforming growth factor-β isoforms
      during ovine excisional and incisional wound repair. *Wound Rep Reg* 3: 141–156

48    Yang L, Qiu CX, Ludlow A, Ferguson MWJ, Brunner G (1999) Active TGF-β in wound
      repair. Determination using a new assay. *Am J Pathol* 154: 105–111

49    Whitby DJ, Ferguson MW (1991) Immunohistochemical localization of *Growth Factors*
      in fetal wound healing. *Dev Biol* 147: 207–215

50    Martin P, Dickson MC, Millan FA, Akhurst RJ (1993) Rapid induction and clearance of
      TGF beta 1 is an early response to wounding in the mouse embryo. *Dev Genet* 14:
      225–238

51    Hubner G, Hu Q, Smola H, Werner S (1996) Strong induction of activin expression after
      injury suggests an important role of activin in wound repair. *Dev Biol* 173: 490–496

52    Stelnicki EJ, Longaker MT, Holmes D, Vanderwall K, Harrison MR, Largman C, Hoff-

man WY (1998) Bone morphogenetic protein-2 induces scar formation and skin maturation in the second trimester fetus. *Plast Reconstruct Surg* 101: 12–19

53   Kaiser S, Schirmacher P, Philipp A, Protschka M, Moll I, Nicol K, Blessing M (1998) Induction of bone morphogenetic protein-6 in skin wounds. Delayed reepitheliazation and scar formation in BMP-6 overexpressing transgenic mice. *J Invest Dermatol* 111: 1145–1152

54   Kulkarni AB, Ward JM, Yaswen L, Mackall CL, Bauer SR, Huh CG, Gress RE, Karlsson S (1995) Transforming growth factor-beta 1 null mice. An animal model for inflammatory disorders. *Am J Pathol* 146: 264–275

55   Boivin GP, O'Toole BA, Orsmby IE, Diebold RJ, Eis MJ, Doetschman T, Kier AB (1995) Onset and progression of pathological lesions in transforming growth factor-beta 1-deficient mice. *Am J Path* 146: 276–288

56   Letterio JJ, Geiser AG, Kulkarni AB, Roche NS, Sporn MB, Roberts AB (1994) Maternal rescue of transforming growth factor-beta 1 null mice. *Science* 264: 1936–1938

57   Brown RL, Ormsby I, Doetschman TC, Greenhalgh DG (1995) Wound helaing in the transforming growth factor-$\beta_1$-deficient mouse. *Wound Rep Reg* 3: 25–36

58   Sanford L, Ormsby I, Gittenberger-de Groot A, Sariola H, Friedman R, Boivin G, Cardell E, Doetschman T (1997) TGFbeta2 knockout mice have multiple developmental defects that are non-overlapping with other TGFbeta knockout phenotypes. *Development* 124: 2659–2670

59   Kaartinen V, Voncken JW, Shuler C, Warburton D, Bu D, Heisterkamp N, Groffen J (1995) Abnormal lung development and cleft palate in mice lacking TGF-beta 3 indicates defects of epithelial-mesenchymal interaction. *Nature Genet* 11: 415–421

60   Qiu CX, Brunner G, Ferguson MWJ (2001) Abnormal wound healing and scarring in the TGF-$\beta$3 null mouse embryo. *Development; in press*

61   Sanderson N, Factor V, Nagy P, Kopp J, Kondaiah P, Wakefield L, Roberts A, Sporn M, Thorgeirsson S (1995) Hepatic expression of mature transforming growth factor beta 1 in transgenic mice results in multiple tissue lesions. *Proc Natl Acad Sci USA* 92: 2572–2576

62   Shah M, Revis Jr D, Herrick S, Baillie R, Thorgeirson S, Ferguson M, Roberts A (1999) Role of elevated plasma transforming growth factor-$\beta$1 levels in wound healing. *Am J Pathol* 154: 1115–1124

63   Proetzel G, Pawlowski S, Wiles M, Yin M, Boivin G, Howles P, Ding J, Ferguson M, Doetschman T (1995) Transforming growth factor-beta 3 is required for secondary palate fusion. *Nat Genet* 11: 409–414

64   Romer J, Bugge TH, Pyke C, Lund LR, Flick MJ, Degen JL, Dano K (1996) Impaired wound healing in mice with a disrupted plasminogen gene. *Nature Med* 2: 287–292

65   Bugge TH, Kombrinck KW, Flick MJ, Daugherty CC, Danton MJ, Degen JL (1996) Loss of fibrinogen rescues mice from the pleiotropic effects of plasminogen deficiency. *Cell* 87: 709–719

66   Polverini PJ, DiPietro LA, Dixit VM, Hynes RO, Lawler J (1995) Thrombospondin 1

knockout mice show delayed organisation and prolonged neovascularisation of skin wounds. *FASEB J* 9: A272

67   DiPietro LA, Nissen NN, Gamelli RL, Koch AE, Pyle JM, Polverini PJ (1996) Thrombospondin 1 synthesis and function in wound repair. *Am J Pathol* 148: 1851–1860

68   Savill J, Fadok V, Henson P, Haslett C (1993) Phagocyte recognition of cells undergoing apoptosis. *Immunol Today* 14: 131–136

69   Kyriakides TR, Zhu YH, Smith LT, Bain SD, Yang Z, Lin MT, Danielson KG, Iozzo RV, LaMarca M, McKinney CE et al (1998) Mice that lack thrombospondin 2 display connective tissue abnormalities that are associated with disordered collagen fibrillogenesis, an increased vascular density, and a bleeding diathesis. *J Cell Biol* 140: 419–430

70   Kyriakides TR, Tam JWY, Bornstein P (1999) Accelerated wound healing in mice with a disruption of the thrombospondin 2 gene. *J Invest Dermatol* 113: 782–787

71   Huang X, Griffiths M, Wu J, Farese RVJ, Sheppard D (2000) Normal development, wound healing, and adenovirus susceptibility in beta5-deficient mice. *Mol Cell Biol* 20: 755–759

72   Ludwig T, Eggenschiler J, Fisher P, D'Ercole AJ, Davenport ML, Efstratiadis A (1996) Mouse mutants kacking the type 2 IGF receptor (IGF2R) are rescued from perinatal lethality in Igf2 and Igf1r null backgrounds. *Dev Biol* 177: 517–535

73   Bowness JM, Tarr AH, Wong T (1988) Increased transglutaminase activity during skin wound healing in rats. *Biochim Biophys Acta* 17: 234–240

74   Munz B, Smola H, Engelhardt F, Bleuel K, Brauchle M, Lein I, Evans LW, Huylebroeck D, Balling R, Werner S (1999) Overexpression of activin A in the skin of transgenic mice reveals new activities of activin in epidermal morphogenesis, dermal fibrosis and wound repair. *EMBO J* 18: 5205–5215

75   Zhang H, Bradley A (1996) Mice deficient for BMP2 are nonvariable and have defects in amnion/chorion and cardiac development. *Development* 122: 2977–2986

76   Katagiri T, Boorla S, Frendo JL, Hogan BL, Karsenty G (1998) Skeletal abnormalities in doubly heterozygous Bmp4 amd Bmp7 mice. *Dev Genet* 22: 340–348

77   Sellers RS, Peluso D, Morris EA (1997) The effect of recominant human bone morphogenetic protein-2 (rhBMP-2) on the healing of full-thickness defects of articular cartilage. *J Bone Joint Surg Am* 79: 1452–1463

78   Weinstein M, Yang X, Li C, Xu X, Gotay J, Deng CX (1998) Failure of egg cylinder elongation and mesoderm induction in mouse embryos lacking the tumor suppressor smad2. *Proc Natl Acad Sci USA* 95: 9378–9383

79   Nomura M, Li E (1998) Smad2 role in mesoderm formation, left-right patterning and craniofacial development. *Nature* 393: 786–790

80   Datto MB, Frederick JP, Pan L, Borton AJ, Zhuang Y, Wang XF (1999) Targeted disruption of Smad3 reveals an essential role in transforming growth factor beta-mediated signal transduction. *Mol Cell Biol* 4: 2495–2504

81   Yang X, Castilla LH, Xu X, Li C, Gotay J, Weinstein M, Liu PP, Deng CX (1999) Angiogenesis defects and mesenchymal apoptosis in mice lacking SMAD5. *Development* 126: 1571–1580

82    Yang X, Letterio JJ, Lechleider RJ, Chen L, Hayman R, Gu H, Roberts AB, Deng C (1999) Targeted disruption of SMAD3 results in impaired mucosal immunity and diminished T cell responsiveness to TGF-beta. *EMBO J* 18: 1280–1291

83    Takaku K, Oshima M, Miyoshi H, Matsui M, Seldin MF, Taketo MM (1998) Intestinal tumorigenesis in compound mutant mice of both Dpc4 (Smad4) and Apc genes. *Cell* 92: 645–656

84    Yang X, Li C, Xu X, Deng C (1998) The tumor suppressor SMAD4/DPC4 is essential for epiblast proliferation and mesoderm induction in mice. *Proc Natl Acad Sci USA* 95: 3667–3672

85    Serra R, Johnson M, Filvaroff EH, LaBorde J, Sheehan DM, Derynck R, Moses HL (1997) Expression of a truncated, kinase-defective TGF-beta type II receptor in mouse skeletal tissue promotes terminal chondrocyte differentiation and osteoarthritis. *J Cell Biol* 139: 541–552

86    Ashcroft G, Yang X, Glick A, Weinstein M, Letterio J, Mizel D, Anzano M, Greenwell-Wild T, Wahl S, Deng C et al (1999) Mice lacking Smad3 show accelerated wound healing and an impaired local inflammatory response. *Nat Cell Biol* 1: 260–266

87    Massague J (1999) Wounding Smad. *Nat Cell Biol* 1: E117–E119

88    Shah M, Foreman DM, Ferguson MWJ (1994) Neutralising antibody to TGF-$\beta_{1,2}$ reduces cutaneous scarring in adult rodents. *J Cell Sci* 107: 1137–1157

89    Shah M, Foreman DM, Ferguson MWJ (1995) Neutralisation of TGF-$\beta$1 and TGF-$\beta$2 or exogenous addition of TGF-$\beta$3 to cutaneous rat wounds reduces scarring. *J Cell Sci* 108: 985–1002

90    Cordeiro MF, Gay JA, Khaw PT (1999) Human anti-transforming growth factor-beta2 antibody: a new glaucoma anti-scarring agent. *Invest Ophthalmol Vis Sci* 40: 2225–2234

91    Ernst H, Konturek P, Hahn EG, Brzozowski T, Konturek SJ (1996) Acceleration of wound healing in gastric ulcers by local injection of neutralising antibody to transforming growth factor beta 1. *Gut* 39: 172–175

92    Choi BM, Kwak HJ, Jun CD, Park SD, Kim KY, Kim HR, Chung HT (1996) Control of scarring in adult wounds using antisense transforming growth factor-beta 1 oligodeoxynucleotides. *Immunol Cell Biol* 74: 144–150

93    Logan A, Berry M, Gonzalez AM, Frautschy SA, Sporn MB, Baird A (1994) Effects of transforming growth factor beta 1 on scar production in the injured central nervous system of the rat. *Eur J Neurosci* 1: 355–363

94    Lucas PA, Warejcka DJ, Young HE, Lee BY (1996) Formation of abdominal adhesions is inhibited by antibodies to transforming growth factor-beta1. *J Surg Res* 65: 135–138

95    Shah M, Whitby DJ, Ferguson MWJ (1996) Fetal wound healing and scarless surgery. In: IT Jackson, BC Somerlad (eds): *Recent advances in plastic surgery*. Churchill Livingstone, Edinburgh, 1–12

96    Adzick NS, Lorenz HP (1994) Cells, matrix, *Growth Factors*, and the surgeon. The biology of scarless fetal wound repair. *Ann Surg* 220: 10–18

97    Beck LS, DeGuzman L, Lee WP, Xu Y, Siegel MW, Amento EP (1993) One systemic

administration of transforming growth factor-beta 1 reverses age- or glucocorticoid-impaired wound healing. *J Clin Invest* 92: 2841–2849

98    Pierce GF, Mustoe TA, Lingelbach J, Masakowski VR, Gramates P, Deuel TF (1989) Transforming growth factor beta reverses the glucocorticoid-induced wound-healing deficit in rats: possible regulation in macrophages by platelet-derived growth factor. *Proc Natl Acad Sci USA* 86: 2229–2233

99    Beck LS, Deguzman L, Lee WP, Xu Y, McFatridge LA, Amento EP (1991) TGF-beta 1 accelerates wound healing: reversal of steroid-impaired healing in rats and rabbits. *Growth Factors* 5: 295–304

100   Bernstein EF, Harisiadis L, Salomon G, Norton J, Sollberg S, Uitto J, Glatstein E, Glass J, Talbot T, Russo Aea (1991) Transforming growth factor-beta improves healing of radiation-impaired wounds. *J Invest Dermatol* 97: 430–434

101   Oshima M, Oshima H, Taketo MM (1996) TGF-β receptor type II deficiency results in defects of yolk sac hematopoiesis and vasculogenesis. *Dev Biol* 179: 297–302

102   Jhaveri S, Erzurumlu RS, Chiaia N, Kumar TR, Matzuk MM (1998) Defective whisker follicles and altered brainstem patterns in activin and follistatin knockout mice. *Mol Cell Neuros* 12: 206–219

103   Vassalli A, Matzuk MM, Gardner HA, Lee KF, Jaenisch R (1994) Activin/inhibin beta B subnunit gene disruption leads to defects in eyelid development and female reproduction. *Genes Dev* 8: 414–427

104   Gu Z, Reynolds EM, Song J, Lei H, Feijen A, Yu L, He W, MacLaughlin DT, van den Eijnden-van Raaij J, Donahoe PK et al (1999) The type I serine/threonine kinase receptor ActRIA (ALK2) is required for gastrulation of the mouse embryo. *Development* 126: 2551–2561

105   Song J, Oh SP, Schrewe H, Nomura M, Lei H, Okano M, Gridley T, Li E (1999) The type II activin receptors are essential for egg cylinder growth, gastrulation, and rostral head development in mice. *Dev Biol* 213: 157–169

106   Matzuk MM, Kumar TR, Bradley A (1995) Different phenotypes for mice deficient in either activins or activin receptor type II. *Nature* 374: 356–360

107   Matzuk MM, Lu N, Vogel H, Sellheyer K, Roop DR, Bradley A (1995) Multiple defects and perinatal death in mice deficient in follistatin. *Nature* 374: 360–363

108   Matzuk MM, Finegold MJ, Mather JP, Krummen L, Lu H, Bradley A (1994) Development of cancer cachexia-like syndrome and adrenal tumors in inhibin-deficient mice. *Proc Natl Acad Sci USA* 91: 8817–8821

109   Coerver KA, Woodruff TK, Finegold MJ, Mather J, Bradley A, Matzuk MM (1996) Activin signaling through activin receptor type II causes the cachexia-like symptoms in inhibin-deficient mice. *Mol Endocrinol* 5: 534–543

110   Solloway MJ, Dudley AT, Bikoff EK, Lyons KM, Hogan BL, Robertson EJ (1998) Mice lacking Bmp6 function. *Dev Genet* 22: 321–339

111   Solloway MJ, Robertson EJ (1999) Early embryonic lethality in Bmp6:Bmp7 double mutant mice suggests functional redundancy within the 60A subgroup. *Development* 126: 1753–1768

112 Zhao GQ, Liaw L, Hogan BL (1998) Bone morphogenetic proetin 8A plays a role in the maintenance of spermatogenesis and the integrity of the epidermis. *Development* 125: 1103–1112

113 Zhao GQ, Deng K, Labosky PA, Liaw L, Hogan BL (1996) The gene encoding bone morphogenetic protein 8B is required for the initiation and maintenance of spermatogenesis in the mouse. *Genes Dev* 10: 1657–1669

114 Furuta Y, Hogan BLM (1998) BMP4 is essential for lens inducation in the mouse embryo. *Genes Dev* 12: 3764–3775

115 Lawson KA, Dunn NR, Roelen BAJ, Zeinstra LM, Davis AM, Wright CVE, Korving JPWFM, Hogan BLM (1999) Bmp4 is required for the generation of primordial germ cells in the mouse embryo. *Genes Dev* 13: 424–436

116 Mishina Y, Suzuki A, Ueno N, Behringer RR (1995) Bmpr encodes a type I bone morphogenetic protein receptor that is essential for gastrulation during mouse embryogenesis. *Genes Dev* 9: 3027–3037

117 Chang H, Huylebroeck D, Verschueren K, Guo Q, Matzuk MM, Zwijsen A (1999) Smad5 knockout mice die at mid-gestation due to multiple embryonic and extraembryonic defects. *Development* 126: 1631–1642

118 Chang H, Zwijsen A, Vogel H, Huylebroeck D, Matzuk MM (2000) Smad5 is essential for left-right asymmetry in mice. *Dev Biol* 219: 71–78

# Index

# The PIR-Series
# Progress in Inflammation Research

Homepage: http://www.birkhauser.ch

Up-to-date information on the latest developments in the pathology, mechanisms and therapy of inflammatory disease are provided in this monograph series. Areas covered include vascular responses, skin inflammation, pain, neuroinflammation, arthritis cartilage and bone, airways inflammation and asthma, allergy, cytokines and inflammatory mediators, cell signalling, and recent advances in drug therapy. Each volume is edited by acknowledged experts providing succinct overviews on specific topics intended to inform and explain. The series is of interest to academic and industrial biomedical researchers, drug development personnel and rheumatologists, allergists, pathologists, dermatologists and other clinicians requiring regular scientific updates.

**Available volumes:**

*T Cells in Arthritis*, P. Miossec, W. van den Berg, G. Firestein (Editors), 1998
*Chemokines and Skin*, E. Kownatzki, J. Norgauer (Editors), 1998
*Medicinal Fatty Acids*, J. Kremer (Editor), 1998
*Inducible Enzymes in the Inflammatory Response*, D.A. Willoughby, A. Tomlinson (Editors), 1999
*Cytokines in Severe Sepsis and Septic Shock*, H. Redl, G. Schlag (Editors), 1999
*Fatty Acids and Inflammatory Skin Diseases*, J.-M. Schröder (Editor), 1999
*Immunomodulatory Agents from Plants*, H. Wagner (Editor), 1999
*Cytokines and Pain*, L. Watkins, S. Maier (Editors), 1999
In Vivo *Models of Inflammation*, D. Morgan, L. Marshall (Editors), 1999
*Pain and Neurogenic Inflammation*, S.D. Brain, P. Moore (Editors), 1999
*Anti-Inflammatory Drugs in Asthma*, A.P. Sampson, M.K. Church (Editors), 1999
*Novel Inhibitors of Leukotrienes*, G. Folco, B. Samuelsson, R.C. Murphy (Editors), 1999
*Vascular Adhesion Molecules and Inflammation*, J.D. Pearson (Editor), 1999
*Metalloproteinases as Targets for Anti-Inflammatory Drugs*, K.M.K. Bottomley, D. Bradshaw, J.S. Nixon (Editors), 1999
*Free Radicals and Inflammation*, P.G. Winyard, D.R. Blake, C.H. Evans (Editors), 1999
*Gene Therapy in Inflammatory Diseases*, C.H. Evans, P. Robbins (Editors), 2000
*New Cytokines as Potential Drugs*, S. K. Narula, R. Coffmann (Editors), 2000
*High Throughput Screening for Novel Anti-inflammatories*, M. Kahn (Editor), 2000
*Immunology and Drug Therapy of Atopic Skin Diseases*, C.A.F. Bruijnzeel-Komen, E.F. Knol (Editors), 2000
*Novel Cytokine Inhibitors*, G.A. Higgs, B. Henderson (Editors), 2000
*Inflammatory Processes. Molecular Mechanisms and Therapeutic Opportunities*, L.G. Letts, D.W. Morgan (Editors), 2000
*Cellular Mechanisms in Airways Inflammation*, C. Page, K. Banner, D. Spina (Editors), 2000
*Inflammatory and Infectious Basis of Atherosclerosis*, J.L. Mehta (Editor), 2001
*Muscarinic Receptors in Airways Diseases*, J. Zaagsma, H. Meurs, A.F. Roffel (Editors), 2001